Vascular Challenges in Skull Base Surgery

Paul A. Gardner, MD
Professor and Peter J. Jannetta Endowed Chair
Department of Neurological Surgery
University of Pittsburgh School of Medicine;
Co-Director, Center for Cranial Base Surgery
University of Pittsburgh Medical Center
Pittsburgh, Pennsylvania, USA

Carl H. Snyderman, MD, MBA
Professor
Department of Otolaryngology
University of Pittsburgh School of Medicine;
Co-Director, Center for Cranial Base Surgery
University of Pittsburgh Medical Center
Pittsburgh, Pennsylvania, USA

Brian T. Jankowitz, MD
Associate Professor
Director, Cerebrovascular Surgery
Department of Neurological Surgery
Perelman School of Medicine at the University of Pennsylvania
Philadelphia, Pennsylvania, USA

410 illustrations

Thieme
New York • Stuttgart • Delhi • Rio de Janeiro

Library of Congress Cataloging-in-Publication Data is available with the publisher.

Thieme Publishers New York
333 Seventh Avenue, 18th Floor
New York, NY 10001, USA
www.thieme.com
+1 800 782 3488, customerservice@thieme.com

Cover design: © Thieme
Cover image source: © Penny Oliver
Typesetting by TNQ Technologies, India

Printed in Germany by Beltz Grafische Betriebe   5 4 3 2 1

ISBN 978-1-68420-068-9

Also available as an e-book:
eISBN (PDF): 978-1-68420-069-6
eISBN (epub): 978-1-63853-646-8

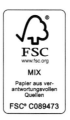

This book is dedicated to:

My greatest contributions to the future, my children, Emma and Ella.

Paul A. Gardner, MD

My family for their unwavering support.

Carl H. Snyderman, MD, MBA

My children, Kathleen, Liam, and Julian, all that's sacred comes from youth.

Brian T. Jankowitz, MD

Contents

1 Vascular Anatomy of the Head and Neck/Circle of Willis 1

Aneek Patel, Hussam Abou-Al-Shaar, Maximiliano A. Nuñez, Georgios A. Zenonos, Paul A. Gardner, and Juan C. Fernandez-Miranda

2 Evaluation of Tumor-Involved Vasculature (Including Balloon Test Occlusion) 10

Joao Alves Rosa, Becky Hunt, and Shelley Renowden

3 Embolization of Skull Base Tumors 20

Daniel A. Tonetti and Brian T. Jankowitz

Contents

10 Dealing with Major Intraoperative Vascular Injury 89

Sean P. Polster, Paul A. Gardner, and Juan C. Fernandez-Miranda

11 Dealing with Major Vascular Injuries During Endonasal Posterior Fossa Surgery 105

Pierre-Olivier Champagne, Thibault Passeri, Eduard Voormolen, Anne-Laure Bernat, Rosaria Abbritti, and Sébastien Froelich

Contents

16   Perforator Injury During Open Skull Base Surgery 141

Nicholas T. Gamboa and William T. Couldwell

17   Endovascular Options to Treat Iatrogenic Vascular Injury and Tumor Involvement of the Skull Base.. 151

Jacob F. Baranoski, Colin J. Przybylowski, Bradley A. Gross, Felipe C. Albuquerque, and Andrew F. Ducruet

18   Extracranial Anterior Cranial Base Surgery for Vascular Tumors............................ 161

Carl H. Snyderman

Contents

Videos

Preface

The cranial base is one of the most inaccessible regions of the human body and consequently presents a complex surgical challenge. Every cranial nerve and intracranial artery and vein pass through foramina, concentrically splayed around the central skull base. Cranial nerve injury can impact quality of life, but injury to arteries or veins poses the greatest potential to devastate a patient. This makes vascular damage the most feared complication for both patients and surgeons. Outcomes range from headache to loss of senses or function to irreversible stroke, vegetative state, or even death.

The understanding of the anatomy, surgical techniques for avoidance and management of injury, and endovascular adjuncts have advanced dramatically over the past decade. These advances, in addition to new surgical techniques and approaches, from endoscopic and minimally invasive to creative bypass techniques, have revolutionized the practice of skull base surgery.

This book was designed to learn from masters of each of these facets with careful consideration of all possible vascular challenges. No single practitioner or specialty can develop all aspects of intra- and extracranial vascular control alone, but through a conglomeration of knowledge, the basic tenets for avoidance and management strategies for vascular injury can be set forth for all skull base surgeons to apply.

Many of the chapters and all of the authors were chosen to further our own practice and, not surprisingly, formulating and editing this text has dramatically advanced our understanding of the challenges facing our subspecialty as it relates to the management of these critical structures.

Paul A. Gardner, MD
Carl H. Snyderman, MD, MBA
Brian T. Jankowitz, MD

Acknowledgment

We extend our gratitude to Mary Jo Tutchko, without whom nothing would get done.

Paul A. Gardner, MD
Carl H. Snyderman, MD, MBA
Brian T. Jankowitz, MD

Contributors

Rosaria Abbritti, MD
Department of Neurosurgery
Lariboisière Hospital
Paris, France

Hussam Abou-Al-Shaar, MD
Department of Neurological Surgery
University of Pittsburgh
Pittsburgh, Pennsylvania, USA

Felipe C. Albuquerque, MD
Department of Neurosurgery
Barrow Neurological Institute
Phoenix, Arizona, USA

Ossama Al-Mefty, MD
Department of Neurosurgery
Brigham and Women's Hospital
Harvard Medical School
Boston, Massachusetts, USA

Rami O. Almefty, MD
Department of Neurosurgery
Temple University
Philadelphia, Pennsylvania, USA

Katherine Anetakis, MD
Department of Neurological Surgery
University of Pittsburgh
Pittsburgh, Pennsylvania, USA

Jeffrey R. Balzer, PhD
Department of Neurological Surgery
University of Pittsburgh
Pittsburgh, Pennsylvania, USA

Nicholas C. Bambakidis, MD
Department of Neurological Surgery
University Hospitals of Cleveland
Cleveland, Ohio, USA

Jacob F. Baranoski, MD
Department of Neurosurgery
Barrow Neurological Institute
Phoenix, Arizona, USA

Carolina Benjamin, MD
Department of Neurosurgery
University of Miami
Miami, Florida, USA

Anne-Laure Bernat, MD
Department of Neurosurgery
Lariboisière Hospital
Paris, France

Pierre-Olivier Champagne MD, PhD,
Department of Neurosurgery
Laval University Hospital Center
Quebec, Canada

Ananth Chintapalli, MS
Department of ENT- Head & Neck Surgery
Kamineni Academy of Medical Sciences and
   Research Center
Hyderabad, India

William T. Couldwell, MD, PhD
Department of Neurosurgery
University of Utah
Salt Lake City, Utah, USA

Donald J. Crammond, PhD
Department of Neurological Surgery
University of Pittsburgh
Pittsburgh, Pennsylvania, USA

Amir R. Dehdashti, MD
Department of Neurosurgery
North Shore University Hospital
Zucker School of Medicine at Hofstra/Northwell
Manhasset, New York, USA

Matheus F. de Oliveira, MD, PhD
Department of Neurosurgery
São Paulo Skull Base Center
São Paulo, Brazil

Vincent Dodson, MD
Department of Neurological Surgery
Rutgers New Jersey Medical School
Newark, New Jersey, USA

Andrew F. Ducruet, MD
Department of Neurosurgery
Barrow Neurological Institute
Phoenix, Arizona, USA

Jean Anderson Eloy, MD
Department of Otolaryngology
Rutgers New Jersey Medical School
Newark, New Jersey, USA

Juan C. Fernandez-Miranda, MD
Department of Neurosurgery
Stanford University
Stanford, California, USA

Carla J.A. Ferreira, MD
Department of Neurological Surgery
University of Pittsburgh
Pittsburgh, Pennsylvania, USA

Sébastien Froelich MD
Department of Neurosurgery
Lariboisière Hospital
Paris, France

Nicholas T. Gamboa, MD
Department of Neurosurgery
University of Utah
Salt Lake City, Utah, USA

Paul A. Gardner, MD
Professor and Peter J. Jannetta Endowed Chair
Department of Neurological Surgery
University of Pittsburgh School of Medicine;
Co-Director, Center for Cranial Base Surgery
University of Pittsburgh Medical Center
Pittsburgh, Pennsylvania, USA

Bradley A. Gross, MD
Department of Neurological Surgery
University of Pittsburgh
Pittsburgh, Pennsylvania, USA

Wayne D. Hsueh, MD
Department of Otolaryngology
Rutgers New Jersey Medical School
Newark, New Jersey, USA

Becky Hunt, MBChB, FRCR
Department of Neuroradiology
North Bristol NHS Trust
Bristol, United Kingdom

Brian T. Jankowitz, MD
Associate Professor
Director, Cerebrovascular Surgery
Department of Neurological Surgery
Perelman School of Medicine at the
University of Pennsylvania
Philadelphia, Pennsylvania, USA

Gurkirat Kohli, MD
Department of Neurological Surgery
Rutgers New Jersey Medical School
Newark, New Jersey, USA

Kevin Kwan, MD
Department of Neurosurgery
North Shore University Hospital
Zucker School of Medicine at Hofstra/Northwell
Manhasset, New York, USA

Philippe Lavigne, MD
Department of Otolaryngology
University of Montreal
Montreal, Quebec, Canada

James K. Liu, MD
Department of Neurological Surgery
Rutgers New Jersey Medical School
Newark, New Jersey, USA

Neil Majmundar, MD
Department of Neurological Surgery
Rutgers New Jersey Medical School
Newark, New Jersey, USA

João Mangussi-Gomes, MD
Department of Otolaryngology
São Paulo Skull Base Center
São Paulo, Brazil

Michael M. McDowell, MD
Department of Neurological Surgery
University of Pittsburgh
Pittsburgh, Pennsylvania, USA

Michael A. Mooney, MD
Department of Neurosurgery
Brigham and Women's Hospital
Harvard Medical School
Boston, Massachusetts, USA

Anil Nanda, MD, MPH, FACS
Department of Neurosurgery
Rutgers-New Jersey Medical School and
Rutgers-Robert Wood Johnson Medical School
Newark, New Jersey, USA

Vinayak Narayan, MD
Department of Neurosurgery
Rutgers-Robert Wood Johnson Medical School and
University Hospital
New Brunswick, New Jersey, USA

Kosumo Noda, MD
Department of Neurosurgery
Sapporo Teishinkai Hospital
Sapporo, Hokkaido, Japan

Maximiliano A. Nuñez, MD
Department of Neurosurgery
Stanford University
Stanford, California, USA

Aneek Patel, BS
School of Medicine
New York University
New York, New York, USA

Thibault Passeri, MD
Department of Neurosurgery
Lariboisière Hospital
2Paris, France

David L. Penn, MD, MS
Department of Neurological Surgery
University Hospitals of Cleveland
Cleveland, Ohio, USA

Ivo Peto, MD
Department of Neurosurgery
North Shore University Hospital
Zucker School of Medicine at Hofstra/Northwell
Manhasset, New York, USA

Sean P. Polster, MD
Department of Neurological Surgery
University of Pittsburgh
Pittsburgh, Pennsylvania, USA

Sampath Chandra Prasad Rao, MS, DNB, FEB-ORLHNS
Department of ENT- Skull Base Surgery
Manipal Hospital
Bangalore, India

Colin J. Przybylowski, MD
Department of Neurosurgery
Barrow Neurological Institute
Phoenix, Arizona, USA

Zeeshan Qazi, MBBS, MS, MCh
Department of Neurological Surgery
Mayo Clinic
Phoenix, Arizona, USA

Shelley Renowden, BSc, MBChB, MRCP, FRCR
Department of Neuroradiology
North Bristol NHS Trust
Bristol, United Kingdom

Joao Alves Rosa, MD, MRCP, FRCR
Department of Neuroradiology
North Bristol NHS Trust Bristol
Bristol, United Kingdom

Julia R. Schneider, DO
Department of Neurosurgery
North Shore University Hospital
Zucker School of Medicine at Hofstra/Northwell
Manhasset, New York, USA

Laligam N. Sekhar, MD, FACS, FAANS
Department of Neurological Surgery
University of Washington
Seattle, Washington, USA

Chandranath Sen, MD
Department of Neurosurgery
NYU Langone Health
New York, New York, USA

Carl H. Snyderman, MD, MBA
Professor
Department of Otolaryngology
University of Pittsburgh School of Medicine;
Co-Director, Center for Cranial Base Surgery
University of Pittsburgh Medical Center
Pittsburgh, Pennsylvania, USA

Aldo C. Stamm, MD
Department of Otolaryngology
São Paulo Skull Base Center
São Paulo, Brazil

Rokuya Tanikawa, MD
Department of Neurosurgery
Sapporo Teishinkai Hospital
Sapporo, Hokkaido, Japan

Parthasarathy D. Thirumala, MD, MS
Department of Neurological Surgery
University of Pittsburgh
Pittsburgh, Pennsylvania, USA

Daniel A. Tonetti, MD
Department of Neurological Surgery
University of Pittsburgh
Pittsburgh, Pennsylvania, USA

Rowan Valentine, MBBS, PhD
Department of Surgery-Otorhinolaryngology,
   Head and Neck Surgery
University of Adelaide
Adelaide, Australia

Marte Van Keulen, MD
Department of Neurological Surgery
University Hospitals of Cleveland
Cleveland, Ohio, USA

Ananth K. Vellimana, MD
Department of Neurological Surgery
Washington University
St. Louis, Missouri, USA

Eduardo A.S. Vellutini, MD
Department of Neurosurgery
São Paulo Skull Base Center
São Paulo, Brazil

Eduard Voormolen, PhD, MD
Department of Neurosurgery
Lariboisière Hospital
Paris, France

Eric W. Wang, MD
Department of Otolaryngology
University of Pittsburgh
Pittsburgh, Pennsylvania, USA

Peter-John Wormald, MD
Department of Surgery-Otorhinolaryngology,
    Head and Neck Surgery
University of Adelaide
Adelaide, Australia

Georgios A. Zenonos, MD
Department of Neurological Surgery
University of Pittsburgh School of Medicine
Pittsburgh, Pennsylvania, USA

1 Vascular Anatomy of the Head and Neck/Circle of Willis*

Aneek Patel, Hussam Abou-Al-Shaar, Maximiliano A. Nuñez, Georgios A. Zenonos, Paul A. Gardner, and Juan C. Fernandez-Miranda

Summary

This chapter reviews the pertinent anatomy of head and neck vasculature as it relates to skull base and cerebrovascular surgery. Understanding this anatomy is a foundational step to selecting surgical approaches and treatment modalities, knowing the clinical consequences of intraoperative decisions, and avoiding complications. In this chapter, we will break down the head and neck circulatory system into anterior and posterior circulation and review the major branches, common variants, and their clinical significance.

Keywords: Internal carotid artery, vertebral artery, anterior cerebral artery, middle cerebral artery, basilar artery, posterior cerebral artery, posterior communicating artery

1.1 Key Learning Points

- The vasculature of the head and neck can have a considerable level of anatomic variability, including variations in origin points, origin vessels, collateralization, and trajectories in relation to other anatomical landmarks.
- An understanding of the origins, courses, and variants of head and neck vessels is essential for the successful planning of skull base and cerebrovascular surgery, including the selection of the optimal approach, visualization of vital structures, proximal and distal vascular control, and limitations.
- The cavernous internal carotid artery (ICA) has the following components: short vertical or ascending segment, posterior genu, horizontal segment, and anterior genu.
- The communicating segment of the ICA carries the largest numbers of perforators to the anterior perforated substance and optic tracts. Injury to these small vessels that lie posterior to the carotid bifurcation will cause a dense contralateral motor deficit.
- The second division of the anterior cerebral artery (A2) gives off the recurrent artery of Heubner after the anterior communicating artery, which is the most common site of intracranial aneurysms. It is critical to preserve this branch whose occlusion typically results in a caudate infarct.
- The M1 segment of the middle cerebral artery delivers the lateral lenticulostriate arteries as well as the anterior temporal artery. Temporary clipping of M1 should be done as distally as possible to avoid occluding these critical M1 perforators.
- The ophthalmic artery and other branches of the ICA commonly anastomose with extracranial vessels, including the internal maxillary artery and ethmoidal arteries.
- Access to the basilar apex often requires a posterior clinoidectomy and/or transcavernous corridor; for low-lying apical aneurysms, an endoscopic endonasal approach may be an option.

---

* The relevant venous anatomy is covered in depth in Chapter 20

1.2 Introduction

The vasculature of the head and neck consists of an anterior and a posterior circulations that give off branches as they travel up the neck and partially anastomose at the circle of Willis to provide blood supply throughout the brain. The circle of Willis sits in the center of the cranial base and can be accessed through a variety of skull base and cerebrovascular surgical techniques, each one with its advantages and limitations. The circle of Willis plays a vital role in providing adequate collateral supply to both hemispheres through communicating arterial trees both anteriorly and posteriorly. A comprehensive understanding of head and neck vasculature is fundamental for the treatment of vascular and skull base lesions as well as for preventing complications and identifying surrounding critical structures. However, this anatomic understanding must also remain fluid, as head and neck vasculature can often include natural variations or distortions because of pathology which should be taken into account preoperatively and adapted to intraoperatively. In this chapter, we will review the anatomy of the head and neck vasculature, and discuss the major anatomical variants and clinical significance of the vasculature in the head and neck as they are pertinent to skull base and cerebrovascular surgery.

1.3 Anterior Circulation

1.3.1 Cervical Carotid Artery

The internal carotid artery (ICA) has seven segments: cervical (C1), petrous (C2), lacerum (C3), cavernous (C4), clinoid (C5), ophthalmic (C6), and communicating (C7) segments (▶ Fig. 1.1).

The common carotid artery (CCA) branches directly off the aortic arch on the left and the brachiocephalic artery on the right, which then becomes the right subclavian artery. This brachiocephalic bifurcation most commonly occurs posterior to the sternoclavicular joint.[1] The most common anatomical variation is known as a "bovine aortic arch," in which both the left and right CCAs originate from the brachiocephalic artery.[2] Most often incidentally found, this variation has a prevalence of 11 to 27%.[3] Bilaterally, the CCAs travel up the neck within the fibrous carotid sheath, which is made up of deep fascial layers and also contains the internal jugular vein (IJ) and vagus nerve (▶ Fig. 1.2). Within the carotid sheath, the CCA runs medial to the IJ and anterior to the vagus nerve in most individuals.[4] The CCA then bifurcates into the ICA and external carotid artery (ECA). The level of this bifurcation varies and is most commonly at the level of C3, approximately 1 to 2 cm above the superior border of the thyroid lamina, although it can also bifurcate as low as the level of the cricoid cartilage or as high as the hyoid cartilage.[5,6,7] High-bifurcating CCAs become clinically important because they serve as cautionary surgical landmarks for a nearby hypoglossal nerve and marginal mandibular nerve.[8,9] For this reason, carotid stenting may be preferable over carotid endarterectomy in cases of high-bifurcating CCAs.[10]

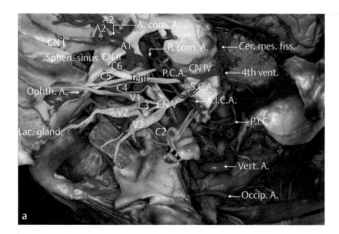
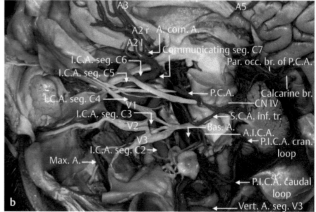
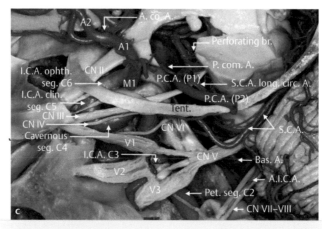

Fig. 1.1 (a–c) Left-sided lateral dissection demonstrating the circle of Willis and the relationship of the vasculature to surrounding neural structures. Note the segments of the internal carotid artery (ICA) as it courses superiorly through the skull base. A., artery; A. Com. A., anterior communicating artery; A.I.C.A., anterior inferior cerebellar artery; Bas. A., basilar artery; Br., branch; Cer. Mes. Fiss., cerebellomesencephalic fissure; Clin., clinoidal; CN., cranial nerve; Cran., cranial; I.C.A., internal carotid artery; Inf., inferior; L., left; Lac., lacrimal; Max., maxillary; Occip. A., occipital artery; Opth., ophthalmic; Par. Occ. Br. of P.C.A., parieto-occipital branches of the posterior cerebral artery; P.C.A., posterior cerebral artery; P. Com. A., posterior communicating artery; Pet., petrous; P.I.C.A., posterior inferior cerebellar artery; R., right; S.C.A., superior cerebellar artery; Seg., segment; Sphen., sphenoid; Tr., trunk; Tent., tentorium; Vent., ventricle; Vert., vertebral.

After the carotid bifurcation, the ECA exits the carotid sheath and the ICA continues within the sheath. The origin of the superior thyroid artery (STA), the first branch of the ECA, varies widely between the CCA, the carotid bifurcation, and the ECA, and studies largely disagree on which variant is most prevalent.[7,8,11] After potentially giving off the STA, the ECA then gives off the ascending pharyngeal artery, which supplies the larynx, after which it gives off the lingual artery.[9] The other branches of the ECA in order include the facial, occipital, and posterior auricular arteries (▶ Fig. 1.2). The ECA ends as the internal maxillary and superficial temporal artery, both of which are readily utilized during bypass surgery. After the bifurcation, the ICA continues within the carotid sheath toward the skull base, where it enters the carotid canal of the temporal bone.

It should be noted that the common classification system used for the segments of the ICA was made to describe the course of the ICA based on pertinent anatomical landmarks as they are encountered from an open, microsurgical perspective. However, with the increasing applications of endoscopic endonasal approaches to skull base lesions, the standard classification scheme for the ICA will also be compared to a classification scheme that is more suitable for endonasal surgery (▶ Table 1.1). As such, what has been described microscopically as the cervical segment of the ICA, C1, can also be classified as the parapharyngeal segment of the ICA; through an endoscopic corridor, this segment is defined as the portion of ICA found behind the lateral cartilaginous eustachian tube spanning to the external opening of the carotid canal.[12]

1.3.2 Petrous and Lacerum Carotid Artery

The petrous segment of the ICA, C2, describes the portion of the ICA that courses first vertically and then horizontally through the carotid canal of the temporal bone, entirely encased in bone; however, the superior aspect of the canal may be dehiscent, placing the ICA at risk of inadvertent injury during middle fossa approaches. Within the carotid canal, the ICA is surrounded by periosteum and gives off no branches.[13] While coursing anteromedially, C2 runs deep and medial to

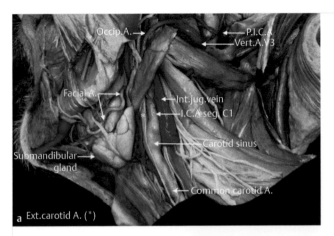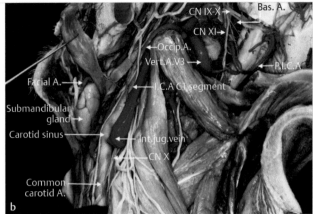
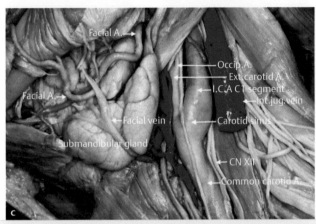

Fig. 1.2 (a–c) Left posterolateral dissection showing the course of the common carotid artery after its origin ascending in the carotid sheath until its bifurcation into the external and internal carotid arteries. Note the branches of the external carotid artery depicted in the figure including the facial and occipital arteries. The internal jugular vein lies lateral to the internal carotid artery (ICA) in the carotid sheath. A., artery; Bas.A., basilar artery; CN., cranial nerve; Common carotid A., common carotid artery; Ext., external; Facial A, facial artery; I.C.A., internal carotid artery; Int. Jug., internal jugular; Occip.A., occipital artery; P.I.C.A., posterior inferior cerebellar artery; Vert. A., vertebral artery; V3, 3rd segment vertebral artery.

Table 1.1 Correlating traditional ICA segments to their nearest anatomic counterparts from an endoscopic endonasal ICA classification scheme

Microscopic ICA segments	Endoscopic ICA segment correlates
Cervical (C1)	Parapharyngeal
Petrous (C2)	Petrous
Lacerum (C3)	Lacerum (Paraclival origin)
Cavernous (C4)	Paraclival/Parasellar
Clinoid (C5)	Parasellar
Ophthalmic (C6)	Intradural/Supraclinoidal
Communicating (C7)	

Abbreviation: ICA, internal carotid artery.

the greater and lesser superficial petrosal nerves and to the tensor tympani and eustachian tube.[14]

Upon exiting the petrous carotid canal, the ICA courses along the superior aspect of the foramen lacerum. This lacerum or C3 segment describes the stretch of ICA that bends and courses medial to the petrolingual ligament and lingual process to enter

the cavernous sinus (▶ Fig. 1.1 and ▶ Fig. 1.3). Throughout this segment, the ICA continues to be surrounded by periosteum and has a constant anatomic relationship with the pterygosphenoidal fissure and vidian nerve.[14,15] In fact, the pterygosphenoidal fissure represents a highly reliable landmark to identify and expose the lacerum ICA during endonasal endoscopic approaches.

1.3.3 Paraclival and Cavernous Carotid Artery

After exiting the carotid canal of the petrous temporal bone and passing through foramen lacerum, the ICA courses parallel to the clivus before entering the cavernous sinus (▶ Fig. 1.1 and ▶ Fig. 1.4). At this level, the ICA runs within the carotid sulcus or groove, which is located in the lateral aspect of the body of the sphenoid. In cases of well-pneumatized sphenoid sinuses, the carotid grooves are readily identified at the lateral aspect of the clival recess; that is why this ICA segment has been classically named "paraclival." This ICA segment also courses medial to V2 and the inferior aspect of gasserian ganglion for which it has also been called "paratrigeminal."[16]

The upper petroclival fissure runs just behind the ICA at the carotid groove, with the petrous apex laterally and the petrosal process of the sphenoid bone medially; the top of this process can be used as a reliable landmark to identify the floor of the cavernous sinus where the abducens nerve enters from Dorello's canal.[17,18]

The cavernous ICA has the following components: short vertical or ascending segment, posterior genu, horizontal segment, and anterior genu (▶ Fig. 1.4). The posterior genu commonly serves as the origin of the meningohypophyseal trunk (or the inferior hypophyseal, tentorial, and dorsal meningeal arteries separately), which supplies the posterior pituitary gland, dorsum sella, clival dura, and tentorium, while

the lateral aspect of the proximal horizontal segment is typically the origin of the inferolateral trunk that gives off branches to the lateral wall of the cavernous sinus and related cranial nerves (▶ Fig. 1.4).[19] The horizontal segment of the cavernous ICA delimits the venous compartments of the cavernous sinus into: superior, inferior, posterior, and lateral;[20] each compartment has distinct boundaries and dural and neurovascular relationships: the superior compartment relates to the interclinoidal ligament and oculomotor nerve, the posterior compartment bears the gulfar segment of the abducens nerve and inferior hypophyseal artery, the inferior compartment contains the sympathetic nerve and distal cavernous abducens nerve, and the lateral compartment includes all cavernous cranial nerves and the inferolateral arterial trunk.

The ICA then ascends lateral to the medial wall of the cavernous sinus and medial to V1, trochlear, and oculomotor nerves as it continues superiorly until it reaches the proximal dural ring, which is formed ventrally by the carotido-clinoidal ligament and dorsally by the carotid-oculomotor membrane.[21] Thus, cavernous ICA aneurysms are extradural and their rupture does not lead to subarachnoid hemorrhage but may lead to the formation of spontaneous carotid-cavernous fistulae.

The segment between the proximal and distal dural rings is known as the clinoid segment (▶ Fig. 1.4). It is not uncommon to have bony dehiscence over the ventral aspect of the clinoid segment of the carotid artery, which is vital to identify during endoscopic endonasal surgery to avoid ICA injury. Identifying the clinoid segment is particularly important in the surgical management of paraclinoidal aneurysms because this segment is the site of proximal control. Microsurgically, it can be accessed by performing an anterior clinoidectomy and distal annulectomy. Endoscopically, this segment is entered by transecting the carotido-clinoidal ligament, which forms the ventral aspect of the proximal dural ring.[17] This ligament can also be calcified, connecting the middle clinoid to the anterior clinoid, making its removal significantly more difficult. The aforementioned bony dehiscence and calcified

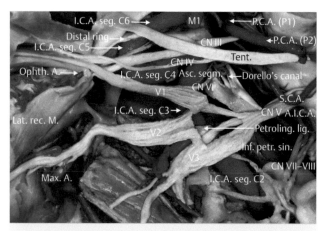

Fig. 1.3 The left-sided petrous internal carotid artery (ICA) courses through the petrous bone to become the C3 segment after traversing the petrolingual ligament to enter the cavernous sinus. A., artery; A.I.C.A., anterior inferior cerebellar artery; Asc. Segm., ascending segment of cavernous ICA; CN., cranial nerve; I.C.A., internal carotid artery; Inf. Pet. Sin., inferior petrosal sinus; Lat. Rect.M., lateral rectus muscle; Max. A, internal maxillary artery; P.C.A., posterior cerebral artery; Petroling. Lig., petrolingual ligament; S.C.A., superior cerebellar artery; Seg(m)., segment; Tent. tentorium.

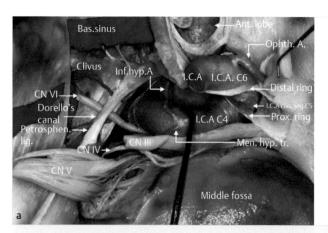

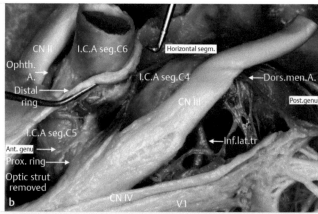

Fig. 1.4 (a, b) Cadaveric dissection showing the right cavernous (C4), clinoidal (C5), and ophthalmic (C6) segments of the internal carotid artery (ICA). Note the different branches of the cavernous ICA segment. Additionally, note the course of the ICA as it traverses through the proximal and distal dural rings and the different turns that the cavernous ICA takes. A., artery; Ant. Lobe, anterior lobe of pituitary gland; CN., cranial nerve; Clin., clinoidal; Dors.Men.A., dorsal meningeal artery; Inf.Hyp.A., inferior hypophyseal artery; Inf.Lat.Tr., inferolateral trunk; Men.Hyp.Tr., meningohypophyseal trunk; Opth.A., ophthalmic artery; Petrosphen.Lig., petrosphenoid ligament; Post., posterior; Prox., proximal dural; Seg(m)., segment.

rings make studying the preoperative imaging and computed tomography scans as well as meticulous dissection intraoperatively of paramount importance. After passing through the distal dural ring, the ICA enters the intradural space.

1.3.4 Supraclinoid Internal Carotid Artery

After passing through the distal dural ring, the ICA runs posteriorly and then superiorly until it bifurcates into the anterior cerebral artery (ACA) and middle cerebral artery (MCA) at the circle of Willis. Before this bifurcation, the ICA gives off several critical branches: the superior hypophyseal artery, the ophthalmic artery, the posterior communicating artery, and the anterior choroidal artery.

The first major branch of the ICA is the ophthalmic artery (OphA), which arises from the medial surface of the ICA (▶ Fig. 1.5). The OphA is responsible for supplying the muscles of the orbit as well as several facial muscles. It runs inferior to the optic nerve to enter the optic canal in the lesser wing of the sphenoid bone. The OphA branches into the critical central retinal artery (usually medial to the ciliary ganglion), which supplies the retina.[22] The OphA typically branches off the inferior surface of the ICA, near the distal dural ring, and therefore risk of OphA occlusion needs to be taken into account when deciding between flow diversion and clipping for proximal ICA aneurysms.[23] However, it should be noted that the distal ophthalmic artery has significant collateral from the ethmoidal arteries, making occlusion of the proximal ophthalmic artery often asymptomatic.[24]

The medial aspect of the ophthalmic segment of the ICA may give off one or more superior hypophyseal arteries (SHAs) that supply the inferior and anterior aspects of the chiasm, stalk, and pituitary gland. A recent study, however, has shown that the origin of the SHA is often at the clinoidal ICA segment.[25] The anatomy and potential displacement of the SHAs become particularly important during suprasellar surgery, as their displacement over the superolateral aspect of tumors such as meningiomas and craniopharyngiomas dispose them to a greater risk of injury from an "open," lateral approach in comparison to an endonasal one. There are many variations in the branching pattern of the SHAs, but most commonly there are three branches: infundibular anastomotic, which supplies the stalk and universally anastomoses with its counterpart; optic or recurrent, which vascularizes the inferior and anterior aspects of the precanalicular optic nerve and chiasm; and the descending or diaphragmatic, which irrigates the dural diaphragm and/or the upper surface of the gland. The SHA branches supplying the chiasm and stalk should be preserved in every instance while SHA branches that supply the sellar diaphragm can be more readily sacrificed if necessary. It is important to note that craniopharyngiomas and other suprasellar lesions will often get vascular supply from the SHA branches, and selective cauterization is mandatory to preserve the critical main trunks.

The ICA next gives off the posterior communicating artery (PComA) either posteriorly or laterally. The PComA runs posteromedially to reach the posterior cerebral artery (PCA) above the oculomotor nerve, which is most commonly medial, although it can occasionally run lateral, to the nerve (▶ Fig. 1.1c). Due to this proximity, PComA aneurysms can often present with third nerve palsies.[26] Approximately 4 to 15 perforating vessels can be found throughout the length of the PComA, the largest of which is designated the anterior thalamoperforating artery. Perforator injury can be avoided closer to the PCA, where the frequency of PComA perforators decreases substantially.[27,28] Not uncommonly the PComA terminates as the PCA, without a distinct PCA originating from the basilar artery (BA), termed fetal PCA. Thus, aneurysms of a fetal PCA should be dealt with high caution as occlusion of the vessel can lead to catastrophic PCA stroke. The PComA or proximal PCA is frequently adherent to the posterior or lateral aspect of suprasellar lesions, especially craniopharyngiomas, and should be carefully identified and preserved.

The anterior choroidal artery (AChA) arises from the inferolateral aspect of the ICA and runs inferior to the optic chiasm, crossing the optic tract first medially and then laterally. Branches of the AChA supply the uncus of the temporal lobe (unco-hippocampal artery), optic tract, and choroid plexus of the temporal horn. They also go through the anterior perforated substance to supply the posterior limb of the internal capsule. Hence, injury to this artery may result in hemianopia and contralateral hemiparesis.[29] After entering the choroid plexus via the anterior choroidal point, the AChA may still give off branches to the pulvinar of thalamus and other relevant areas of the central core.

The communicating segment of the ICA carries the largest numbers of perforators to the anterior perforated substance and optic tracts. Injury to these small vessels that lie posterior to the carotid bifurcation will cause a dense contralateral motor deficit. Importantly, AChA aneurysms commonly occur at the branch points between the parent AChA vessel and a perforator; these aneurysms are difficult to treat both endovascularly and microsurgically due to the proximity of perforating vessels and limited surgical corridor.[30,31]

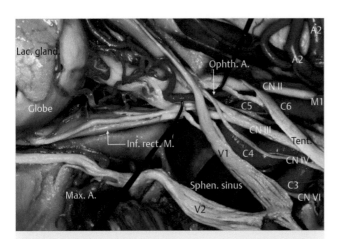

Fig. 1.5 The left ophthalmic artery branches anteromedially from the internal carotid artery (ICA) and courses anteriorly into the orbit along with and inferolaterally to the optic nerve in the optic canal. A., artery; CN., cranial nerve; Inf. Rec. M., inferior rectus muscle; Lac., lacrimal; Max. A., internal maxillary artery; Ophth. A., ophthalmic artery; Sphen., sphenoid; Tent. tentorium.

1.3.5 Anterior Cerebral Artery (A1 and A2 Segments)

The anterior branch of the ICA bifurcation is the ACA, which travels anterior, medial, and superior to the optic tract to reach the anterior communicating artery (AComA) (▶ Fig. 1.1). The ACA is divided into five segments, the first two of which are important to understand their course and branches for skull base and cerebrovascular surgery. The most proximal segment, A1, is defined as the segment between the origin of the ACA from the ICA and the branching point of the AComA. The medial lenticulostriate arteries originate from the medial aspect of A1 to enter the anterior perforated substance. The AComA can also carry perforators to the superior aspect of the chiasm and hypothalamus. The subcallosal artery emerges from the posterior or posterosuperior surface of the AComA to supply the septal region and one or both fornices and is most commonly encountered inferior to the AComA through an endonasal approach.[32] Damage to this vessel can result in acute, severe memory loss.[33]

The proximal segment of A2 gives off one or more recurrent arteries of Heubner (RAH), which run parallel and lateral to A1 in opposite directions and end anterior to the carotid bifurcation where they enter the anterior perforated substance. In approximately half of the patients, the RAH can run anterior to the A1, which is particularly salient during the surgical treatment of AComA aneurysms. Damage to the RAH, which supplies portions of the basal ganglia, caudate, and internal capsule, can lead to hemiparesis and/or aphasia.[34]

The A2 segment also gives rise more distally to the frontoorbital artery (FOA), which runs along the inferior surface of the frontal lobe and supplies the olfactory bulb and olfactory tract along with adjacent fronto-basal gyri. It courses anteriorly along the frontal lobe, crossing the olfactory tract, and enters the olfactory sulcus. As such, it is commonly involved in olfactory groove meningiomas (OGMs) and must be carefully dissected away from the resected tumor.[34]

The AComA itself, a small anastomosis between the A1 segments of the ACAs bilaterally, is the most common intracranial site of aneurysms.[35] Although endovascular treatment of these aneurysms is possible, it can be difficult in some instances due to the tortuosity of A1 and wide involvement of the A1/A2 bifurcation.[36] In such instances, surgical clipping may be indicated; medially projecting aneurysms may be rarely considered for endoscopic endonasal surgery, but these are generally best treated with microsurgical clipping. The A3 and A4 segments correspond to the callosomarginal artery at the superior surface of the corpus callosum and the pericallosal artery, respectively, followed by A5 terminal branches of the ACA.

1.3.6 Middle Cerebral Artery (M1 Segment)

After giving off the ACA, the ICA becomes the MCA, which supplies the majority of the lateral cerebral cortex as well as parts of the basal temporal and occipital lobes, and insula (▶ Fig. 1.1c). The origin of MCA is commonly found medial to the sylvian fissure and lateral to the chiasm.[37] The MCA is made up of four segments; the first segment, M1, is most relevant to skull base and cerebrovascular surgery. The M1 segment courses within the sylvian vallecula along the proximal or sphenoidal sylvian fissure, running posterior and parallel to the lesser sphenoid wing, superior and medial to the uncus, and inferior to the anterior perforated substance to which it delivers the lateral lenticulostriate arteries before becoming M2. However, in instances of a short M1 segment that ends before traversing the vallecula of the sylvian fissure, the perforating branches can originate from the proximal M2 as well. The lateral lenticulostriate arteries supply deep structures of the basal ganglia (the lentiform nucleus, portions of the internal capsule, and caudate) as well as the insular cortex, and their occlusion can lead to motor, cognitive, and speech impairments. Infarcts in lateral lenticulostriate arteries tend to present with more severe motor deficits than those in anterior lenticulostriate arteries.[38,39]

The M1 segment of the MCA also gives off the anterior temporal artery (ATA), which supplies the temporal pole and is responsible for semantic and social processing. The M1 segment ends at the limen insulae, where the MCA typically bifurcates into a superior and inferior division.

It is important to note that M1 perforators, predominantly branching off the dorsolateral surface of the M1 segment, are present throughout the length of the segment as it crosses through the sylvian fissure. Therefore, temporary proximal clipping of M1 risks occlusion of these critical perforators; if necessary, clipping should be done as distally and as close to the lesion as possible to minimize unnecessary vessel occlusion.[40] The M2 starts after the bifurcation to enter the distal or opercular sylvian fissure and circular sulcus of the insula, followed by the opercular (M3) and cortical (M4) segments of the MCA.[41] The cortical segments of the MCA are the common recipients of anastomosis in bypass surgery, given their ease of access, size match with donor and arterial interposition grafts, and avoidance of even transient M1 occlusion.

1.4 Posterior Circulation

1.4.1 Vertebral and Basilar Arteries

The vertebral arteries (VAs) provide posterior cerebral blood supply, ultimately anastomosing with the anterior carotid supply at the circle of Willis. The VA originates from the subclavian arteries bilaterally and has a short extraosseous segment before entering the transverse foramen of C6 (in 15–20% C7) as the V1 segment. As it travels in the transverse foramina, it becomes V2, giving off several muscular branches on its way. At the level of C3, V2 exits the transverse foramen and loops along the vertebral artery groove posterosuperiorly and then exits the C2 transverse foramen to become the V3 segment.[46] V3 then enters the transverse foramen of C1 and exits, which gives off the posterior meningeal and sometimes the accessory meningeal arteries. It then turns medially in the sulcus arteriosus of C1 before heading anteriorly and superiorly to enter the dura as V4 (▶ Fig. 1.2b, c).[47]

The V4 segment is divided by the preolivary sulcus into lateral and anterior medullary segments. Intracranially, V4 gives off the posterior inferior cerebellar artery (PICA), which is responsible for supplying part of the cerebellum as well as the lateral aspect of the medulla (▶ Fig. 1.1a, b). The origin of PICA commonly occurs approximately 2 cm superior to the dural entrance of V4, although this origin can vary, occurring anywhere from the V3 segment to the BA.[48] Occlusion of the PICA can lead to a lateral medullary syndrome, which is characterized by ipsilateral face and contralateral body hemisensory deficit, ipsilateral Horner's syndrome, and cerebellar signs (ataxia, dysmetria, dysdiadokinesia, nystagmus, slurred speech, and intention tremor).[49]

Continuing superiorly, the VA then gives off the anterior spinal artery bilaterally and then courses between the lower cranial nerves to reach the contralateral VA and forms the BA. The anterior spinal artery most commonly originates approximately 5 to 10 mm proximal to the vertebrobasilar junction (VBJ).[50] The VBJ occurs medial and most commonly immediately inferior to the origin of cranial nerve VI (CN VI) in the pontomedullary sulcus, although it can often occur superior to the sulcus as well.[50,51] As such, the VBJ is a good landmark for the origin of CN VI.

The first major branch of the BA, if the PICA has already originated from the VA, is the anterior inferior cerebellar artery (AICA), which originates from the more inferior half of the BA in over 90% of individuals (▶ Fig. 1.1b, c). Rarely, as mentioned when discussing the PICA, the AICA can originate from a common AICA-PICA trunk stemming off the BA as well.[52] The BA then gives off multiple pontine perforating vessels bilaterally before branching into the superior cerebellar artery (SCA) followed closely by the PCA.[53] This bifurcation, known as the basilar apex, is significant because it is a relatively common site for aneurysms and can be difficult to access microsurgically; it can often require posterior clinoidectomy and/or a transcavernous corridor (for both open and endonasal approaches). For this reason, the position of the basilar apex is important; low-lying basilar apex aneurysms (as well as low-lying AICA aneurysms, which are less common but similarly challenging to access microsurgically) can be accessed through the endoscopic endonasal approach if clipping is indicated. The third cranial nerve courses between the PCA and SCA, a reliable and important localizing relationship.

1.4.2 Posterior Cerebral Artery (P1 and P2 Segments)

The PCA is the terminal branch of the BA, originating from the basilar apex (▶ Fig. 1.1). The first segment, P1, runs from the basilar bifurcation up to the anastomosis with the PComA. Posterior thalamoperforators branch off the PCA and go into the interpeduncular cistern and the posterior perforated substance. Long and short circumflex arteries originate in this segment to supply the mesencephalon. The origins of these branches and the trunk of P1 can be accessed through a lateral frontotemporal or cranio-orbital approach with or without a posterior clinoidectomy, or endoscopically through a transclival (pituitary transposition) approach although endovascular intervention is often a first-line treatment modality for P1 aneurysms.[54]

The critical P2 segment begins after the anastomosis with the PComA, courses around the midbrain along the ambient cistern, and gives off one to three cortical branches or inferior temporal arteries (▶ Fig. 1.1c and ▶ Fig. 1.3). The thalamogeniculate artery arises from this segment and enters the geniculate body to supply the thalamus and optic radiations.

Occlusion of the thalamogeniculate artery moreover leads to thalamic symptoms, which are marked by severe pain and pure sensory loss in the face, arm, and legs.[55] It then gives off the middle and lateral posterior choroidal arteries. While the middle posterior choroidal artery supplies the thalamus, pineal gland, and choroid plexus in the third ventricle, the lateral posterior choroidal artery enters the choroidal fissure to supply the choroid plexus in the posterior temporal horn and atrium. A PCA bifurcation was identified in 89% of hemispheres, typically at the middle segment of the medial temporal region, just before the quadrigeminal cistern. The most common pattern of bifurcation was by division into posteroinferior temporal and parieto-occipital arterial trunks.[56] P3 originates distal to the inferior temporal arteries and ends at the beginning of the calcarine fissure, followed by P4 ending as the splenial artery.

1.4.3 Extracranial-Intracranial Anastomoses

Together, the ICA and vertebral artery supply the entire intracranial (IC) circulation, while the ECA is responsible for the entire extracranial (EC) circulation. Although predominantly two separate circulatory systems, the two circulations anastomose in several locations, commonly at the skull base. Branches of the OphA are often involved in EC-IC anastomoses. The proximal lacrimal branch commonly anastomoses with the middle meningeal artery (MMA), a major branch of the internal maxillary artery (IMax); this variant is found in approximately 40% of individuals. When present, this anastomosis typically occurs between the superior orbital fissure and the posterior wall of the orbit.[24] The distal lacrimal branch of the OphA also commonly anastomoses extracranially, interfacing in many cases with the deep temporal artery within the orbit. Other frequently encountered OphA anastomoses include the anastomosis of the anterior and posterior ethmoidal arteries with the sphenopalatine, septal, greater palatine, or middle meningeal arteries within the ethmoid sinus, as well as potential connections between the supraorbital artery with the STA.[42]

Direct branches of the ICA also commonly anastomose with other branches of the IMax. The inferolateral trunk can connect with the IMax within the cavernous sinus, and the arteries of foramen ovale and lacerum (from the ICA) can anastomose with the accessory meningeal artery of the IMax and the ascending pharyngeal artery, respectively. The meningohypophyseal trunk and vertebral artery, too, can occasionally anastomose with clival branches of the ascending pharyngeal artery.[42] In the neck, muscular branches of the ascending and deep cervical arteries can connect with vertebral arteries spanning from the level of C1 to C7.[43]

Several key collaterals between intracranial vessels are important to consider as well. Leptomeningeal collateralization has been observed in a majority of individuals and, through varying courses, comprises a network of leptomeningeal vessels that connect major vessels of the circle of Willis. These connections often go unnoticed, but can become critical during acute ischemic events.[44] Much more rarely, an embryologically persistent trigeminal artery can remain and connect the intracavernous segment of the ICA to the BA, providing another anastomosis between anterior and posterior intracranial circulations.[45]

1.5 Conclusion

The vasculature of the head and neck consists of a system of circulation that centers on the collaterals of the circle of Willis at the skull base. Both the anterior and posterior circulations supply blood to the head and neck branch directly or indirectly from the aorta and travel superiorly. The CCA travels up the neck in the carotid sheath before giving off the ECA and entering the skull base as the ICA, which then gives off several major branches before splitting into the ACA and the MCA at the circle of Willis. The vertebral arteries also travel up the neck posteriorly, giving off branches and perforators, before merging to become the BA, which then also bifurcates as it enters the circle of Willis. The bilateral anterior circulations variably anastomose and collateralize via the AComA and the anterior and posterior circulations can have significant collateral supply via the PComA. However, other variants, including ECA-ICA anastomotic variants, can be equally or more important and should be carefully studied and understood in each individual.

Anterior and posterior circulation consists of a series of common variants that must be anticipated and accounted for in successful skull base surgery. For vascular surgeries, an anatomical and clinical understanding of the vasculature allows for approach planning as well as a dynamic understanding of what should and cannot be occluded or sacrificed based on the patient's anatomy. For all other skull base surgeries, a strong understanding of the anatomy allows for the prevention of intraoperative complications and is useful in planning safe surgical corridors.

References

[1] Johnson MH, Thorisson HM, Diluna ML. Vascular anatomy: the head, neck, and skull base. Neurosurg Clin N Am. 2009; 20(3):239–258

[2] Layton KF, Kallmes DF, Cloft HJ, Lindell EP, Cox VS. Bovine aortic arch variant in humans: clarification of a common misnomer. AJNR Am J Neuroradiol. 2006; 27(7):1541–1542

[3] Goldsher YW, Salem Y, Weisz B, Achiron R, Jacobson JM, Gindes L. Bovine aortic arch: prevalence in human fetuses. J Clin Ultrasound. 2020; 48(4):198–203

[4] Garner DH, Kortz MW, Baker S. Anatomy, head and neck, carotid sheath. In: StatPearls. Treasure Island, FL: StatPearls Publishing; 2020

[5] Klosek SK, Rungruang T. Topography of carotid bifurcation: considerations for neck examination. Surg Radiol Anat. 2008; 30(5):383–387

[6] Mirjalili SA, McFadden SL, Buckenham T, Stringer MD. Vertebral levels of key landmarks in the neck. Clin Anat. 2012; 25(7):851–857

[7] Al-Rafiah A, EL-Haggagy AA, Aal IH, Zaki AI. Anatomical study of the carotid bifurcation and origin variations of the ascending pharyngeal and superior thyroid arteries. Folia Morphol (Warsz). 2011; 70(1):47–55

[8] Lo A, Oehley M, Bartlett A, Adams D, Blyth P, Al-Ali S. Anatomical variations of the common carotid artery bifurcation. ANZ J Surg. 2006; 76(11):970–972

[9] Michalinos A, Chatzimarkos M, Arkadopoulos N, Safioleas M, Troupis T. Anatomical considerations on surgical anatomy of the carotid bifurcation. Anat Res Int. 2016; 2016:6907472

[10] Kolkert JL, Meerwaldt R, Geelkerken RH, Zeebregts CJ. Endarterectomy or carotid artery stenting: the quest continues part two. Am J Surg. 2015; 209 (2):403–412

[11] Natsis K, Raikos A, Foundos I, Noussios G, Lazaridis N, Njau SN. Superior thyroid artery origin in Caucasian Greeks: a new classification proposal and review of the literature. Clin Anat. 2011; 24(6):699–705

[12] Labib MA, Prevedello DM, Carrau R, et al. A road map to the internal carotid artery in expanded endoscopic endonasal approaches to the ventral cranial base. Neurosurgery. 2014; 10 Suppl 3:448–471, discussion 471

[13] Nutik SL. Removal of the anterior clinoid process for exposure of the proximal intracranial carotid artery. J Neurosurg. 1988; 69(4):529–534

[14] Bouthillier A, van Loveren HR, Keller JT. Segments of the internal carotid artery: a new classification. Neurosurgery. 1996; 38(3):425–432, discussion 432–433

[15] Wang W-H, Lieber S, Mathias RN, et al. The foramen lacerum: surgical anatomy and relevance for endoscopic endonasal approaches. J Neurosurg. 2018; 131(5):1–12

[16] Marcati E, Andaluz N, Froelich SC, et al. Paratrigeminal, paraclival, precavernous, or all of the above? A circumferential anatomical study of the C3–C4 transitional segment of the internal carotid artery. Oper Neurosurg (Hagerstown). 2018; 14(4):432–440

[17] Abdulrauf SI, Ashour AM, Marvin E, et al. Proposed clinical internal carotid artery classification system. J Craniovertebr Junction Spine. 2016; 7(3):161–170

[18] Borghei-Razavi H, Truong HQ, Fernandes Cabral DT, et al. Endoscopic endonasal petrosectomy: anatomical investigation, limitations, and surgical relevance. Oper Neurosurg (Hagerstown). 2019; 16(5):557–570

[19] Reisch R, Vutskits L, Patonay L, Fries G. The meningohypophyseal trunk and its blood supply to different intracranial structures. An anatomical study. Minim Invasive Neurosurg. 1996; 39(3):78–81

[20] Fernandez-Miranda JC, Zwagerman NT, Abhinav K, et al. Cavernous sinus compartments from the endoscopic endonasal approach: anatomical considerations and surgical relevance to adenoma surgery. J Neurosurg. 2018; 129(2):430–441

[21] Truong HQ, Lieber S, Najera E, Alves-Belo JT, Gardner PA, Fernandez-Miranda JC. The medial wall of the cavernous sinus. Part 1: Surgical anatomy, ligaments, and surgical technique for its mobilization and/or resection. J Neurosurg. 2018; 131(1):122–130

[22] Baldoncini M, Campero A, Moran G, et al. Microsurgical anatomy of the central retinal artery. World Neurosurg. 2019; 130:e172–e187

[23] Puffer RC, Kallmes DF, Cloft HJ, Lanzino G. Patency of the ophthalmic artery after flow diversion treatment of paraclinoid aneurysms. J Neurosurg. 2012; 116(4):892–896

[24] Bertelli E, Regoli M, Bracco S. An update on the variations of the orbital blood supply and hemodynamic. Surg Radiol Anat. 2017; 39(5):485–496

[25] Truong HQ, Najera E, Zanabria-Ortiz R, et al. Surgical anatomy of the superior hypophyseal artery and its relevance for endoscopic endonasal surgery. J Neurosurg. 2018; 131(1):154–162

[26] Etame AB, Bentley JN, Pandey AS. Acute expansion of an asymptomatic posterior communicating artery aneurysm resulting in oculomotor nerve palsy. BMJ Case Rep. 2013; 2013:bcr2013010134

[27] Avci E, Bademci G, Oztürk A. Posterior communicating artery: from microsurgical, endoscopic and radiological perspective. Minim Invasive Neurosurg. 2005; 48(4):218–223

[28] Kim S-H, Yeo D-K, Shim J-J, Yoon S-M, Chang J-C, Bae H-G. Morphometric study of the anterior thalamoperforating arteries. J Korean Neurosurg Soc. 2015; 57(5):350–358

[29] Drábek P. [Anterior choroidal artery syndromes]. Cesk Neurol Neurochir. 1991; 54(4):208–211

[30] Hendricks BK, Spetzler RF. Surgical challenges associated with anterior choroidal artery aneurysm clipping: 2-dimensional operative video. Oper Neurosurg (Hagerstown). 2020; 19(3):E289

[31] Cho MS, Kim MS, Chang CH, Kim SW, Kim SH, Choi BY. Analysis of clip-induced ischemic complication of anterior choroidal artery aneurysms. J Korean Neurosurg Soc. 2008; 43(3):131–134

[32] Najera E, Alves Belo JT, Truong HQ, Gardner PA, Fernandez-Miranda JC. Surgical anatomy of the subcallosal artery: implications for transcranial and endoscopic endonasal surgery in the suprachiasmatic region. Oper Neurosurg (Hagerstown). 2019; 17(1):79–87

[33] Pardina-Vilella L, Pinedo-Brochado A, Vicente I, et al. The goblet sign in the amnestic syndrome of the subcallosal artery infarct. Neurol Sci. 2018; 39(8):1463–1465

[34] Najera E, Truong HQ, Belo JTA, Borghei-Razavi H, Gardner PA, Fernandez-Miranda J. Proximal branches of the anterior cerebral artery: anatomic study and applications to endoscopic endonasal surgery. Oper Neurosurg (Hagerstown). 2019; 16(6):734–742

[35] Brzegowy P, Kucybała I, Krupa K, et al. Angiographic and clinical results of anterior communicating artery aneurysm endovascular treatment. Wideochir Inne Tech Malo Inwazyjne. 2019; 14(3):451–460

[36] Elhadi AM, Kalani MYS, McDougall CG, Albuquerque FC. Endovascular treatment of aneurysms. In: Aminoff MJ, Daroff RB, eds. Encyclopedia of the Neurological Sciences. 2nd ed. Oxford: Academic Press; 2014:57–62

[37] Gibo H, Carver CC, Rhoton AL, Jr, Lenkey C, Mitchell RJ. Microsurgical anatomy of the middle cerebral artery. J Neurosurg. 1981; 54(2):151–169

[38] Horie N, Morofuji Y, Iki Y, et al. Impact of basal ganglia damage after successful endovascular recanalization for acute ischemic stroke involving lenticulostriate arteries. J Neurosurg. 2019; 132(6):1880–1888

[39] Kumral E, Evyapan D, Balkir K. Acute caudate vascular lesions. Stroke. 1999; 30(1):100–108

[40] Pai SB, Varma RG, Kulkarni RN. Microsurgical anatomy of the middle cerebral artery. Neurol India. 2005; 53(2):186–190

[41] Wen HT, Rhoton AL, Jr, de Oliveira E, Castro LH, Figueiredo EG, Teixeira MJ. Microsurgical anatomy of the temporal lobe: part 2—sylvian fissure region and its clinical application. Neurosurgery. 2009; 65(6) Suppl:1–35, discussion 36

[42] Harbaugh R, Shaffrey CI, Couldwell WT. Neurosurgery Knowledge Update: A Comprehensive Review. Thieme; 2015

[43] Geibprasert S, Pongpech S, Armstrong D, Krings T. Dangerous extracranial-intracranial anastomoses and supply to the cranial nerves: vessels the neurointerventionalist needs to know. AJNR Am J Neuroradiol. 2009; 30(8): 1459–1468

[44] Tariq N, Khatri R. Leptomeningeal collaterals in acute ischemic stroke. J Vasc Interv Neurol. 2008; 1(4):91–95

[45] Alcalá-Cerra G, Tubbs RS, Niño-Hernández LM. Anatomical features and clinical relevance of a persistent trigeminal artery. Surg Neurol Int. 2012; 3:111–111

[46] Cacciola F, Phalke U, Goel A. Vertebral artery in relationship to C1-C2 vertebrae: an anatomical study. Neurol India. 2004; 52(2):178–184

[47] Abd el-Bary TH, Dujovny M, Ausman JI. Microsurgical anatomy of the atlantal part of the vertebral artery. Surg Neurol. 1995; 44(4):392–400, discussion 400–401

[48] Delion M, Dinomais M, Mercier P. Arteries and veins of the cerebellum. Cerebellum. 2017; 16(5-6):880–912

[49] Day GS, Swartz RH, Chenkin J, Shamji AI, Frost DW. Lateral medullary syndrome: a diagnostic approach illustrated through case presentation and literature review. CJEM. 2014; 16(2):164–170

[50] Akar ZC, Dujovny M, Slavin KV, Gomez-Tortosa E, Ausman JI. Microsurgical anatomy of the intracranial part of the vertebral artery. Neurol Res. 1994; 16 (3):171–180

[51] Songur A, Gonul Y, Ozen OA, et al. Variations in the intracranial vertebrobasilar system. Surg Radiol Anat. 2008; 30(3):257–264

[52] Hou K, Li G, Luan T, Xu K, Xu B, Yu J. Anatomical study of anterior inferior cerebellar artery and its reciprocal relationship with posterior inferior cerebellar artery based on angiographic data. World Neurosurg. 2020; 133: e459–e472

[53] Marinković SV, Gibo H. The surgical anatomy of the perforating branches of the basilar artery. Neurosurgery. 1993; 33(1):80–87

[54] Sanai N, Tarapore P, Lee AC, Lawton MT. The current role of microsurgery for posterior circulation aneurysms: a selective approach in the endovascular era. Neurosurgery. 2008; 62(6):1236–1249, discussion 1249–1253

[55] Li S, Kumar Y, Gupta N, et al. Clinical and neuroimaging findings in thalamic territory infarctions: a review. J Neuroimaging. 2018; 28(4): 343–349

[56] Fernández-Miranda JC, de Oliveira E, Rubino PA, Wen HT, Rhoton AL, Jr. Microvascular anatomy of the medial temporal region: Part 1: its application to arteriovenous malformation surgery. Neurosurgery. 2010; 67(3) Suppl Operative:ons237–ons276, discussion ons276

2 Evaluation of Tumor-Involved Vasculature (Including Balloon Test Occlusion)

Joao Alves Rosa, Becky Hunt, and Shelley Renowden

Summary

The most common tumors to involve the skull base are meningiomas and the most common vascular tumors are paragangliomas (glomus tympanic and glomus jugulare lesions) and juvenile nasopharyngeal angiofibromas. Adequacy and safety of tumor resection will depend upon the extent of disease, arterial supply, and the ability to perform safe preoperative embolization. Radical resection may rarely also require sacrifice of the internal carotid or vertebral artery. Reduction in morbidity associated with sacrifice of the internal carotid artery is achieved by balloon test occlusion.

Keywords: Skull base, tumor, vascular, angiography, balloon test occlusion

2.1 Key Learning Points

- Digital subtraction angiography remains the gold standard for vascular assessment of skull base tumors and their suitability for embolization.
- Six vessel angiography and assessment of collateral blood flow are often required.
- Diagnostic digital subtraction angiography can help identify dangerous anastomoses and venous drainage patterns.
- Internal carotid artery sacrifice without prior balloon occlusion testing carries significant morbidity/mortality.

2.2 Introduction

The skull base is anatomically complex, involving osseous, soft tissue, neural, and vascular components which give rise to a diverse range of benign and malignant tumors. Tumors arising from the extracranial head and neck may also involve the skull base by direct extension. Paragangliomas (glomus tumors) (▶ Fig. 2.1, ▶ Fig. 2.2, and ▶ Fig. 2.3), after skull base meningiomas, are the most frequent vascular tumors arising directly from the skull base, and juvenile nasal angiofibromas (JNAs) are the most frequent vascular tumors to involve the skull base, extending from their site of origin in the pterygopalatine fossa/sphenopalatine foramen (▶ Fig. 2.4). Other vascular skull base tumors include hemangiomas, hemangiopericytomas, esthesioneuroblastomas, endolymphatic sac tumors, and vascular metastases.

2.3 Arterial and Venous Anatomy

Although variations are expected, the commonest skull base tumor types have well-described typical arterial supply patterns.

Glomus jugulare tumors (▶ Fig. 2.1, ▶ Fig. 2.2, and ▶ Fig. 2.3) arise from paraganglia located along either Jacobson's or Arnold's nerve, around the jugular bulb and the vascular supply is well reported.[1,2] The inferior tympanic branch of the ascending pharyngeal artery supplies the inferomedial portion of the tumor at jugular foramen. The posterolateral component derives a supply

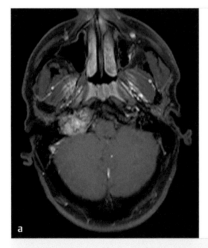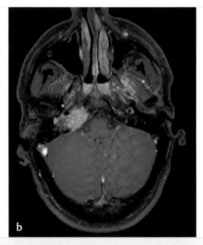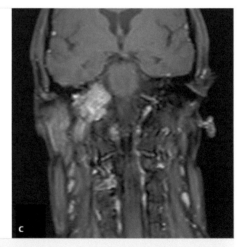

Fig. 2.1 A 35-year-old man with an extensive right-sided glomus jugulare tumor (also bilateral carotid body tumors—not demonstrated). Gadolinium-enhanced T1 W axial (**a, b**) and coronal (**c**) magnetic resonance (MR) images with fat saturation demonstrate an enhancing mass centered at the right jugular foramen, with intradural extension. Additional sequences (not shown) demonstrated the typical "salt and pepper" appearance of a vascular skull base tumor in keeping with a glomus jugulare tumor. The glomus jugulare tumor extended below the skull base in the carotid space and involved the hypoglossal canal, horizontal petrous carotid canal, internal auditory canal, and petrous apex.

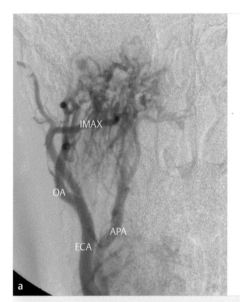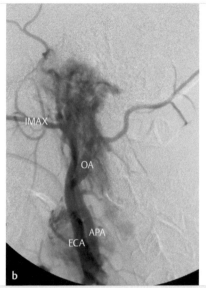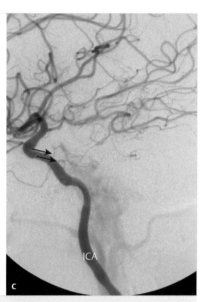

Fig. 2.2 Same patient as ▶ Fig. 2.1. Frontal **(a)** and lateral **(b)** projections of a right external carotid artery (ECA) angiogram confirm the presence of an intensely vascular tumor centered on the jugular foramen, supplied predominantly by an enlarged ascending pharyngeal artery (APA). Further supply is demonstrated from the stylomastoid artery arising from an enlarged occipital artery (OA) and anterior tympanic and accessory meningeal branches arising from the internal maxillary artery (IMax), with arteriovenous shunting. (The stylomastoid, anterior tympanic, and accessory meningeal supply were optimally demonstrated at the time of embolization although the selective runs are not provided here.) A right internal carotid artery (ICA) angiogram **(c)** shows additional dural clival supply (*black arrows*).

from the stylomastoid artery, a branch of either the occipital or posterior auricular arteries. Anteriorly, the tumor is supplied by the anterior tympanic branch of the internal maxillary artery and the superior compartments from the middle and accessory meningeal arteries. Cerebellar arteries contribute to the intradural extension of the tumor.

Juvenile nasopharyngeal angiofibromas (▶ Fig. 2.4) are benign but locally aggressive tumors commonly arising from the nasopharynx in the sphenopalatine foramen/pterygopalatine fossa. They expand anteriorly into the nasal cavity, ethmoid and maxillary sinuses, and laterally into the infratemporal fossa. Further expansion along skull base foramina or by direct bone erosion of the greater sphenoid wing or lateral wall of the sphenoid sinus results in intracranial extension.

The primary arterial supply is from the distal internal maxillary artery,[3,4] mainly the sphenopalatine artery, descending palatine arteries, and ascending pharyngeal artery but with accessory supply from the anterior and posterior deep temporal arteries and accessory meningeal artery. As the tumor grows, it recruits additional supply from the ascending palatine branch of the facial artery, ethmoidal branches from the ophthalmic artery, and branches of the internal carotid artery (ICA) (mandibulovidian, pterygovaginal artery, inferolateral trunk, and meningohypophyseal trunk). Arterial supply may be bilateral even if the tumor is lateralized.

The arterial anatomy of skull base meningiomas is given in ▶ Table 2.1. Hemangiopericytomas may be confused with meningiomas but are even more vascular, have corkscrew-like vessels, and receive their dominant supply from the internal carotid or vertebrobasilar circulation. Endolymphatic sac tumors are supplied by the ascending pharyngeal and stylomastoid arteries.

Assessment of venous structures is particularly useful in skull base meningiomas, although sites of arteriovenous shunting are also often present in JNAs.[5,6]

In meningiomas (▶ Fig. 2.6), an early arterial phase blush persisting into the late venous phase is characteristic and the presence of arteriovenous shunting has been associated with more aggressive tumors.[7] It has been demonstrated that skull base meningiomas change the pattern of venous circulation by exerting mass effect and obstructing the surrounding venous structures, causing drainage to be diverted toward collateral venous routes.[8,9]

This is particularly relevant in petroclival meningiomas (PCMs) as particular patterns of drainage of the superficial middle cerebral vein (SMCV), such as drainage into the pterygoid plexus through a sphenobasal vein or into the transverse sinus (TS) through a sphenopetrosal sinus, are more prevalent in this population and have been associated with intraoperative and postoperative venous complications.[10,11]

Invasion of the dural sinuses by the tumor can cause a similar pattern of dural sinus occlusion and alternative pattern of venous drainage on the cerebral angiogram. Magnetic resonance (MR) is invaluable in distinguishing simple mass effect on the venous structures from invasion of the dural sinus.

Therefore, detailed assessment of the drainage pattern will impact on outcomes and chosen surgical approach. For example, if an anterior petrosal approach is considered, the presence of a sphenobasal vein should prompt consideration of strategies to avoid injuring this vein in the region of the foramen ovale.[12] If there is drainage through a sphenopetrosal sinus, a tentorial incision that preserves drainage during a transpetrosal approach are needed.[11]

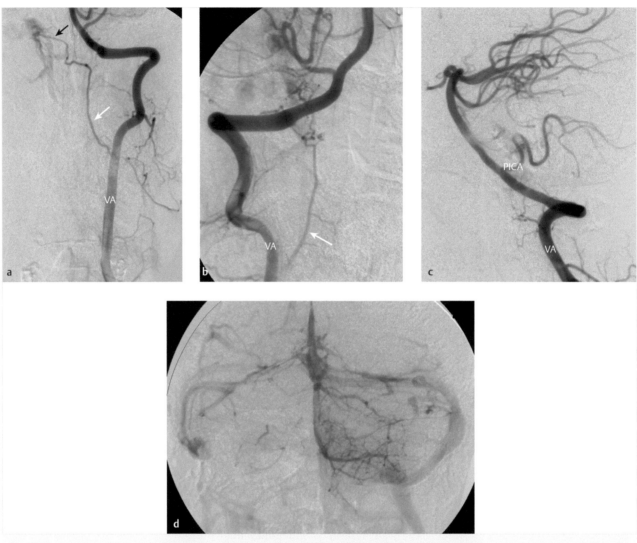

Fig. 2.3 Same patient as ► Fig. 2.1 and ► Fig. 2.2. Frontal projections of left (a) and right (b) vertebral artery (VA) angiograms show supply from the right hypoglossal branch of the neuromeningeal trunk of the ascending pharyngeal artery (*black arrow*) via an anastomosis from both VA C3 radicular branches (*white arrow*) and the odontoid arcade. Lateral projection of a right VA angiogram (c) demonstrates pial supply from the right posterior inferior cerebellar artery (PICA). Occlusion of the right jugular bulb is shown on a venous phase image of a right VA angiogram (d).

Venous drainage characterization is also important in anterior clinoid meningiomas. If drainage of the SMCV into the pterygoid plexus or directly into the cavernous sinus (CS) is present, a tailored surgical strategy is required.[13]

2.4 Imaging of Skull Base Vascular Tumors

Clinical assessment is limited by the inaccessible location of most skull base neoplasms and, as such, evaluation is predominantly radiological. Computed tomography (CT), including high-resolution bone reconstructions and CT angiography (CTA) and venography (CTV), and magnetic resonance imaging (MRI), including postcontrast sequences and magnetic resonance angiography (MRA) and magnetic resonance venography (MRV), are the primary imaging modalities for the initial evaluation and diagnosis of skull base pathologies.

Cross-sectional imaging allows for the assessment of the primary lesion as well as involvement of adjacent tissue, bone infiltration, perineural spread, and distortion or direct invasion of vascular structures. Although vascular anatomy, gross tumoral vascularity, and the patency of involved blood vessels are adequately evaluated using CTA/CTV and MRA/MRV, these modalities cannot accurately assess the arterial feeding vessels, venous drainage, collateral blood flow, and complex vascular architecture of the lesion. Dynamic CTA can provide noninvasive high-resolution four-dimensional radiographic information of tumor vasculature but currently its clinical use is yet to be defined and does not yet replace formal angiography.[14]

Digital subtraction angiography (DSA) remains the "gold standard" for preoperative evaluation of tumor-involved vasculature. Comprehensive angiography of the internal and external carotid arteries, vertebral arteries, and (depending upon tumor location and extent) the thyrocervical and costocervical

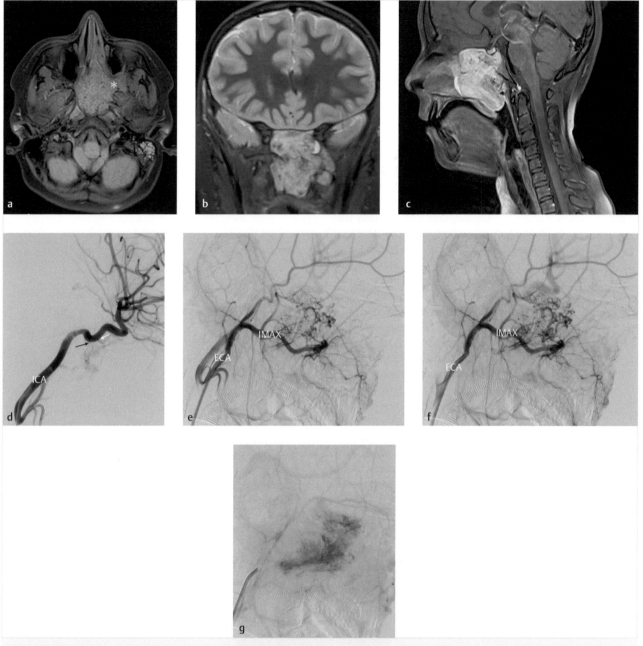

Fig. 2.4 A 10-year-old boy presenting with a 6-month history of epistaxis has a diagnosis of a left-sided juvenile nasopharyngeal angiofibroma: Magnetic resonance (MR) images: axial T1 W with fat saturation (**a**), coronal Short Tau Inversion Recovery (STIR) (**b**), and sagittal gadolinium-enhanced T1 W with fat saturation (**c**) demonstrate a vascular enhancing nasopharyngeal mass widening the sphenopalatine foramen ([a], *white asterisk*), extending into the nasal cavity and sphenoid sinus. There was primarily a unilateral supply from the inferolateral trunk (*white arrow*) and mandibulovidian branch (*black arrow*) of the left internal carotid artery (ICA) (**d**) and distal branches of the left internal maxillary artery, primarily the sphenopalatine artery, as seen on external carotid angiograms (**e, f**). Angiography demonstrates minimally dilated feeding arteries and an intense vascular blush persisting into the late venous phase (**g**). There was a very small contribution from the right sphenopalatine artery (not shown).

trunks provides essential preoperative information regarding the tumoral vascular anatomy, identifies the dominant feeding arteries that may be considered for preoperative embolization, and assesses the anatomy of and adequacy of the circle of Willis (COW), the degree of collateralization, and adequacy of the posterior circulation and venous patency and dominance. Head and neck tumors may parasitize regional pial blood supply as they enlarge and extend intracranially. Arterial displacement, distortion, and encasement may be identified (▶ Fig. 2.6). It is also important to define the arterial supply to the retina as preoperative embolization may involve arterial connections with the central artery of the retina. Dangerous anastomoses, however, may not reveal themselves on an initial angiogram but may only become obvious when changes in blood flow occur during embolization. These are, therefore, more appropriately discussed elsewhere.

Table 2.1 Arterial supply to skull base meningiomas

Anatomical region	Location	Common vascular supply
Anterior skull base meningioma	Olfactory groove and planum sphenoidale	• Ethmoidal branches of the ophthalmic artery; recurrent meningeal branch of lacrimal artery
Middle fossa meningioma	Cavernous sinus and clinoid region	• Inferolateral and meningohypophyseal trunk • Cavernous branch of middle meningeal artery; accessory meningeal artery of foramen rotundum; recurrent meningeal branch of ophthalmic artery
	Sphenoid wing	• Sphenoidal branch of middle meningeal artery (lateral tumors) • Internal carotid artery (medial tumors)
Posterior fossa meningioma	Petroclival region and cerebellar pontine angle	• Internal carotid artery via meningohypophyseal trunk • Middle meningeal and accessory meningeal arteries • Ascending pharyngeal artery • Occipital and posterior auricular arteries

The primary aim of surgery is to achieve the greatest resection with minimal complications. On occasion, total or maximal resection may only be achievable with permanent occlusion of the ICA or other parent vessel. In this context, DSA in combination with balloon test occlusion (BTO) is necessary to evaluate whether the patient will tolerate occlusion/sacrifice of the ICA. Assessing the safety of vertebral artery (VA) occlusion will depend upon VA dominance and adequacy of the posterior communicating arteries, which can also be assessed with a VA BTO.

2.4.1 Digital Subtraction Angiography (DSA)

A standard cerebral angiogram involves selective injection of the internal and external carotid arteries and vertebral arteries bilaterally (occasionally the thyrocervical and costocervical trunks as well). When embolization is being considered, superselective injection of tumor feeding vessels can be performed using smaller microcatheters. Collateral blood flow and the adequacy of the COW can be assessed with carotid cross compression (Matas maneuver) or compression of the ipsilateral ICA during a VA injection (Allcock maneuver).

By extending each fluoroscopic "run" into the late venous phase, it is possible to characterize not only the pattern of tumor enhancement but also its venous drainage pattern, mass effect, and eventual obstruction of intracranial venous structures.

Careful characterization of the venous anatomy and existing collateral routes will help plan the best surgical approach and minimize perioperative venous complications.

Complications

DSA confers a low risk of complication,[15,16,17] which may occur at the site of puncture or within the cervicocerebral circulation. Puncture site complications include localized hematoma, vessel dissection, pseudoaneurysm formation, and retroperitoneal hematoma. Cervicocerebral complications include vessel dissection and distant emboli with the associated risk of transient ischemic attack (TIA) and stroke. The risk of neurological complication associated with DSA varies in the published literature, but the larger, more recent studies report a rate of 0 to 0.7% for transient neurological symptoms, and 0 to 0.5% for permanent

neurological deficits. In experienced hands, DSA is therefore a safe procedure with a very low risk of significant associated morbidity.

2.5 Balloon Test Occlusion (BTO) (▶ Fig. 2.5 and ▶ Fig. 2.6)

The ability to achieve gross total resection or significant debulking of tumors which were previously considered inoperable has come with the advancement of skull base surgical technique over the past two decades. These neoplasms frequently involve the ICA and maximum resection can sometimes only be obtained with preoperative permanent occlusion of the vessel, if surgery carries a significant risk of vessel rupture and requires intraprocedural ICA ligation. Untested vessel sacrifice carries a significant risk of neurological morbidity secondary to immediate or delayed hypoperfusion. Historic data demonstrates a 17 to 49%[18,19,20,21] incidence of stroke (many fatal) following permanent occlusion of the ICA and around 28% for common carotid artery occlusion without preoperative trial of temporary occlusion.

The use of BTO in differentiating patients who will tolerate permanent vessel occlusion and those who require a bypass or vessel preservation significantly reduces the risk of stroke and the associated neurological morbidity but does not eliminate it completely. Standard BTO with clinical monitoring only will identify the cohort of patients for whom vessel sacrifice without bypass will **not** be tolerated, as these patients develop neurological symptoms during the procedure while the balloon is inflated and the ICA occluded. It will not identify those patients with impaired cerebrovascular reserve who are at risk of developing neurological deficits secondary to delayed hypoperfusion, which can occur hours to days following ICA occlusion. Numerous adaptations and adjuncts have therefore been developed to improve the sensitivity of BTO, but the underlying principle in all is to assess the efficacy of the collateral circulation, predominantly primary collaterals, in maintaining perfusion of the affected vascular territory. Primary collaterals include the anterior and posterior communicating arteries. Secondary collaterals from the external carotid and leptomeningeal collaterals may take longer to develop.

Approximately 10% of patients develop symptoms during the occlusion. Up to 20% who tolerate occlusion clinically will develop infarction after parent vessel occlusion (PVO); in 20% of these the onset may be after 48 hours sometimes up to 2 weeks later.[22]

Adjunctive techniques to evaluate regional cerebral blood flow (CBF) and perfusion include BTO which are primarily delayed in venous phase[23] and technetium-99 m hexamethylpropylene-amine oxime single photon emission computed tomography (SPECT, ▶ Fig. 2.3 and ▶ Fig. 2.4).[24,25,26] Other methods reported include transcranial Doppler ultrasonography,[27] perfusion CT,[28] xenon CT,[29] and measurement of arterial stump pressure.[30] Although these reduce the risk of delayed cerebral ischemia down to 3 to 8%, they cannot predict embolic stroke and may also fail to identify some patients with limited reserve. No adjunctive technique is clearly superior.

2.5.1 Balloon Test Occlusion Protocol

Numerous protocols for performing BTO exist,[31] and the exact procedure will be dependent on the facilities and experience of individual departments. In our institution, BTO is performed under local anesthetic in the awake patient, and the adequacy of CBF evaluated by a combination of clinical assessment, venous delay, and SPECT using the metastable radio-isotope 99m Tc hexamethylpropylene-amine oxime (HMPAO).

Systemic blood pressure is measured continuously noninvasively. Sheaths are placed in the common femoral arteries bilaterally and 5,000 units of heparin administered intravenously. Due to the risk of thromboembolic events, adequate anticoagulation should be ensured with Activated Coagulation Times >250. A double lumen balloon catheter (which allows distal perfusion of the ICA, with heparinized saline, to avoid a standing column of blood) is navigated into the ipsilateral upper cervical ICA, around C1–C3 (▶ Fig. 2.5). Inflation at a lower level, in the bulb, risks the carotid sinus reflex which can result in significant bradycardia. Common carotid artery occlusion is not recommended because it decreases perfusion pressure in the carotid sinus and, by reflex, increases arterial blood pressure and so may diminish test reliability.

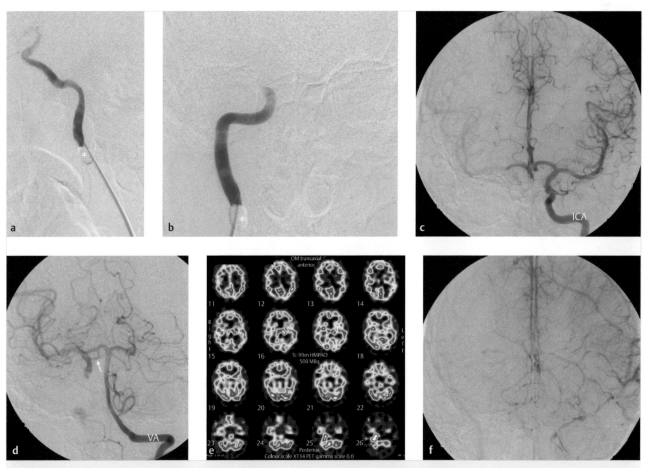

Fig. 2.5 Balloon test occlusion (BTO) **right** internal carotid artery (ICA). Same patient as ▶ Fig. 2.1, ▶ Fig. 2.2, and ▶ Fig. 2.3. Lateral **(a)** and frontal **(b)** projections of a **right** ICA angiogram demonstrate a balloon inflated (*white asterisk*) in the cervical ICA in a heparinized patient and injection through the double lumen balloon catheter with stagnation of contrast due to flow arrest. The patient experienced no neurological deficit. Frontal projections of a **left** ICA **(c)** and left vertebral artery **(d)** angiograms, with maintained **right** ICA occlusion, demonstrate cross flow from the left ICA via the anterior communicating artery and excellent cross flow from the right posterior cerebral artery via the posterior communicating artery (**[d]**, *white arrow*). Single photon emission computed tomography (SPECT) axial projection **(e)** showed symmetric perfusion at the time of balloon occlusion without evidence of a perfusion delay suggesting that ICA occlusion would be tolerated. Venous phase image of the left ICA angiography **(f)** showed no significant delay in venous filling between hemispheres. Right hemisphere venous contrast is diluted due to excellent flow and wash out of contrast from the right posterior cerebral artery across the posterior communicating artery.

The balloon is inflated under fluoroscopic control and the timer started. Occlusion is confirmed by injection of contrast through the catheter showing stasis. The patient is neurologically assessed over a 20 to 30 minutes time period, evaluating motor, sensory, memory, and analytical skills. If at any stage the patient develops a neurological deficit, the balloon is immediately deflated as the patient has failed the test occlusion. In addition to clinical evaluation, angiography is performed via the contralateral ICA and VA, assessing venous delay in the "occluded" hemisphere. Additional secondary collaterals may be assessed by injections into the external carotid artery. It is assumed that patients who have symmetry within the venous phase have sufficient collateral circulation to tolerate ICA sacrifice. The appearance of the first cortical veins is the start of the venous phase. A delay in excess of 0.5 second is considered to indicate risk of hemodynamic ischemic stroke. Toward the end of the study, approximately 20 to 25 minutes after balloon inflation, 99 m Tc HMPAO 500 to 600 MBq is injected via a peripheral intravenous cannula. After a further 2 to 3 minutes, the balloon is then deflated and the catheters removed. The patient is transferred to the nuclear medicine suite and SPECT performed, evaluating perfusion in the axial, coronal, and sagittal planes (▶ Fig. 2.5 and ▶ Fig. 2.6).

99 m Tc HMPAO shows rapid cerebral uptake and distributes proportionately to regional CBF. The tracer is converted intracellularly to a hydrophilic compound and remains fixed in the brain for a prolonged period allowing delayed imaging after injection. Cerebral uptake of tracer reflects not only perfusion but also the metabolic status of cerebral tissue; hence, when injected during BTO, its distribution is an indicator of both regional perfusion and metabolism. 99 m Tc HMPAO SPECT scans are analyzed comparing a minimum of four hemispheric regions of interest in the occluded hemisphere and with the contralateral side. Greater than 10% reduction in activity in a region of interest is regarded as significant and may indicate suboptimal cerebrovascular reserve. Baseline SPECT scans

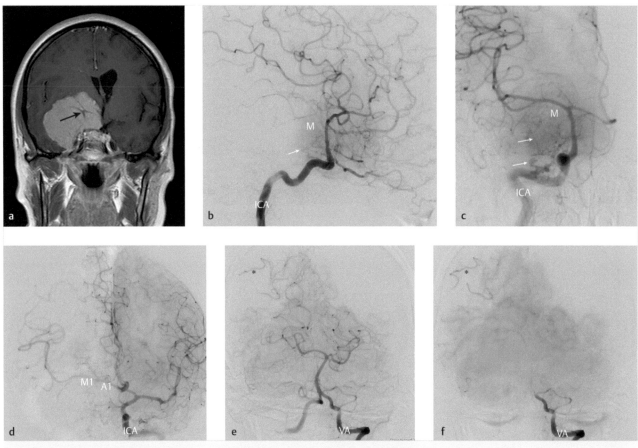

Fig. 2.6 Large right paraclinoid meningioma. Coronal projection, gadolinium-enhanced T1-weighted magnetic resonance (MR) image **(a)** demonstrates a large right paraclinoid meningioma encasing and narrowing the distal internal carotid artery (ICA), M1, and A1 arteries (*black arrow*). Due to its significant mass effect, the tumor was also causing distortion of the optic chiasm and ipsilateral pons (not shown). Lateral **(b)** and frontal **(c)** projections of a right ICA angiogram confirm that the meningioma is supplied by dural branches (*white arrows*) of the right ICA. The supraclinoid ICA and right anterior cerebral artery are encased, distorted, and narrowed by the tumor. The right middle cerebral artery is displaced superiorly. "M" indicates the tumor blush. Balloon test occlusion **right** ICA: Frontal projection of left ICA injection **(d)** demonstrates very little anterior communicating arterial cross flow to the A1 and M1 segments of the right Anterior Cerebral Artery (ACA) and MCA, respectively. Associated poor filling of the right hemispheric distal cortical branches. Frontal projection of the left vertebral artery injection **(e)** shows no posterior communicating artery cross flow and very slow pial leptomeningeal collateralization (*black asterisk*) with arterial flow persisting well into the venous phase **(f)**. There was no neurological deficit but the patient was obviously at risk from delayed cerebral ischemia and this was further confirmed by photon emission computed tomography (SPECT).

(Continued)

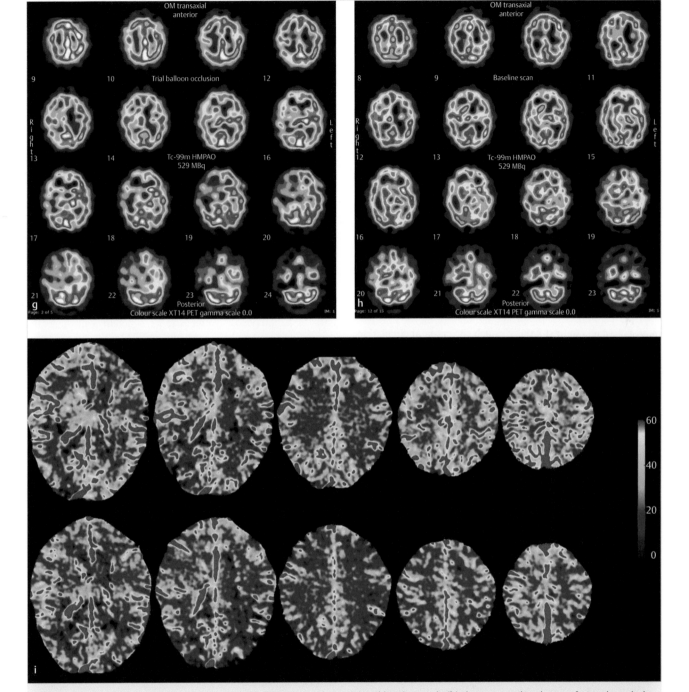

Fig. 2.6 *(Continued)* Axial projections at the time of balloon test occlusion **(g)** and baseline study **(h)** show very striking hypoperfusion through the right middle cerebral artery territory and also the right anterior cerebral artery territory during temporary balloon occlusion, with little abnormality visible on the baseline study. The percentage difference in perfusion through the middle cerebral arteries is of the order of 25 to 40% and appearances suggest very strongly that the patient will not tolerate permanent carotid occlusion without a bypass procedure. Perfusion computed tomography (CT) **(i)** performed in the angiography suite, showing cerebral blood volume at the time of balloon test occlusion (top row) and baseline (bottom row), demonstrates relative increase in cerebral blood volume during balloon occlusion of the right ICA (refer to color scale on the right). Elevation of cerebral blood volume suggests that the patient may be near the limits of cerebral autoregulation and confirms that the patient may be at risk of delayed cerebral ischemia.

obtained after an interval of a few days may be necessary to exclude pre-existing asymmetry.

BTO SPECT has the advantage that it avoids patient transfer to another room with the balloon in situ. Its main disadvantage is that it is only semi-quantitative.

BTO is associated with procedural complications in approximately 3.5% of patients and permanent deficits are described in 0.5 to 1.7%.[32,33] However, this is likely to vary significantly with operator and center experience.

2.5.2 Alternative Common Adjuncts

In some institutions, BTO may be performed under general anesthesia, although this is increasingly uncommon and unnecessary. General anesthesia is associated with a drop in mean arterial blood pressure by as much as 26%. In this situation a venous delay of 2 seconds is regarded as safe for parent vessel ICA occlusion. A delay of >4 seconds is an absolute contraindication to ICA occlusion. A venous delay of 2 to 4 seconds signifies borderline reserve.[24]

Neurophysiological monitoring in the form of Somatosensory Evoked Potentials (SSEPs) and electroencephalography (EEG), although not validated for BTO under general anesthesia can provide an indirect measure of CBF and may ultimately be the most sensitive predictor of intolerance to blood vessel occlusion.

Transcranial Doppler ultrasound (TCD), which is noninvasive but operator dependent, assesses CBF velocity in the ipsilateral middle cerebral artery. A reduction in mean velocity and pulsatility index of <30% is reported to be a good predictor of clinical tolerance to ICA occlusion.[28]

CT perfusion (CTP) is performed by monitoring the first pass of an iodinated contrast bolus through the cerebral circulation. The contrast agent passes through the cerebral parenchyma causing a transient increase in density directly proportional to the amount of contrast in the vessels and blood in that region. Time attenuation curves are generated for an arterial region of interest (ROI), venous ROI, and each pixel. Color-coded perfusion maps showing cerebral blood volume (CBV), CBF, and mean transit time (MTT) are generated. Although dependent on user interpretation, qualitative visual assessment of these maps has shown to be an effective way of identifying areas at risk of ischemia.[29] Calculation of quantitative parameters (CBV – $mL \times 100 \ g^{-1}$, CBF – $mL \times 100 \ g^{-1} \times min^{-1}$, MTT – seconds) can also be used to demonstrate areas at risk.[29] However, differences in hardware and software may affect quantified metrics and visual interpretation of the color-coded maps will suffice.

This can also be combined with an acetazolamide challenge.[34]

The traditional disadvantage of CTP has been the necessity to transfer the patient from the angiography suite to the CT scanner with the catheters in place in the ICA, re-inflating the balloon in a blind fashion, and risking vessel trauma.[29] (Xenon-enhanced CT also confers this disadvantage but remains the most accurate quantitative study.)

However, perfusion CT imaging assessing CBV may now be performed in the angiography suite (▶ Fig. 2.6i) following an intravenous injection of contrast both before and during BTO. Hence, no patient transfer is required during BTO.[35] No change in relative CBV infers adequate collateral flow and low risk of delayed cerebral ischemia. Patients who have marginal collaterals and are at the limits of cerebral autoregulation may show an increase in CBV and may be at risk of delayed cerebral ischemia.

It is likely that assessment of the venous phase and angiography suite CTP will be the most practically useful means of assessment of cerebrovascular reserve and ability to tolerate ICA occlusion, but the validity of the latter is yet to be reported.

Pharmacological hypotensive challenge, in addition to neurological examination during BTO, is considered unlikely to improve efficacy, may have a false positive rate, and may mean that some patients undergo unnecessary bypass procedures. Hypotension may be induced using nitroprusside or labetalol, lowering the mean arterial blood pressure by 30%. This may identify an additional 20% who have limited collateral reserve but is also associated with a false negative rate 5 to 15%.[36]

Balloon Test Occlusion in the Vertebrobasilar Circulation

Assessment here is purely clinical. BTO in the vertebrobasilar circulation should only be performed if bilateral VA occlusion is considered unless the patient has only one VA or the other is hypoplastic. BTO in these cases should be performed above the level of occipital artery collaterals. It has been argued that bilateral VA occlusion can be tolerated with two slim posterior communicating arteries or a single posterior communicating artery, meaning that the anatomy of the COW is not always predictable of the clinical outcome.[37] A bilateral VA BTO should always be performed prior to such a radical undertaking. TCD may be used to assess Posterior Cerebral Artery (PCA) flow—in the presence of a functional PcomA, the P1 segment will show increased and reversed flow velocity and P2 will show a drop in velocity. If this is not demonstrated, an incomplete balloon occlusion should be suspected, which may produce a false-negative test. Unfortunately, the limit for the P2 velocity drop with respect to tolerating a bilateral VA or when basilar artery occlusion is not established.[37] As a result, the risks and possible unfavorable outcomes of a vertebrobasilar circulation occlusion should be carefully considered and weighted against the potential benefits.

2.6 Conclusion

The ability to adequately and safely resect vascular skull base tumors depends upon the extent of disease, arterial supply, and ability to perform safe preoperative embolization. Radical resection may also require sacrifice of the internal carotid or VA. Reduction in morbidity associated with sacrifice of the ICA is achieved by balloon test occlusion. Many BTO protocols are reported with the aim of improving the predictability of safe occlusion but all have advantages and disadvantages and none are currently clearly superior.

References

[1] Jindal G, Miller T, Raghavan P, Gandhi D. Imaging evaluation and treatment of vascular lesions at the skull base. Radiol Clin North Am. 2017; 55(1): 151–166

[2] Woolen S, Gemmete JJ. Paragangliomas of the head and neck. Neuroimaging Clin N Am. 2016; 26(2):259–278

[3] Ballah D, Rabinowitz D, Vossough A, et al. Preoperative angiography and external carotid artery embolization of juvenile nasopharyngeal angiofibromas in a tertiary referral paediatric centre. Clin Radiol. 2013; 68 (11):1097–1106

[4] Mehan R, Rupa V, Lukka VK, Ahmed M, Moses V, Shyam Kumar NK. Association between vascular supply, stage and tumour size of juvenile nasopharyngeal angiofibroma. Eur Arch Otorhinolaryngol. 2016; 273(12): 4295–4303

[5] Valavanis A. Embolisation of intracranial and skull base tumours. In: Valavanis A, ed. Interventional Neuroradiology. Berlin, Heidelberg: Springer Berlin Heidelberg; 1993

[6] Schroth G, Haldemann AR, Mariani L, Remonda L, Raveh J. Preoperative embolization of paragangliomas and angiofibromas. Measurement of intratumoral arteriovenous shunts. Arch Otolaryngol Head Neck Surg. 1996; 122(12):1320–1325

[7] Wilson G, Weidner W, Hanafee W. The demonstration and diagnosis of meningiomas by selective carotid angiography. Am J Roentgenol Radium Ther Nucl Med. 1965; 95(4):868–873

[8] Adachi K, Hasegawa M, Hirose Y. Evaluation of venous drainage patterns for skull base meningioma surgery. Neurol Med Chir (Tokyo). 2017; 57(10): 505–512

[9] DiMeco F, Li KW, Casali C, et al. Meningiomas invading the superior sagittal sinus: surgical experience in 108 cases. Neurosurgery. 2004; 55(6):1263–1272, discussion 1272–1274

[10] Fukuda M, Saito A, Takao T, Hiraishi T, Yajima N, Fujii Y. Drainage patterns of the superficial middle cerebral vein: effects on perioperative managements of petroclival meningioma. Surg Neurol Int. 2015; 6:130

[11] Adachi K, Hayakawa M, Ishihara K, et al. Study of changing intracranial venous drainage patterns in petroclival meningioma. World Neurosurg. 2016; 92:339–348

[12] Shibao S, Toda M, Orii M, Fujiwara H, Yoshida K. Various patterns of the middle cerebral vein and preservation of venous drainage during the anterior transpetrosal approach. J Neurosurg. 2016; 124(2):432–439

[13] Nagata T, Ishibashi K, Metwally H, et al. Analysis of venous drainage from sylvian veins in clinoidal meningiomas. World Neurosurg. 2013; 79(1):116–123

[14] Gupta S, Bi WL, Mukundan S, Al-Mefty O, Dunn IF. Clinical applications of dynamic CT angiography for intracranial lesions. Acta Neurochir (Wien). 2018; 160(4):675–680

[15] Johnston DC, Chapman KM, Goldstein LB. Low rate of complications of cerebral angiography in routine clinical practice. Neurology. 2001; 57(11): 2012–2014

[16] Willinsky RA, Taylor SM, TerBrugge K, Farb RI, Tomlinson G, Montanera W. Neurologic complications of cerebral angiography: prospective analysis of 2,899 procedures and review of the literature. Radiology. 2003; 227(2): 522–528

[17] Dawkins AA, Evans AL, Wattam J, et al. Complications of cerebral angiography: a prospective analysis of 2,924 consecutive procedures. Neuroradiology. 2007; 49(9):753–759

[18] Schorstein J. Carotid ligation in saccular intracranial aneurysms. Br J Surg. 1940; 28(109):50–70

[19] Olivecrona H. Ligature of the carotid artery in intracranial aneurysms. Acta Chir Scand. 1944; 91:353–368

[20] Norlen G, Falconer M, Jefferson G, Johnson R. The pathology, diagnosis and treatment of intracranial saccular aneurysms. Proc R Soc Med. 1952; 45(5): 291–302

[21] Moore O, Baker HW. Carotid-artery ligation in surgery of the head and neck. Cancer. 1955; 8(4):712–726

[22] Schneweis S, Urbach H, Solymosi L, Ries F. Preoperative risk assessment for carotid occlusion by transcranial Doppler ultrasound. J Neurol Neurosurg Psychiatry. 1997; 62(5):485–489

[23] Abud DG, Spelle L, Piotin M, Mounayer C, Vanzin JR, Moret J. Venous phase timing during balloon test occlusion as a criterion for permanent internal carotid artery sacrifice. AJNR Am J Neuroradiol. 2005; 26(10):2602–2609

[24] Mathews D, Walker BS, Purdy PD, et al. Brain blood flow SPECT in temporary balloon occlusion of carotid and intracerebral arteries. J Nucl Med. 1993; 34 (8):1239–1243

[25] Zhong J, Ding M, Mao Q, Wang B, Fu H. Evaluating brain tolerability to carotid artery occlusion. Neurol Res. 2003; 25(1):99–103

[26] Lorberboym M, Pandit N, Machac J, et al. Brain perfusion imaging during preoperative temporary balloon occlusion of the internal carotid artery. J Nucl Med. 1996; 37(3):415–419

[27] Eckert B, Thie A, Carvajal M, Groden C, Zeumer H. Predicting hemodynamic ischemia by transcranial Doppler monitoring during therapeutic balloon occlusion of the internal carotid artery. AJNR Am J Neuroradiol. 1998; 19(3): 577–582

[28] Lui YW, Tang ER, Allmendinger AM, Spektor V. Evaluation of CT perfusion in the setting of cerebral ischemia: patterns and pitfalls. AJNR Am J Neuroradiol. 2010; 31(9):1552–1563

[29] Linskey ME, Jungreis CA, Yonas H, et al. Stroke risk after abrupt internal carotid artery sacrifice: accuracy of preoperative assessment with balloon test occlusion and stable xenon-enhanced CT. AJNR Am J Neuroradiol. 1994; 15(5):829–843

[30] Wang AY-C, Chen C-C, Lai H-Y, Lee S-T. Balloon test occlusion of the internal carotid artery with stump pressure ratio and venous phase delay technique. J Stroke Cerebrovasc Dis. 2013; 22(8):e533–e540

[31] Chaudhary N, Gemmete JJ, Thompson BG, Pandey AS. Intracranial endovascular balloon test occlusion—indications, methods, and predictive value. Neurosurg Clin N Am. 2009; 20(3):369–375

[32] Tarr RW, Jungreis CA, Horton JA, et al. Complications of preoperative balloon test occlusion of the internal carotid arteries: experience in 300 cases. Skull Base Surg. 1991; 1(4):240–244

[33] Mathis JM, Barr JD, Jungreis CA, et al. Temporary balloon test occlusion of the internal carotid artery: experience in 500 cases. AJNR Am J Neuroradiol. 1995; 16(4):749–754

[34] Okudaira Y, Arai H, Sato K. Cerebral blood flow alteration by acetazolamide during carotid balloon occlusion: parameters reflecting cerebral perfusion pressure in the acetazolamide test. Stroke. 1996; 27(4):617–621

[35] Struffert T, Deuerling-Zheng Y, Engelhorn T, et al. Monitoring of balloon test occlusion of the internal carotid artery by parametric color coding and perfusion imaging within the angio suite: first results. Clin Neuroradiol. 2013; 23(4):285–292

[36] Dare AO, Chaloupka JC, Putman CM, Fayad PB, Awad IA. Failure of the hypotensive provocative test during temporary balloon test occlusion of the internal carotid artery to predict delayed hemodynamic ischemia after therapeutic carotid occlusion. Surg Neurol. 1998; 50(2):147–155, discussion 155–156

[37] Sorteberg A. Balloon occlusion tests and therapeutic vessel occlusions revisited: when, when not, and how. AJNR Am J Neuroradiol. 2014; 35(5): 862–865

3 Embolization of Skull Base Tumors

Daniel A. Tonetti and Brian T. Jankowitz

Summary

This chapter will review the different methods of embolizing skull base tumors including common pitfalls and perils.

Keywords: Embolization, particles, PVA, liquid embolic, Onyx, NBCA, coils

3.1 Key Learning Points

- Preoperative tumor embolization can decrease intraoperative blood loss and increase the chance of successful tumor resection.
- Embolization is predicated entirely on the avoidance of complications.
- There should be a clear understanding of the goals of tumor embolization agreed upon between the surgeon and the neurointerventionalist.
- Safe embolization requires knowledge of patient-specific anastomotic connections and the risk/benefit profile of available embolysates, given the relevant anatomy.

3.2 Introduction

Endovascular embolization can be utilized in conjunction with surgery to improve chances for successful skull base tumor resection by decreasing tumor vascularity. Significant advances have been made in technique and embolic materials since the first descriptions of such procedures in 1973.[1] The most common agents currently used are ethylene vinyl alcohol copolymer (Onyx), n-butyl cyanoacrylate (NBCA), coils, particles, ethanol, or a combination of the above.[2]

Of paramount importance to the clinical team caring for a patient with a skull base tumor is the awareness that the primary goal of tumor embolization is to enhance the chances of a successful surgical resection. Tumors of the skull base can be exceedingly vascular and may have difficult-to-access vascular pedicles; therefore, embolization can play a direct role in decreasing the difficulty of the resection for the surgeon. Ideally this allows for increased surgical field visualization with decreased morbidity of the surgical procedure.[3] However, tumor embolization should be approached with extreme caution as it will rarely significantly influence the overall outcome of surgery, and, though prior literature has supported the efficacy of tumor embolization to reduce both intraoperative blood loss[4,5,6] and recurrence,[7] there are no tumors that absolutely require preoperative embolization.

Commonly treated, highly vascular tumors of the skull base include some meningiomas, hemangiopericytomas, juvenile nasopharyngeal angiofibromas (JNAs), hemangioblastomas, and paragangliomas (glomus tumors). Although this list is not exhaustive, these are the most common vascular skull base tumors and represent the majority of a neurointerventionalist's referrals for tumor embolization.

Direct intratumoral puncture techniques have been described for skull base tumors accessible percutaneously or via natural orifices.[8] This technique may be of use in patients with superficial, easily accessible, hypervascular tumors, but is not without risk of major complications.[9] The most useful application of this technique is for previously embolized, recurrent JNAs. When all safe arterial pathways to a tumor have been surgically occluded or embolized, direct puncture may be the only method of access. This has been described in small case series for certain carotid body, glomus jugulare, and glomus vagale paragangliomas.[10,11,12] This chapter will focus on the role of preoperative transarterial embolization in the management of vascular skull base tumors, as transarterial embolization is more common and the role for direct tumoral puncture has yet to be well established. However, many of the same guidelines, risks, and recommendations with regard to procedural safety apply for direct tumor techniques.

3.3 Goal of Embolization and Injury Avoidance

Prior to skull base tumor embolization, it is of critical importance to identify patient-specific vascular anatomy including anastomotic connections and have a complete understanding of the following:

- Tumoral blood supply.
- Involved cerebral and cranial nerve blood supply.
- Associated blood supply of end-organs including skin and retina.

Common arterial feeders of skull base tumors can arise from branches of the internal carotid arteries (ICAs), the external carotid arteries (ECAs), the vertebral arteries (VAs), or any combination of these arteries and/or their branches. Tumors arising from the skull base meninges are classically supplied by dural feeders at the site of dural attachment, which may include branches from the ECA/ICA/VA, and by cortical or pial branches at the tumor's periphery. Blood supply to dural tumors has been well described in the literature;[13] a complete understanding of a given patient's specific anatomy prior to embolization is a prerequisite to avoid complication from errant embolization.

We advocate for a presurgical diagnostic cerebral angiogram for most skull base tumors, even if there is no plan for embolization. The benefit is multifold. The vascularity of these tumors can be hard to predict, even with extensive noninvasive imaging such as magnetic resonance imaging (MRI) or computed tomography (CT). Knowing about aberrant parasitized feeding arteries, overall vascularity, collateral flow through the circle of Willis, and venous drainage patterns and involvement can aid in the operative approach, prepare for blood loss, and help predict the safety of vessel sacrifice. A balloon test occlusion can be easily planned in conjunction with the diagnostic angiogram when deemed necessary. If embolization is planned, a separate diagnostic procedure in an awake patient can avoid the embarrassment of putting someone under general anesthesia only to discover the absence of accessible arterial feeders. Furthermore, some straight-forward pedicles may be amenable to an awake embolization, which then allows for provocative Wada testing—selective injection of a temporary neuroanesthetic agent such as sodium amytal, propofol, or lidocaine—to simulate neurologic deficit.

Super-selective catheterization of ECA and ICA branches is needed to define the blood supply to any given tumor and to identify any potential intracranial-extracranial anastomoses which may prove dangerous if misunderstood and embolized. Combination blood supply of some skull base tumors from complex ICA and ECA anastomoses of the meninges can often make embolization both challenging and risky. Anastomotic pathways between intracranial and extracranial circulations are well-described.[14] Generally, there are three regions that serve as major extracranial-to-intracranial anastomotic connections: the orbital region via the ophthalmic artery, the petrous-cavernous region, and the upper cervical region with the posterior circulation.

Special attention should be paid to any potential anastomoses with the ophthalmic artery, a common source of ICA–ECA anastomosis. Although the ophthalmic artery typically anastamoses with ethmoidal arteries, it may arise from the middle meningeal artery (MMA);[15] in this circumstance, MMA sacrifice can lead to visual loss. The occipital artery can anastomose with the vertebral artery via C1 and C2 radicular branches, as can ascending and deep cervical arteries with the C3–C7 radicular branches. Key ICA–ECA anastomoses in the petrous-cavernous region include the vidian artery of the petrous ICA with the internal maxillary artery, and anastomoses between the inferolateral trunk (ILT) and meningohypophyseal trunk (MHT) with the ascending pharyngeal artery (APA). Careful consideration should also be paid to the ILT, MHT, and APA because of their complicated supply to the cranial nerves at the base of the skull; in our experience, it is generally unwise to embolize major branches of these vessels.

The decision to embolize a skull base tumor prior to surgical resection requires a holistic team-based approach with all parties involved taking an active role in the decision. There should be a clear understanding of the goals of tumor embolization, and these goals and the timing of embolization should be agreed upon by both the surgical team and the neurointerventionalist prior to any intervention. Specific goals of tumor embolization may include:

- Occlusion of a deep feeding artery on the side opposite to the surgical trajectory.
- Deep penetration with small particles to soften and induce necrosis within surgically hard-to-reach tumors, augmenting ease of tumor resection.
- Proximal occlusion of select dominant feeding artery/arteries with coils to reduce blood loss during operative exposure or debulking.

It is advantageous for the endovascular team to know the surgeon's specific requirements and how embolization specifically can influence the outcome of a proposed surgery, and the goals of both teams should be aligned and congruent. For example, special attention must be paid to preserving the septal branch of the sphenopalatine artery (SPA) if a nasoseptal flap will be necessary for skull base reconstruction during an endonasal tumor. Nasoseptal flaps are frequently pedicled on the posterior septal artery, the terminal branch of the SPA,

and the preservation or sacrifice of this branch should be discussed with the entire surgical team prior to embolization.

It is common for an overzealous interventionalist at the time of embolization to pursue the often-unreachable "perfect" radiographic outcome. In light of this aspect of human nature, we have found it useful to have a predetermined embolization stopping point, beyond which represents deteriorating gains and rapidly increasing risk to the patient. Knowing when to quit is a skill gained through experience, and we have found predetermined stopping points useful for complication avoidance. Specific stopping points that we have used in our practice include:

- Surpassing a predefined amount of radiation (*>5* Gy) or fluoro time (*>60* min).
- Reflux of liquid embolic into feeding arteries, with careful attention to avoid bilateral internal maxillary artery reflux and occlusion if the harvest of a nasoseptal flap is necessary.
- Following occlusion of deep, surgically inaccessible feeding arteries.
- Following occlusion of a single dominant feeder.

Skull base tumors often have a dominant feeding artery that offers the best chance of meaningful devascularization. These are frequently dural-based, and in most cases vessel sacrifice conveys very low risk to the patient. In contrast, most occipital artery or cavernous carotid branches supplying a given skull base tumor rarely provide large conduits and are typically not worth the risk of embolization.

3.4 Available Embolysates

Choice of embolysate can have a major impact on injury avoidance. We have found the following agents, listed in decreasing order of safety, to be beneficial: coils, large particles (e.g., poly-vinyl alcohol [PVA]), Onyx, NBCA, small particles (e.g., embospheres), and ethanol. The size of embolysate matters, both in terms of efficacy and complication rates.[16,17] In general, liquid embolics and small particles can penetrate tumor capillary beds more distally than coils or large particles; this allows for reduced surgical vascularity but increases the chance of complication from intracranial-extracranial anastomoses or nerve palsy from occlusion of cranial nerve vasa nervorum. Coils or large particles may be sufficient for proximal pedicle embolization and generally are safer due to their increased ability for control. The choice of embolysate should be carefully considered to avoid complications and should address the goal of embolization. Pros and cons of certain commercial embolysates are outlined in ▶ Table 3.1.

3.5 Case Examples

Case 1. A 15-year-old boy with a new diagnosis of a large JNA was referred for preoperative tumor embolization (▶ Fig. 3.1). Preprocedure anteroposterior (AP) and lateral right ECA injection demonstrated intense tumor blush from the distal internal maxillary artery (▶ Fig. 3.2), and this vessel was selected for embolization with Onyx18. Intraprocedural, super-selective right distal internal maxillary artery injection demonstrated extensive tumor blush (▶ Fig. 3.3). Postembolization AP and

Table 3.1 Advantages and disadvantages of commercial embolysates

Embolysate type (examples)	Advantages	Disadvantages
Coils • Tornado® (Cook Medical, Bloomington, IN) • Axium™ (Medtronic, Santa Rosa, CA) • Target® (Stryker Neurovascular, Fremont, CA) • Barricade™ (Balt USA, Irvine, CA)	• Simple to use and deploy • Very controllable in low- or moderate-flow states • Proximal flow arrest	• No distal penetration
Large particles • Polyvinyl alcohol (PVA)	• Relatively safe • Proximal flow arrest • Causes significant inflammatory reaction and vessel fibrosis	• No distal penetration • Significant recanalization rate • Clumping/aggregation may occur, occluding vessel more proximal than expected based on size
n-Butyl cyanoacrylate (NBCA)	• Excellent distal penetration • Forms permanent cast of the vessel, progressing to chronic inflammation and fibrosis	• Difficult to control in high-flow fistulae • Requires experience to aid in tailoring an NBCA/Ethiodol mixture ratio resulting in an appropriate polymerization time • Recanalization can occur if only partial embolization is achieved
Ethylene vinyl alcohol copolymer (Onyx) • Onyx18 • Onyx34	• Easy to control • Excellent distal penetration • Used commonly, well-understood • Nonadhesive, allowing for longer injection times and temporarily suspending injection if necessary • Provides body to the tumor and delineates operative margins to facilitate surgical manipulation and resection	• High radiation exposure and time commitment • Dimethyl sulfoxide (DMSO) can be neurotoxic and rapid injection may cause vasospasm and necrosis, which may increase chances of cranial neuropathy • Can cause sparking with electrocautery during surgery
Small particles • Tris-acryl Gelatin Microspheres (Embospheres)	• Excellent distal penetration • Generally won't aggregate/clump • Causes significant inflammatory reaction and vessel fibrosis • Consistent particle size	• Need for intermittent agitation to maintain suspension • Can be difficult to control • High risk of capillary penetration which may cause ischemia and cranial neuropathy
Ethanol	• Excellent distal penetration	• Rarely used • Difficult to control, disseminates widely • Rapidly diluted by vascular inflow

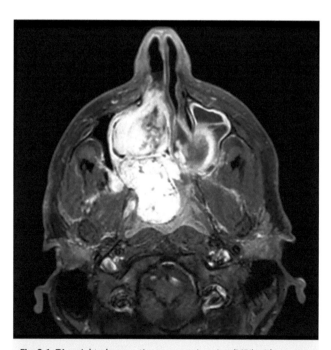

Fig. 3.1 T1-weighted magnetic resonance imaging (MRI) with contrast demonstrates a large heterogeneously enhancing tumor of the nasopharynx in this 15-year-old boy.

lateral digital subtraction angiography (DSA) of the right ECA demonstrates no residual tumor supply from the right ECA (► Fig. 3.4); however, ICA injection reveals persistent tumor blush from several cavernous carotid branches (► Fig. 3.5). Given the elevated risk with super-selective catheterization and embolization of these intracranial cavernous ICA branches, the embolization procedure was terminated. The patient underwent successful endonasal surgical resection with resultant gross total resection the following day.

Case 2. A 54-year-old man presented to his otolaryngologist with 3 months of right-sided hearing loss and facial hemiparesis and was found on MRI to have an avidly-enhancing posterior fossa tumor in the region of the right cerebellopontine angle (► Fig. 3.6) with a presumed diagnosis of hemangiopericytoma. At the request of his neurosurgeon he underwent preoperative embolization. Right ECA injection revealed multiple feeding arteries (► Fig. 3.7, *red arrows*) to the tumor (*black arrow*) from the right internal maxillary and middle meningeal arteries. Super-selective injection of the right MMA revealed significant tumor blush (*black arrow*, ► Fig. 3.8), and the patient then underwent Onyx18 and Barricade coil embolization of the right MMA with no residual filling from the MMA at the end of the procedure (► Fig. 3.9).

Additional tumor vascular supply was identified from cavernous branches of the right ICA (► Fig. 3.10) and from the right

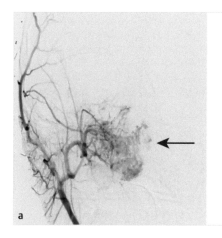
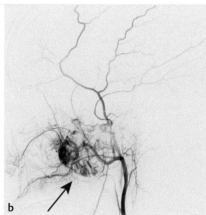

Fig. 3.2 **(a)** Anteroposterior (AP) and **(b)** lateral right external carotid artery (ECA) angiography demonstrates dense tumor blush (*black arrows*) from the distal internal maxillary artery.

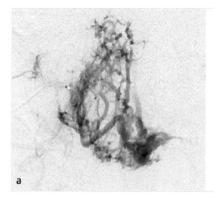
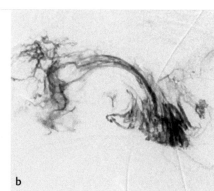

Fig. 3.3 Super-selective **(a)** anteroposterior (AP) and **(b)** lateral angiography of the internal maxillary artery during embolization.

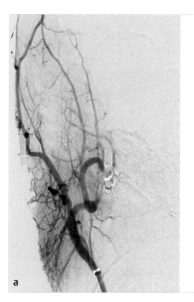
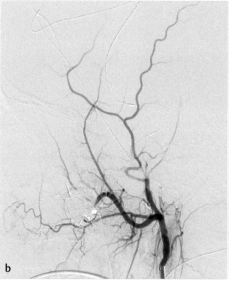

Fig. 3.4 **(a, b)** Right external carotid artery (ECA) injection post embolization shows no residual tumor blush from the internal maxillary artery.

superior cerebellar artery (SCA) and anterior inferior cerebellar artery (AICA) (▶ Fig. 3.11). The right SCA was super-selectively catheterized and embolized with Onyx18. Postembolization angiography of the posterior circulation demonstrated no residual tumor filling from the right SCA; residual filling from AICA remained (▶ Fig. 3.12). At this point two large pedicles supplying the tumor had been successfully embolized and total fluoroscopy time had exceeded 60 minutes; the neurointerventionalist and the neurosurgeon jointly elected to end the embolization procedure. The patient awoke from the procedure with no new neurologic deficits, and he underwent gross total tumor resection the following day. The pathology revealed that the tumor was a hemangioblastoma rather than the presumed diagnosis of hemangiopericytoma.

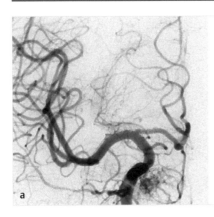
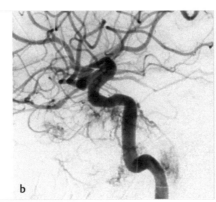

Fig. 3.5 Right (a) anteroposterior (AP) and (b) lateral internal carotid artery (ICA) injection reveals persistent tumor blush from the right cavernous ICA.

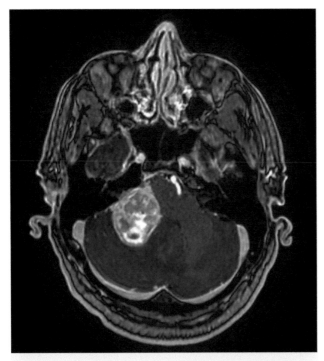

Fig. 3.6 T1-weighted contrast-enhanced axial magnetic resonance imaging (MRI) demonstrates a right cerebellopontine angle heterogeneously enhancing tumor with intratumoral cysts.

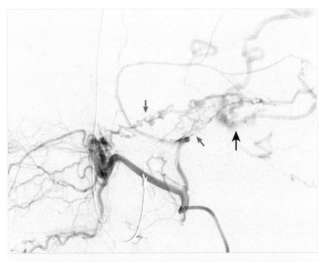

Fig. 3.7 Right lateral external carotid artery (ECA) injection revealed tumor vascular supply from the distal internal maxillary artery and the middle meningeal artery (*red arrows*) with resultant tumor blush (*black arrow*).

3.6 Management Strategy

Histopathologic tumoral changes after embolization of skull base tumors are dynamic, with recently devascularized tumors undergoing infarction and necrosis followed by thrombus formation and edema. Postembolization inflammation can lead to transient swelling of the tumor, and tumors with significant mass effect may cause worsening neurologic deficit, hydrocephalus, or herniation; if mass effect is a concern, it is a preference at our institution to start these patients on high-dose steroids and perform resection within 24 hours or less of embolization. However, performing embolization at least several days before surgery may increase the ease of resection for the surgeon by promoting tumor necrosis, particularly for meningiomas.[18] After 7 days post embolization, partial revascularization and recanalization of embolized pedicles may

occur.[19] Maximizing the benefits and limiting the inadequacies of preoperative embolization is made on a case-by-case basis; our institutional preference for the majority of skull base tumors, given the surrounding elegant anatomy and propensity for postembolization infarction and edema, is for very early (<24 hours) surgical resection.

Four-vessel angiography may prove useful in patients who have undergone prior surgery to identify any prior vascular injury (e.g., pseudoaneurysm, vascular occlusion). General anesthesia is typically preferred for these procedures to eliminate patient movement, which may improve technical feasibility and increase safety. In this scenario, intraoperative neurophysiologic monitoring of somatosensory evoked potentials and electroencephalography allows for monitoring of some cerebral function when a neurologic examination is unobtainable. Many of these procedures can also be performed with the patient awake; however, the benefit of avoiding general anesthesia has to be balanced against increased movement, difficulty in visualizing the embolization material, urinary retention, patient discomfort, and pain at the injection site due to physical distension or drug irritation (particularly with dimethyl sulfoxide [DMSO]). Anecdotally, local irritation from DMSO injection can

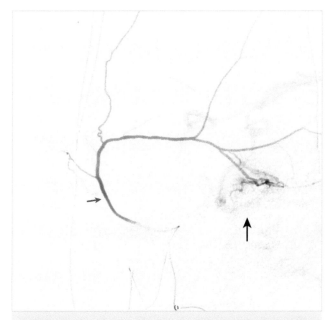

Fig. 3.8 Lateral view of a super-selective injection of the right middle meningeal artery (MMA) (*red arrow*) demonstrates significant tumor blush (*black arrow*). This vessel was embolized with Onyx18 and Barricade coils.

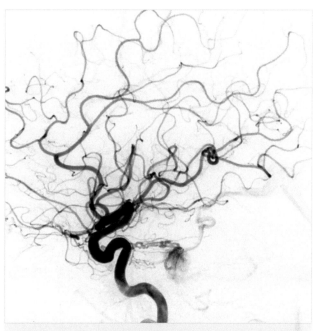

Fig. 3.10 Lateral angiography of the right internal carotid artery (ICA) demonstrates tumor vascular supply from cavernous ICA branches.

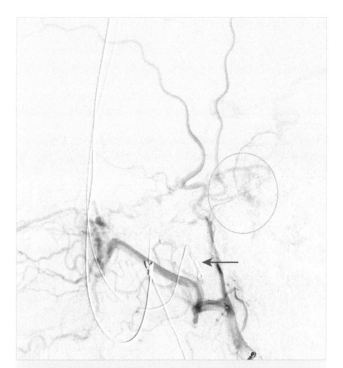

Fig. 3.9 Postembolization lateral angiography of the right external carotid artery (ECA) demonstrates obliteration of the middle meningeal artery (MMA) (*red arrow*) and near disappearance of tumor blush (*orange circle*).

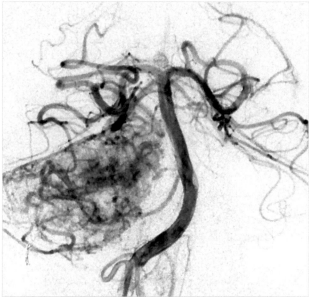

Fig. 3.11 Anteroposterior (AP) angiography of the posterior circulation allows for visualization of tumor filling from the right superior cerebellar artery (SCA) and anterior inferior cerebellar artery (AICA).

be mitigated by injecting 2 to 10 mg of lidocaine intra-arterially immediately prior to embolization.

Amytal, lidocaine, and propofol have been shown to be efficacious in Wada testing and may also be utilized to identify vascular supply to cranial nerves.[20,21,22] Super-selective Wada testing to identify blood supply to the cranial nerves has been described prior to embolization in an attempt to minimize cranial nerve injury. It has been suggested that patients with skull base meningiomas whose tumor-feeding dural arteries arise from the MMA and run posteromedially toward the petrous apex or cavernous sinus are at increased risk of postembolization cranial nerve palsy.[23] Similarly, embolization of

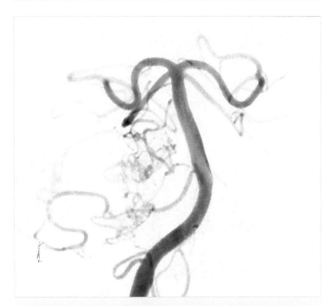

Fig. 3.12 Post–superior cerebellar artery (SCA) embolization demonstrates no residual filling from the right SCA and persistent filling from the right anterior inferior cerebellar artery (AICA).

the ascending pharyngeal artery, which often supplies skull base tumors (e.g., glomus jugulare paragangliomas[24]), can result in facial nerve injury which may be predicted via utilization of super-selective Wada testing.

3.7 Potential Complications

Complications related to tumor embolization can include, in ascending order of seriousness: groin hematoma, temporary or permanent hair loss, contrast nephropathy, cranial nerve palsy, skin or mucosal necrosis, vessel perforation, stroke (ischemic or hemorrhagic), and death. Care must be taken to carefully identify and have a complete understanding of vascular pedicles to the tumor and to normal, healthy tissue. At the time of embolization, selection of appropriate embolysate and flawless procedural technique are required to ensure a satisfactory outcome.

Specific procedural complications are dependent on tumor location. For skull base tumors, embolization of external carotid artery branches is common and risks specific to these tumors include skin and/or mucosal necrosis and cranial nerve palsy. For intracranial tumors or tumors supplied by intracranial vessels, ischemic stroke and death are more common; major complication rates after intracranial embolization have been reported to be as high as 3 to 6%.[17,25] Because preoperative tumor embolization is not absolutely required under any circumstance, avoidance of all major complications is absolutely critical.

It is beneficial to have the surgeon in the angiography suite at the time of embolization to both gauge the success of embolization and to aid in the discussion of surgical approach and identification of the predetermined stopping point. In cases where tumor resection is immediately preceded by embolization, it can be difficult to differentiate postoperative complications attributable to embolization from those attributable to surgical resection. Whenever possible, we recommend obtaining a neurologic examination between embolization and resection to distinguish embolization from surgical complications.

If a complication does occur during an embolization procedure, immediate recognition of the complication and the direct cause is essential. The offending action should be aborted immediately. If the cause of a complication is related to errant embolysate, induced hypertension and intravenous hydration may enhance the perfusion provided by collateral circulation. In the event of cranial nerve palsy, corticosteroids have not been shown to have any benefit. There have been reports of cranial neuropathies after embolization making partial or full recoveries with certain embolysates, which may be related to recanalization.[26]

3.8 Venous Anatomy

Venous anatomic relations to skull base tumors is covered in Chapter 20, Venous Considerations in Skull Base Surgery, but deserves special comment in this section because much information about relevant venous anatomy can be gained and can be extremely helpful in the prospective avoidance of venous injury. Significant surgical morbidity can result from venous infarcts and, although venous anatomy is not directly related to embolization, it is important to ascertain this information during preoperative angiography. The thoughtful neurointerventionalist will obtain angiographic runs during embolization that include the venous phase.

3.9 Conclusion

Preoperative tumor embolization can decrease intraoperative blood loss and potentially enhance the chance of successful surgical resection of skull base tumors. There is no surgical resection that absolutely requires preoperative tumor embolization, and therefore embolization is predicated entirely on the avoidance of complications. Positive outcomes require in-depth knowledge of patient-specific neurovascular anatomy, case and endpoint selection, an excellent understanding and familiarity with neurointerventional equipment and chosen embolysate, and impeccable technique.

References

[1] Djindjian R, Cophignon J, Théron J, Merland JJ, Houdart R. Embolization by superselective arteriography from the femoral route in neuroradiology. Review of 60 cases. 1. Technique, indications, complications. Neuroradiology. 1973; 6(1):20–26

[2] Duffis EJ, Gandhi CD, Prestigiacomo CJ, et al. Society for Neurointerventional Surgery. Head, neck, and brain tumor embolization guidelines. J Neurointerv Surg. 2012; 4(4):251–255

[3] Gupta R, Thomas AJ, Horowitz M. Intracranial head and neck tumors: endovascular considerations, present and future. Neurosurgery. 2006; 59(5) Suppl 3:S251–S260, discussion S3–S13

[4] Chun JY, McDermott MW, Lamborn KR, Wilson CB, Higashida R, Berger MS. Delayed surgical resection reduces intraoperative blood loss for embolized meningiomas. Neurosurgery. 2002; 50(6):1231–1235, discussion 1235–1237

[5] Tikkakoski T, Luotonen J, Leinonen S, et al. Preoperative embolization in the management of neck paragangliomas. Laryngoscope. 1997; 107(6):821–826

[6] LaMuraglia GM, Fabian RL, Brewster DC, et al. The current surgical management of carotid body paragangliomas. J Vasc Surg. 1992; 15(6):1038–1044, discussion 1044–1045

[7] Ungkanont K, Byers RM, Weber RS, Callender DL, Wolf PF, Goepfert H. Juvenile nasopharyngeal angiofibroma: an update of therapeutic management. Head Neck. 1996; 18(1):60–66

[8] Casasco A, Herbreteau D, Houdart E, et al. Devascularization of craniofacial tumors by percutaneous tumor puncture. AJNR Am J Neuroradiol. 1994; 15 (7):1233–1239

[9] Casasco A, Houdart E, Biondi A, et al. Major complications of percutaneous embolization of skull-base tumors. AJNR Am J Neuroradiol. 1999; 20(1): 179–181

[10] Ozyer U, Harman A, Yildirim E, Aytekin C, Akay TH, Boyvat F. Devascularization of head and neck paragangliomas by direct percutaneous embolization. Cardiovasc Intervent Radiol. 2010; 33(5):967–975

[11] Derdeyn CP, Neely JG. Direct puncture embolization for paragangliomas: promising results but preliminary data. AJNR Am J Neuroradiol. 2004; 25(9): 1453–1454

[12] Elhammady MS, Peterson EC, Johnson JN, Aziz-Sultan MA. Preoperative onyx embolization of vascular head and neck tumors by direct puncture. World Neurosurg. 2012; 77(5–6):725–730

[13] Dubel GJ, Ahn SH, Soares GM. Contemporary endovascular embolotherapy for meningioma. Semin Intervent Radiol. 2013; 30(3):263–277

[14] Geibprasert S, Pongpech S, Armstrong D, Krings T. Dangerous extracranial-intracranial anastomoses and supply to the cranial nerves: vessels the neurointerventionalist needs to know. AJNR Am J Neuroradiol. 2009; 30(8): 1459–1468

[15] Liu Q, Rhoton AL, Jr. Middle meningeal origin of the ophthalmic artery. Neurosurgery. 2001; 49(2):401–406, discussion 406–407

[16] Wakhloo AK, Juengling FD, Van Velthoven V, Schumacher M, Hennig J, Schwechheimer K. Extended preoperative polyvinyl alcohol microembolization of intracranial meningiomas: assessment of two embolization techniques. AJNR Am J Neuroradiol. 1993; 14(3):571–582

[17] Carli DF, Sluzewski M, Beute GN, van Rooij WJ. Complications of particle embolization of meningiomas: frequency, risk factors, and outcome. AJNR Am J Neuroradiol. 2010; 31(1):152–154

[18] Kai Y, Hamada J, Morioka M, Yano S, Todaka T, Ushio Y. Appropriate interval between embolization and surgery in patients with meningioma. AJNR Am J Neuroradiol. 2002; 23(1):139–142

[19] Pauw BK, Makek MS, Fisch U, Valavanis A. Preoperative embolization of paragangliomas (glomus tumors) of the head and neck: histopathologic and clinical features. Skull Base Surg. 1993; 3(1):37–44

[20] Patel A, Wordell C, Szarlej D. Alternatives to sodium amobarbital in the Wada test. Ann Pharmacother. 2011; 45(3):395–401

[21] Chiu AH, Bynevelt M, Lawn N, Lee G, Singh TP. Propofol as a substitute for amobarbital in Wada testing. J Clin Neurosci. 2015; 22(11):1830–1832

[22] Horton JA, Kerber CW. Lidocaine injection into external carotid branches: provocative test to preserve cranial nerve function in therapeutic embolization. AJNR Am J Neuroradiol. 1986; 7(1):105–108

[23] Kai Y, Hamada J, Morioka M, et al. Preoperative cellulose porous beads for therapeutic embolization of meningioma: provocation test and technical considerations. Neuroradiology. 2007; 49(5):437–443

[24] White JB, Link MJ, Cloft HJ. Endovascular embolization of paragangliomas: a safe adjuvant to treatment. J Vasc Interv Neurol. 2008; 1(2):37–41

[25] Bendszus M, Monoranu CM, Schütz A, Nölte I, Vince GH, Solymosi L. Neurologic complications after particle embolization of intracranial meningiomas. AJNR Am J Neuroradiol. 2005; 26(6):1413–1419

[26] Valavanis A. Preoperative embolization of the head and neck: indications, patient selection, goals, and precautions. AJNR Am J Neuroradiol. 1986; 7(5): 943–952

4 Vascular Supply of Local-Regional Flaps in Skull Base Surgery

Philippe Lavigne and Eric W. Wang

Summary

With the advent of new technologies and better understanding of the anatomy, skull base defects have become increasingly larger and more complex to reconstruct. Several options now exist from avascular free grafts to large axially perfused local-regional flaps. Some of the vascularized options are harvested traditionally through open approaches, but several endonasal options are available. The concept for both remains the same: a watertight closure to reconstruct the barrier separating the intracranial cavity from external spaces and the aerodigestive tract and prevent postoperative complications. Most vascularized flaps arise from external carotid artery branches, except for the pericranial flap which receives vascular supply from branches of the ophthalmic artery, itself a branch of the internal carotid artery. Reconstructive choice depends on the defect location, size, surgical approach, disease process, patient factors, and surgeon's preference. Ideally, surgeons will be comfortable with several options to offer tailored reconstruction for optimal results.

Keywords: Endoscopic, reconstruction, skull base, vascularized flap

4.1 Key Learning Points

- Reconstruction of skull base defects is needed to create a protective barrier around the cranial cavity.
- Extranasal flap options include: anterior pericranial flap, temporoparietal fascial flap, temporalis muscle flap, facial artery musculomucosal (FAMM) flap, and occipital pericranial flap.
- Endonasal flap options include: nasoseptal flap, inferior turbinate/lateral nasal wall flap, and middle turbinate flap.
- Flap selection depends on the underlying pathology, patient co-morbidities, prior therapy, approach extension, and defect location and size.

4.2 Introduction

Reconstruction of the skull base is critical to re-establish a barrier between the cranial cavity and the sinonasal tract and to prevent postoperative cerebrospinal fluid (CSF) leaks. Failed reconstruction can lead to pneumocephalus, meningitis, abscess formation, and ventriculitis. Significant advances in technology and the advancement of endoscopic endonasal techniques have required endonasal reconstruction of larger and more complex skull base defects. Reconstructive techniques have also evolved, and multiple options are now available to skull base surgeons. The reconstructive algorithm depends on defect size and location, surgical approach, pathologic diagnosis, patient factors, and prior therapy. Small defects (<1 cm) of the ventral skull base can be repaired with >90% success rates with multilayered nonvascularized free grafts.[1] Larger dural defects or those that are exposed to high-flow CSF leaks were found to have CSF leak rates of 16.7 and 16.2% with endoscopic endonasal approaches and open craniofacial resections, respectively.[2,3] Vascularized tissue was found to significantly reduce CSF leak rates in such high risk defects.[4] This chapter presents the most commonly used vascularized reconstructive flaps in transcranial and endoscopic endonasal skull base surgery. ▶ Table 4.1 presents the major characteristics for each flap.

4.3 Extranasal Reconstructive Flaps

For transcranial approaches, vascularized scalp flaps are effective at re-establishing separation of the intracranial space. Preoperative surgical planning of scalp incisions aids in the harvest and preservation of the vascular supply for these reconstructive options. With open approaches, primary repair of the dural defect with suturing of a fascial graft and inset of the flap facilitates a watertight seal. For reconstruction of endonasal skull base defects, extranasal flaps have the advantage of being harvested at distance from the primary pathology. This is most significant for malignant sinus and skull base tumors where involvement of local tissues can jeopardize the vascular supply of a flap or compromise oncologic resection. Furthermore, if the patient has received prior radiation therapy to the nasal cavity or skull base, the flap and its vascular supply are typically beyond the radiation field.[5]

4.3.1 Anterior Pericranial Flap

The anterior pericranial flap (PCF) receives blood flow from the supraorbital and supratrochlear arteries, both branches of the ophthalmic artery. It is the only locoregional skull base reconstructive flap that receives its blood supply from the internal carotid artery (ICA). It can be harvested unilaterally or bilaterally depending on defect size and arc of rotation and can be extended posteriorly beyond the bicoronal skin incision if needed. A standard PCF combines the periosteum and the superficial loose areolar connective tissue. A galeo-pericranial flap also includes the galeal layer but is rarely employed due to increased risk of overlying necrosis. When using anteriorly based scalp flaps, it is advisable to preserve blood supply to the anterior scalp to reduce the risk of skin necrosis, especially in previously irradiated patients. In these patients, the bicoronal scalp incision should be planned to preserve the parietal branch of the superficial temporal artery (STA) for increased vascular supply to the frontal scalp.[6] PCFs are traditionally utilized for skull base defects from the frontal sinus to the planum sphenoidale. This flap can be inserted *intracranially* via a frontal craniotomy, and its utility in endonasal surgery is increasingly noted. It can be transferred endonasally below the plane of the skull base (extracranially) through an osteotomy at the nasion (▶ Fig. 4.1). Care must be taken during this step not to twist the pedicle and compromise the vascular supply to the flap. Endoscopic-assisted harvesting of the PCF has been described

Table 4.1 Intranasal and extranasal reconstructive flaps for skull base reconstruction

Location	Flap name	Vascular supply	Advantage	Disadvantage/Limitations
Extranasal				
	Pericranial flap	Supraorbital and supratrochlear arteries	Large dimension; pliable; technically easy	Risk of injury to frontal branches of facial nerve; delayed endonasal mucosalization; typically large external incision
	Temporoparietal fascia flap	Superficial temporal artery	Consistent vascular anatomy; large dimension; reaches to posterior cranial fossa	Limited reach to anterior cranial fossa; risk of injury to frontal branch of facial nerve; risk of anterior skin necrosis; hair follicle damage; technically challenging
	Temporalis muscle flap	Deep temporal artery	Strong vascular supply; offers significant bulk/volume	Limited arc of rotation; temporal wasting if all the muscle is mobilized
	FAMM flap	Angular artery	No external incision; strong vascular supply	Potential morbidity (trismus, oral cavity harvest site dehiscence); technically challenging; limited reach
	Occipital pericranial flap	Occipital artery	Large reconstructive surface; strong vascular supply	Limited reach to anterior cranial fossa; large flap length to pedicle ratio; additional dissection of neck; access to posterior scalp
Endonasal				
	Nasoseptal flap	Posterior nasoseptal artery	No external incision, long vascular pedicle; reaches all areas of ventral skull base	Potential for microscopic tumor invasion with sinonasal malignancy; potential loss of vascular supply with prior endonasal surgery; limits ipsilateral pterygoid access
	Inferior turbinate/Lateral nasal wall flap	Posterior lateral nasal wall artery	Alternative to NSF when not available	Potential for nasolacrimal duct injury; not as versatile as NSF; short pedicle; lateral nasal wall crusting
	Middle turbinate flap	Middle turbinate artery	Low nasal morbidity; alternative to NSF when not available	Small reconstructive surface; short pedicle and limited arc of rotation

Abbreviations: FAMM, facial artery musculomucosal; NSF, nasoseptal flap; PPF, pterygopalatine fossa.

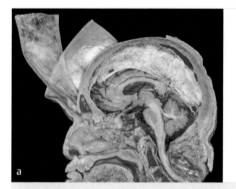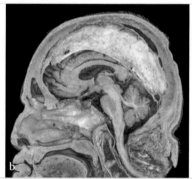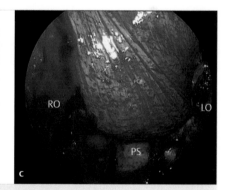

Fig. 4.1 **(a)** Sagittal view of a cadaveric dissection showing transposition of the extracranial pericranial flap (PCF) **(b)** transferred endonasally through an osteotomy at the nasion to cover a defect of the ventral skull base. **(c)** Intraoperative view of endonasal endoscopic PCF inseted through a nasion osteotomy to cover an anterior cranial base defect. PCF, pericranial flap; PS, planum sphenoidale; LO, left orbit; RO, right orbit.

and has the potential for reduced morbidity.[7] Disadvantages of the PCF include the external incision and delayed mucosalization of the flap which leads to prolonged nasal crusting, especially with postoperative radiation therapy (see ▶ Table 4.1).

4.3.2 Temporoparietal Fascial Flap

The STA, a branch of the external carotid artery (ECA), provides blood supply to the temporoparietal fascial flap (TPFF). The STA is accompanied by one or two veins, both superficial or within the temporoparietal fascia. The TPFF extends in a fan-like fashion superficial to the temporalis muscle fascia, and is in continuity with the galea aponeurotica.[8] Preoperative planning of the scalp incision is important to preserve this flap and its STA supply as the flap must be dissected during incision. Significant disadvantages of this flap are risk to hair follicles with subsequent alopecia, the need for transposition through the pterygopalatine fossa to reach the ventral skull base, and risk to the frontal branch of the facial nerve.[9,10] It can also lead to devascularization of the anterior scalp in patients

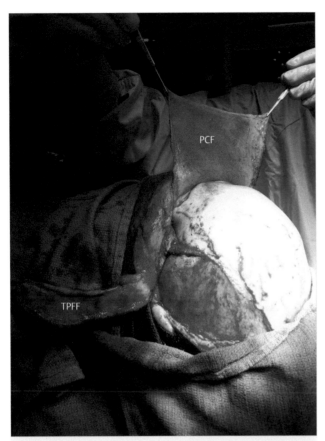

Fig. 4.2 Intraoperative view of a temporoparietal fascia flap (TPFF) and an anterior pericranial flap (PCF) in the same patient for reconstruction of complex skull base defect.

who have had previous surgeries or irradiation. ▸ Fig. 4.2 presents an example of a TPFF and a PCF, both harvested in the same patient for reconstruction of a complex skull base defect.

4.3.3 Temporalis Muscle Flap

The temporalis muscle receives vascular supply from the deep temporal branch of the internal maxillary artery which has a main anterior and posterior division deep to the muscle. This flap provides robust blood supply and bulk but has a limited arc of rotation and is mostly used for reconstruction of lateral skull base and orbital exenteration defects. The entire muscle can be rotated for reconstruction, or it can be divided into an anterior or posterior component to limit cosmetic temporal depression without compromise of its blood supply.

4.3.4 Occipital Pericranial Flap

The occipital artery supplying the pericranium has a convoluted course that usually originates just deep to the insertion of the posterior belly of the digastric muscle. Preserving a wide vascular pedicle base instead of dissecting the artery itself may prevent injury. Reconstructive surface of up to 4 cm × 11 cm can be harvested and transposed to reconstruct lateral and posterior skull base defects. Alternatively, the flap can be rotated below the mastoid tip and tunneled deep to the mandible and through the PPF into the nasal cavity to reconstruct mid-clival defects.[11]

4.3.5 Facial Artery Musculomucosal (FAMM) Flap

Initially described in 1992, the FAMM flap receives vascular supply from retrograde flow of the facial artery.[12] It is harvested intraorally and tunneled through the gingiva-buccal sulcus into a maxillary antrotomy (Caldwell-Luc).[13] Once in the nasal cavity, it can be rotated to reconstruct anterior, middle, or posterior cranial fossa defects.[14,15,16] The strong vascular supply of the FAMM flap makes it ideal to cover areas of skull base osteoradionecrosis. The disadvantages of this flap are its thickness, pliability, and potential for intraoral morbidity (trismus, oronasal fistula, harvest bed dehiscence). Although its use in oral cavity defect reconstruction is well accepted, only limited data supports its use in skull base reconstruction.[5,14,15,16,17]

4.4 Endonasal Reconstructive Flaps

Endonasal skull base defects are conveniently reconstructed using endonasal techniques. Most small, low-flow defects (<1 cm) can be repaired with free nonvascularized grafts with >90% success rate.[1] Larger or high-flow defects are more challenging to reconstruct, and the use of vascularized tissue as a reconstructive barrier has been shown to significantly reduce the risk of postoperative CSF leak when compared to nonvascularized grafts.[4] Although options are limited to the nasoseptal flap (NSF), inferior turbinate/lateral nasal wall flap, and middle turbinate flap, the harvested flap size can be tailored to the surgical approach to optimize dural reconstruction.

4.4.1 Nasoseptal Flap

Also called the Hadad-Bassagasteguy flap, the NSF is vascularized by the posterior septal artery, a branch of the sphenopalatine artery.[18,19] The vascular supply to the flap can be assessed intraoperatively, in both primary and revision surgery, with Doppler ultrasonography or indocyanine green fluorescence angiography (▸ Fig. 4.3 and ▸ Fig. 4.4).[20] Its long, robust, and centrally located pedicle allows it to reach ventral defects of the anterior, middle, and posterior cranial fossa. The flap can be extended to include the nasal floor to increase the reconstructive surface area. This is generally supplied by two arteries that extend from the nasal septum to the nasal floor (▸ Fig. 4.5). Care must be taken during the surgery to protect the flap from traumatic injury, especially when a high-speed drill is used in proximity to the pedicle. The NSF is preferentially elevated on the side opposite to powered instrumentation (drill, ultrasonic curette) to avoid trauma. In some circumstances, the side of flap elevation is dictated by the approach. For example, a transpterygoid approach classically entails lateralization of the pterygopalatine fossa contents and therefore requires elevating the flap on the contralateral side.

The NSF remains the workhorse of endonasal skull base reconstruction as it is versatile, pliable, and has a long pedicle that provides strong vascular supply. The potential disadvantages of this flap are loss of vascular supply from prior endonasal surgery and potential microscopic tumor invasion in cases of endonasal malignancy. In addition, the flap or its pedicle must be harvested or preserved throughout the surgery.

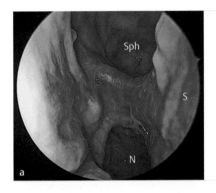
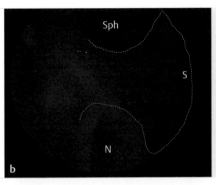

Fig. 4.3 Intraoperative assessment of the vascular supply to a right-side nasoseptal flap in the setting of revision surgery. **(a)** Right nasal cavity endoscopy shows a narrow residual nasoseptal flap pedicle. **(b)** Indocyanine green fluoroscopy filter shows no enhancement of the area of the nasoseptal flap (*dotted line*) suggesting absence of vascular supply. N, nasopharynx; S, septum; Sph, sphenoid.

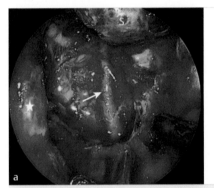
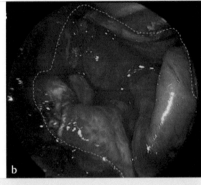
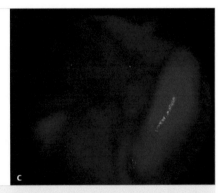

Fig. 4.4 Reconstruction of a clival defect after resection of a clival chordoma. **(a)** Intraoperative view of dural defect: *Arrow*, basilar artery; S, sella; Star, exposed right paraclival carotid artery. **(b)** Nasoseptal flap (*dotted line*) covering the dural defect, right carotid, and sella. **(c)** Indocyanine green fluoroscopy shows strong enhancement of the nasoseptal flap after final reconstruction suggesting good vascular supply.

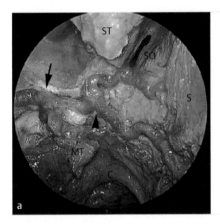
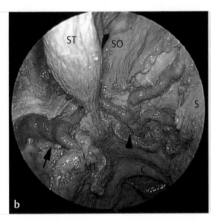

Fig. 4.5 Right nasal cavity endoscopic view of the sphenoidal bifurcation of the posterior septal artery. The sphenoidal bifurcation can be classified into a lateral type **(a)** and a medial type **(b)**. *Black arrow*, sphenopalatine artery bifurcation; *black arrowhead*, sphenoidal bifurcation of the posterior septal artery; C, choana; MT, middle turbinate; S, septum; SO, sphenoid ostium; ST, superior turbinate. (Reproduced with permission from Zhang X, Wang E, Wei H, et al. Anatomy of the posterior septal artery with surgical implications on the vascularized pedicled nasoseptal flap; Head Neck 2015;37(10):1470–1476.)

This places the pedicle at constant risk. The potential for early increased nasal morbidity remains controversial; however, its use in skull base reconstruction was not found to significantly increase long-term postoperative morbidity.[21] Initial concerns of reduced olfaction have been disproved with olfactory mucosa sparing techniques.[22] Several strategies to expedite septal healing have been described: mucosal or fascial grafts, silicone sheet splinting, and reverse septal mucosal flap (Caicedo flap).[17,23,24]

4.4.2 Lateral Nasal Wall Flap

The lateral nasal wall flap receives vascularization from the posterior lateral nasal wall artery, a branch of the sphenopalatine artery. It enters the inferior turbinate at the superior aspect of the posterolateral attachment of the inferior turbinate.[25,26] Initially described as the *inferior turbinate flap*, the reconstructive surface was limited to the mucosa covering the inferior turbinate. Improved understanding of the vascular supply now allows for "extending the flap," increasing the reconstructive surface by including variable amounts of nasal floor and anterior or lateral nasal wall mucosa, hence the more appropriate name: *lateral nasal wall flap*. When dissecting the mucosa from the inferior meatus, the nasolacrimal duct must be identified and transected sharply to prevent scarring and epiphora. This flap has a limited arc of rotation and is most useful for reconstruction of smaller sellar and mid-clival defects when an NSF is not available (▶ Fig. 4.6).

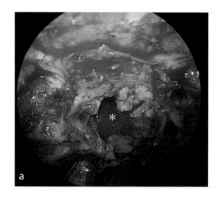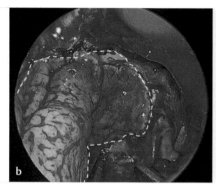

Fig. 4.6 Intraoperative endoscopic view of a right lateral nasal wall flap used to reconstruct a sellar defect after resection of a recurrent pituitary adenoma. **(a)** Dural defect with inlay collagen matrix (*). **(b)** Right lateral nasal wall flap (*dotted line*) covering the dural defect.

4.4.3 Middle Turbinate Flap

The middle turbinate flap is based on the middle turbinate artery of the sphenopalatine artery, and can be used to reconstruct small sellar and planum sphenoidale defects.[27] It is technically challenging to dissect, and premature destabilization of the bony attachment to the skull base increases difficulty and can lead to CSF leak. This flap offers a limited reconstructive area and limited arc of rotation and is therefore rarely used.

4.5 Conclusion

Reconstruction of skull base defects is one of the key challenges in skull base surgery, especially when the ideal reconstructive flap is unavailable. Flap selection depends primarily on the underlying pathology and defect location and size. Multilayered reconstruction using a structured approach following the reconstructive ladder is favored (free grafts, local flaps, regional flaps). An understanding of the blood supply of each flap is critical to ensure preservation and proper pedicle preservation. Skull base surgeons must be able to anticipate challenges in reconstruction and be familiar with several options to reduce the risk of reconstruction failure.

References

[1] Hegazy HM, Carrau RL, Snyderman CH, Kassam A, Zweig J. Transnasal endoscopic repair of cerebrospinal fluid rhinorrhea: a meta-analysis. Laryngoscope. 2000; 110(7):1166–1172

[2] Fraser S, Gardner PA, Koutourousiou M, et al. Risk factors associated with postoperative cerebrospinal fluid leak after endoscopic endonasal skull base surgery. J Neurosurg. 2018; 128(4):1066–1071

[3] Ganly I, Patel SG, Singh B, et al. Complications of craniofacial resection for malignant tumors of the skull base: report of an International Collaborative Study. Head Neck. 2005; 27(6):445–451

[4] Harvey RJ, Parmar P, Sacks R, Zanation AM. Endoscopic skull base reconstruction of large dural defects: a systematic review of published evidence. Laryngoscope. 2012; 122(2):452–459

[5] Zanation AM, Thorp BD, Parmar P, Harvey RJ. Reconstructive options for endoscopic skull base surgery. Otolaryngol Clin North Am. 2011; 44(5): 1201–1222

[6] Snyderman CH, Janecka IP, Sekhar LN, Sen CN, Eibling DE. Anterior cranial base reconstruction: role of galeal and pericranial flaps. Laryngoscope. 1990; 100(6):607–614

[7] Zanation AM, Snyderman CH, Carrau RL, Kassam AB, Gardner PA, Prevedello DM. Minimally invasive endoscopic pericranial flap: a new method for endonasal skull base reconstruction. Laryngoscope. 2009; 119(1):13–18

[8] Brent B, Upton J, Acland RD, et al. Experience with the temporoparietal fascial free flap. Plast Reconstr Surg. 1985; 76(2):177–188

[9] Jaquet Y, Higgins KM, Enepekides DJ. The temporoparietal fascia flap: a versatile tool in head and neck reconstruction. Curr Opin Otolaryngol Head Neck Surg. 2011; 19(4):235–241

[10] Fortes FS, Carrau RL, Snyderman CH, et al. Transpterygoid transposition of a temporoparietal fascia flap: a new method for skull base reconstruction after endoscopic expanded endonasal approaches. Laryngoscope. 2007; 117(6): 970–976

[11] Rivera-Serrano CM, Snyderman CH, Carrau RL, Durmaz A, Gardner PA. Transparapharyngeal and transpterygoid transposition of a pedicled occipital galeopericranial flap: a new flap for skull base reconstruction. Laryngoscope. 2011; 121(5):914–922

[12] Pribaz J, Stephens W, Crespo L, Gifford G. A new intraoral flap: facial artery musculomucosal (FAMM) flap. Plast Reconstr Surg. 1992; 90(3):421–429

[13] Berania I, Lavigne F, Rahal A, Ayad T. Superiorly based facial artery musculomucosal flap: a versatile pedicled flap. Head Neck. 2018; 40(2): 402–405

[14] Xie L, Lavigne P, Lavigne F, Ayad T. Modified facial artery musculomucosal flap for reconstruction of posterior skull base defects. J Neurol Surg Rep. 2016; 77(2):e98–e101

[15] Rivera-Serrano CM, Oliver CL, Sok J, et al. Pedicled facial buccinator (FAB) flap: a new flap for reconstruction of skull base defects. Laryngoscope. 2010; 120(10):1922–1930

[16] Farzal Z, Lemos-Rodriguez AM, Rawal RB, et al. The reverse-flow facial artery buccinator flap for skull base reconstruction: key anatomical and technical considerations. J Neurol Surg B Skull Base. 2015; 76(6):432–439

[17] Kimple AJ, Leight WD, Wheless SA, Zanation AM. Reducing nasal morbidity after skull base reconstruction with the nasoseptal flap: free middle turbinate mucosal grafts. Laryngoscope. 2012; 122(9):1920–1924

[18] Hadad G, Bassagasteguy L, Carrau RL, et al. A novel reconstructive technique after endoscopic expanded endonasal approaches: vascular pedicle nasoseptal flap. Laryngoscope. 2006; 116(10):1882–1886

[19] Zhang X, Wang EW, Wei H, et al. Anatomy of the posterior septal artery with surgical implications on the vascularized pedicled nasoseptal flap. Head Neck. 2015; 37(10):1470–1476

[20] Geltzeiler M, Nakassa ACI, Turner M, et al. Evaluation of intranasal flap perfusion by intraoperative indocyanine green fluorescence angiography. Oper Neurosurg (Hagerstown). 2018; 15(6):672–676

[21] Harvey RJ, Malek J, Winder M, et al. Sinonasal morbidity following tumour resection with and without nasoseptal flap reconstruction. Rhinology. 2015; 53(2):122–128

[22] Harvey RJ, Winder M, Davidson A, et al. The olfactory strip and its preservation in endoscopic pituitary surgery maintains smell and sinonasal function. J Neurol Surg B Skull Base. 2015; 76(6):464–470

[23] Caicedo-Granados E, Carrau R, Snyderman CH, et al. Reverse rotation flap for reconstruction of donor site after vascular pedicled nasoseptal flap in skull base surgery. Laryngoscope. 2010; 120(8):1550–1552

[24] Zeinalizadeh M, Sadrehosseini SM, Barkhoudarian G, Carrau RL. Reconstruction of the denuded nasoseptal flap donor site with a free fascia lata graft: technical note. Eur Arch Otorhinolaryngol. 2016; 273(10):3179–3182

[25] Choby GW, Pinheiro-Neto CD, de Almeida JR, et al. Extended inferior turbinate flap for endoscopic reconstruction of skull base defects. J Neurol Surg B Skull Base. 2014; 75(4):225–230

[26] Fortes FS, Carrau RL, Snyderman CH, et al. The posterior pedicle inferior turbinate flap: a new vascularized flap for skull base reconstruction. Laryngoscope. 2007; 117(8):1329–1332

[27] Prevedello DM, Barges-Coll J, Fernandez-Miranda JC, et al. Middle turbinate flap for skull base reconstruction: cadaveric feasibility study. Laryngoscope. 2009; 119(11):2094–2098

5 Bypass in the Treatment of Skull Base Tumors

Laligam N. Sekhar, Ananth K. Vellimana, and Zeeshan Qazi

Summary

Cerebral revascularization for skull base tumors represents a complex subset of the intracranial bypass procedures with unique challenges compared to revascularization for intracranial aneurysms. Skull base tumors requiring cerebral revascularization may include meningioma, schwannoma, chordoma, chondrosarcoma, and aggressive malignancies (squamous cell carcinoma, adenoid cystic carcinoma, etc.) The decision to perform a bypass could be either pre-operative such as flow augmentation for partial vessel occlusion from tumor invasion and flow replacement for total vessel occlusion by the tumor, or intra-operative to salvage vascular injury during tumor excision. Vascular injury during skull base tumor excision typically occurs due to encasement or invasion of blood vessels, presence of scar tissue, loss of normal arachnoid planes, and unexpected vascular anatomy. This chapter reviews the key management strategies and technical considerations gleaned from the senior author's (LNS) vast experience performing bypass surgery for skull base tumors over three decades. We also use case examples to highlight the decision-making process involved in the optimal management of these lesions.

Keywords: Cerebral revascularization, skull base tumors, EC-IC bypass, high-flow bypass

5.1 Key Learning Points

- Common risk factors for intraoperative vascular injury during skull base tumor surgery are reoperation for previously resected or irradiated tumors, tumor dissection from vessel wall, unexpected vascular anatomy, surgeon disorientation, and use of drills, ultrasonic aspirators, or laser in proximity to vasculature.
- Skull base pathologies that may necessitate flow replacement include meningioma, schwannoma, chordoma, chondrosarcoma, and malignant lesions such as squamous cell carcinoma, adenoid cystic carcinoma, and osteogenic sarcoma.
- Various techniques such as direct suturing, local intracranial-intracranial bypasses, and high-flow bypass exist for vessel reconstruction and replacement. The ability of a patient to tolerate occlusion of a major artery depends on the artery, collateral flow, and patient's age.

5.2 Introduction

Extracranial (EC) to intracranial (IC) bypass for cerebral vascularization was introduced by Yasargil in 1967 in the form of superficial temporal artery (STA) to middle cerebral artery (MCA) bypass for cerebral ischemia in a patient with carotid occlusion.[1] The first high-flow EC-IC bypass was performed a few years later by Lougheed and colleagues utilizing a saphenous vein graft (SVG) between the common carotid artery (CCA) and intracranial internal carotid artery (ICA).[2] Over subsequent decades, new techniques and refinement of existing techniques were introduced by various surgeons in North America, Asia, and Europe. Following the results of the EC-IC bypass trial[3] and Carotid Occlusion Surgery Study (COSS),[4] EC-IC bypass is now seldom performed for flow augmentation in patients with cerebral ischemia due to atherosclerotic steno-occlusive disease. However, an EC-IC bypass continues to be indicated for flow augmentation in select patients with steno-occlusive pathology due to moyamoya disease, and for flow replacement in some patients with complex intracranial aneurysms and skull base tumors.[5,6,7,8,9]

5.3 Vascular Challenge

Skull base tumors can affect various components of the cerebral vasculature including arteries, capillaries, and veins. In this chapter, we will discuss arterial problems that occur during the resection of skull base tumors and the use of bypasses for flow replacement in the event of injury.[7,8,10]

Arterial involvement by tumors may be encasement (partial or complete) or actual wall invasion of vessels varying in size from perforators to major vessels such as ICA, basilar artery (BA), or vertebral artery (VA). In addition to tumor involvement of arteries, iatrogenic injuries during surgical dissection may occur, leading to significant bleeding and brain infarction. When arterial occlusion occurs, an ischemic stroke may result from failure of collateral circulation to maintain adequate blood flow or from thromboembolic complications.

Involvement of small arteries and capillaries may manifest as invasion of pial vasculature by the tumor and cause vasogenic edema of the brain or brainstem. This type of involvement often precludes complete resection of the tumor. Severe neurological deficits could occur when resection of such tumors is attempted in the brainstem or other eloquent brain regions.

Venous involvement can occur from tumor invasion of large dural venous sinuses,[11] or displacement, encasement, or invasion of large cortical veins such as vein of Labbe.[12] Similar to iatrogenic arterial injuries, venous injury may occur during tumor dissection, and could lead to postoperative venous infarction and hemorrhage.

5.4 Injury Avoidance

Injury to arterial structures during skull base tumor resection commonly occurs in the following situations:

- Cases involving reoperation for disease progression, disease recurrence, or inadequate resection during primary surgery. These cases are technically more challenging due to the presence of scar tissue and loss of normal arachnoid planes. A history of prior radiation often adds to the complexity. Awareness of the increased risk of vascular injury during these cases is critical. Extensive preoperative vascular imaging and provocation tests, and preparation for a bypass procedure may be necessary. A T2-weighted magnetic resonance imaging (MRI) can be helpful to assess arachnoid planes and to detect vessel narrowing. Contrast enhancement may not be a reliable indicator of vessel wall invasion.

- Tumor dissection from the vessel wall. Vascular injuries are more common when the artery is encased or invaded by the tumor. When vessels are invaded by a malignant skull base tumor, resection of the tumor and bypass may be needed for oncological reasons. During resection of benign skull base tumors, if arterial narrowing is *not* seen on preoperative imaging, it is reasonable to attempt tumor dissection off the vessel wall. If possible, proximal and distal control of the vessel should be established first. If arterial narrowing is visible on preoperative imaging such as T2-weighted MRI, options include subtotal tumor resection or gross total resection and bypass. Smaller arteries are more prone to injury than larger arteries. To dissect small arteries away from the tumor, microdissection should be attempted after finding an arachnoid plane.
- Unexpected vascular anatomy. The skull base surgeon should thoroughly review preoperative imaging and have a low threshold to obtain additional vascular imaging such as cerebral angiogram.
- Use of drills in proximity to major arteries during bony exposure. We avoid using a cotton patty in the vicinity of the drill to reduce the risk of inadvertent injury to adjacent vascular or neural structures.
- Tumor resection with ultrasonic aspirators or laser. Use of less aggressive tips and low power settings in the vicinity of vascular structures can mitigate this risk.
- Surgeon disorientation, especially in minimally invasive approaches. Use of image guidance can help orient the surgeon to the anatomy when needed.

5.5 Related Pathologies

A variety of skull base tumors can affect adjacent vascular structures. These include:

- Meningioma: This is the most common skull base tumor with vascular involvement. Skull base meningiomas may encase large arteries including the ICA, MCA, ACA (anterior cerebral artery), VA, or BA and their branches. Intradural meningiomas which are virgin lesions usually maintain an arachnoid plane around the tumor which facilitates removal. However, perforators may still be difficult to dissect. Recurrent or progressive tumors after prior surgery and/or radiotherapy and higher grade virgin tumors (WHO grade 2 or 3 meningiomas) may show dense adhesion or invasion of adjacent vasculature making it difficult to dissect without injury to the artery. Extradural meningiomas can often be dissected away from encased arteries; however, when the artery is encased and narrowed this becomes difficult or impossible.
- Schwannoma: Schwannomas very rarely encase arteries. However, dense adhesion to arteries may be seen, especially in previously operated or irradiated tumors, and could result in injury during dissection.
- Chordoma and chondrosarcoma: Encasement of the ICA in the cavernous sinus is common. These tumors can usually be dissected free from adjacent arteries during the first surgery. Recurrent tumors are often densely adherent or invade the

wall of the arteries and there is a high risk of vascular injury during operations for recurrent tumors.

- Aggressive malignancies (e.g., squamous cell carcinoma, osteogenic sarcoma, adenoid cystic carcinoma): When tumor involves the ICA or the VA, arterial resection may be required for oncological reasons to achieve a clean margin.

5.6 Management Strategy

Arterial bypass may be necessary prophylactically or as a salvage strategy in various skull base tumors to reduce the risk of perioperative stroke. Preoperative assessment of vascular flow dynamics is imperative for skull base tumors adjacent to or involving major vascular structures. The ability of patient to tolerate occlusion of a major artery depends on the artery, collateral flow, and patient's age.

5.6.1 Internal Carotid Artery

In our practice, even if the patient has good collaterals and tolerates balloon occlusion test (BOT), we usually reconstruct the parent artery to reduce the risk of recurrent long-term thromboembolic complications from the permanently occluded artery. This is based on our prior reported experience with ICA occlusion following balloon occlusion testing and cerebral blood flow studies.[13] We found that despite the presence of excellent collateral circulation during testing, ICA occlusion caused a major stroke in approximately 13% of the patients.[13] For this reason, we prefer to reconstruct all injured arteries when possible, regardless of the collateral circulation. However, exceptions may be made when the patient is younger than 50 years of age, the preoperative angiogram shows excellent sources of collateral flow, and there are no changes in somatosensory evoked potential (SSEP) and motor evoked potential (MEP) intraoperatively.

5.6.2 Vertebral Artery (VA)

Our preference is to not occlude the VA if possible. However, one VA can be occluded in the extradural portion (V2 or V3 segment) when it is the nondominant VA, the posterior inferior cerebellar artery (PICA) does not arise from the V2 or V3 segment, and the VA has good connection to the BA (i.e., it does not terminate as PICA).

5.6.3 Basilar Artery

An injured BA must always be reconstructed or replaced. The ability to tolerate temporary occlusion depends on flow through posterior communicating artery (PComA) collaterals, and on the presence of important perforating arteries in the temporarily occluded segment.

5.6.4 Middle Cerebral Artery

A significant stroke may occur after MCA occlusion either due to the failure of hemispheric collateral circulation or due to the occlusion of lenticulostriate perforating vessels leading to a capsular infarct. If the M1 segment of the MCA is damaged, direct suturing or an extracranial to intracranial bypass should be performed to revascularize the brain in an expeditious manner. When M2 or M3 segments of MCA are damaged, they can be reconstructed by direct suturing or by EC-IC bypass. If arterial injury is probable such as in recurrent or progressive tumors after prior surgery or radiation, then a bypass using the radial artery (RA) (first preference) or anterior tibial artery (ATA) may be performed as a first-stage surgery prior to tumor resection. Although the ATA has a larger diameter than the RA and therefore less incidence of spasm, RA is preferred over ATA because of ease of graft harvest. ATA is preferred over SV because the vein dilates upon exposure to arterial flow, thereby creating turbulence.

5.6.5 Anterior Cerebral Artery

If necessary, a nondominant ACA can be occluded in the A1 segment without risk of postoperative stroke, provided there is good flow through the anterior communicating artery (AComA) and major perforating arteries such as Heubner's artery are not occluded.

5.6.6 Other Arteries

The PCA and smaller posterior circulation vessels such as anterior inferior cerebellar artery (AICA) and PICA may be reconstructed by direct suturing whenever feasible. If primary repair is not feasible, flow replacement in the basilar and PCA can be provided through a VA or ECA to P2 bypass preferably using a radial artery graft (RAG). For PICA injuries, given the tortuous nature of the vessel, an end-to-end anastomosis is usually attempted first. Alternative options depending on site of injury include side-to-side anastomosis (PICA–PICA, PICA–AICA), PICA reimplantation, occipital artery to PICA bypass, and vessel repair with short interposition graft utilizing occipital artery or RA.

In the case of tumor adherent to or invading small arteries supplying the brainstem or small perforators in the anterior circulation, it is safer to leave a small amount of residual tumor to reduce the risk of infarction.

In cases where the resection site has previously been operated upon or irradiated, or if there is encasement or narrowing of the vessel by tumor, the risk of an intraoperative arterial injury is high and preparation for a bypass may be necessary prior to initiation of tumor resection if preoperative imaging demonstrates lack of adequate collateral circulation. In the case of an unexpected arterial injury, the artery should always be reconstructed or replaced since the surgeon may not know the status of the collateral circulation. In these situations, obtaining adequate proximal and distal vascular control may be challenging.

5.7 Technical Considerations

Three different types of vessel reconstruction and replacement may be considered:

- Direct suturing: This is usually performed using an 8–0 or 9–0 nylon suture. Direct suture repair is suitable for small arteries and small tears in larger arteries.
- Local intracranial to intracranial bypasses: These can be of different types: (1) reimplantation of an artery via end-to-side anastomosis, (2) direct reconnection via end-to-end anastomosis or utilizing a short interposition graft, (3) side-to-side anastomosis (e.g., distal ACA–ACA, PICA–PICA, AICA–PICA).[14] Local bypasses may be suitable for reconstruction of small- or medium-sized arteries.
- EC-IC bypass: The flow rate through an EC-IC bypass depends on baseline flow through the recipient and donor vessels and diameter of the bypass graft. EC-IC bypasses can be categorized as:
  - Low-flow bypass (<50 mL/min): These can be used for flow replacement of small- or medium-sized arteries where the demand is low, or for flow augmentation. Examples include STA–MCA and occipital artery (OA)–PICA bypasses.
  - Moderate-flow bypass (50–99 mL/min): These are typically used for flow replacement in the posterior circulation. An RAG is used as the bypass graft in moderate-flow bypasses.[15]
  - High-flow bypass (>100 mL/min): These are typically used for flow replacement in the anterior circulation in situations of high demand (e.g., ICA replacement in a patient with poor collaterals). RAG is usually the preferred bypass graft followed by anterior tibial artery graft (ATAG)[16] or saphenous vein graft (SVG).[17]
  - Very high flow bypass (>200 mL/min): Use of SVG, ATAG, or large diameter RAG may lead to a very high flow bypass. These bypasses are optimal for flow replacement of the ICA in patients who have absent collateral circulation through the ACom and PCom. A consideration with very high flow bypasses is that turbulent flow at the anastomotic site due to abrupt vessel diameter change, typically at the recipient vessel site, may promote graft thrombosis. Therefore, care should be taken to connect the graft to a large recipient vessel or an arterial bifurcation. Very high flow bypasses must be used with caution in patients with chronic ischemia due to the danger of postoperative hyperemia that could lead to hemorrhage or brain edema.

5.7.1 Technique of High-Flow Bypass

The surgeon, assistant, anesthesiologist, scrub nurse, circulating nurse, and neurophysiologist should all be familiar with their role in the operation and function smoothly as a team.

The patient is administered 325 mg Aspirin before the surgery in order to prevent graft thrombosis. If the patient is allergic to Aspirin, 75 mg clopidogrel may be used. Patient positioning depends on the location and type of pathology, and planned donor and recipient vessels. An arterial sheath should be placed if an intraoperative angiogram is being considered. Type of craniotomy and skull base approach is dictated by lesion location, size, expected pathology, and patient's preoperative symptoms. A subcutaneous tunnel or an open graft channel is created to pass the graft from the intracranial to the extracranial space. With RAG or ATAG, a preauricular or postauricular channel that is superficial to the mandible may be used. With SVG, a postauricular channel is preferred if recipient vessel is the MCA so that the graft is oriented parallel to the sylvian fissure and the MCA prior to its entry into the cranium in order to reduce flow turbulence in the graft. If the recipient vessel is the supraclinoid ICA, then a preauricular channel is preferred for the SVG. A preauricular channel may be created by open dissection after connecting the neck and cranial incisions or via tunneling using a large-bore chest tube. For postauricular channels, we prefer to connect the cranial incision to the neck incision in a curvilinear fashion behind the ear and dissect the subcutaneous space down to the cranium. We also create a groove in the bone along the tunnel with the ultrasonic bone curette to allow more space for the graft to expand and to prevent compression by the skin.

The graft is extracted just prior to the anastomosis and prepared by flushing with heparinized saline followed by pressure distension. The pressure distension technique is very important to prevent postoperative vasospasm (usually occurring by day 3–5 postoperatively), and is utilized for arterial grafts.[15] The distal end of the graft is cut obliquely to create an oval opening and fish-mouthed by spatulation if needed. For bypasses using arterial or venous grafts, 3,000 to 4,000 units of heparin is administered intravenously. We perform the distal anastomosis first because it is technically easier to perform a deeper anastomosis with a mobile graft. Recipient arteries typically used in high-flow bypasses include M2 segment of the MCA, P2 segment of the PCA, supraclinoid ICA, or VA. For venous grafts, it is better to use an M1 or M2 bifurcation. A segment of the recipient vessel devoid of major perforators is identified and temporary clips are placed. The patient is placed in electroencephalographic burst suppression using Propofol, and systolic blood pressure is increased by 20% above baseline by the anesthesiologist prior to temporary clipping. The neurophysiologist should alert the surgeon and anesthesiologist about any changes in SSEP or MEP during clamping. If changes are seen, BP augmentation and expansion of the circulating blood volume via fluid or blood transfusion is performed as necessary. The temporary clip may also be released if possible. A marking pen is used to mark the side wall of the recipient vessel and distal end of the graft. A small arteriotomy is created in the recipient vessel and enlarged into an ovoid opening which is approximately one and a half to two times the recipient vessel diameter. The graft is preferably oriented at a 45-degree angle (donor to recipient) for an end-to-side anastomosis. Suture size depends on size of the vessels and typically 8–0 or 9–0 nylon sutures are used for intracranial vessels. Anchor sutures are placed at opposing ends of the arteriotomy. We prefer to use a running suture for the more difficult side and running or interrupted figure-of-eight sutures for the easier side. Special attention is needed to ensure that suture bites include the intima and media of the artery and are limited to one wall of the vessel. The graft is flushed with heparinized saline before tying the last suture. A temporary clip is placed on the graft and the temporary clips on the recipient artery are removed. The graft is then brought to the donor site via the previously created pre- or postauricular channel.

The donor artery may be the ECA, cervical ICA, V2 or V3 segment of VA, OA near the digastric groove, or, occasionally, STA just inferior to the zygomatic process, or the internal maxillary artery. The size of the donor vessel limits the volume of flow into the graft. An end-to-end or end (graft)-to-side (donor artery) anastomosis is performed. An end-to-side anastomosis is preferred when there is a significant disparity between diameters of graft and donor vessels. When an end-to-side anastomosis is performed, a vascular punch is utilized to create an oval opening in the donor artery, usually 3.5 to 4.5 mm diameter. The anastomosis is usually performed with 8–0 nylon or 7–0 Prolene sutures. Running sutures are used on one side and interrupted figure-of-eight sutures are used on the other side during anastomosis. The graft is placed on slight tension during anastomosis since both arterial and venous grafts expand on resumption of flow. This is especially important with venous grafts. RAGs are back bled to remove air prior to tying the last suture. With SVGs, air is removed through needle puncture or through a side branch since back bleeding is not possible. Temporary clips are opened proximally followed by the distal ones and the graft is inspected for leaks or kinking. Flow in the graft and the recipient vessel is then confirmed using a micro-Doppler probe and an indocyanine green (ICG) angiogram. Generally, the anastomosis time should be less than 45 minutes, and preferably less than 30 minutes. However, for PCA and SCA it can be as long as 50 minutes.

During closure, the dura mater is cut in a circular or cruciate fashion to allow free passage of the graft. The bone flap is subsequently replaced after an opening is created in it to accommodate the graft freely without a kink. The subcutaneous tissues and skin are then approximated. In the case of donor vessels originating in the neck, the neck is closed last. Flow through the graft is checked using micro-Doppler after each step during closure.

In addition to intraoperative Doppler sonography and ICG angiography, an immediate postoperative digital subtraction angiography (DSA) is usually performed to evaluate the entire graft to exclude any areas of significant stenosis or kinking, assess the flow rate, and visualize the distal circulation. If any problems are detected with Doppler sonography or ICG angiography intraoperatively, an intraoperative DSA or computed tomography angiography (CTA) using a portable scanner may be performed.

Postoperatively, Doppler sonography of the graft is performed every hour for the first 24 hours to monitor graft patency. Thereafter, we usually perform Duplex evaluation of the graft and assess flow daily for about 7 days.[18] Good diastolic flow is taken as an indicator of graft patency. Systolic flow is not a reliable indicator as it may be present with a nearly occluded graft. A sharp reduction in flow by 30% or more is a cause for concern and should be investigated with an urgent CTA.[19] Patients are administered Acetylsalicylic Acid = Aspirin 325 mg daily for at least 6 weeks with arterial grafts and lifelong with SVG. Long-term follow-up is performed with annual CTA or magnetic resonance (MR) angiography.

Although rare, problems may be encountered with grafts immediately during or after the procedure. These include thrombosis or other obstruction at either the donor or recipient anastomotic site, focal stenosis of the graft, and obstruction caused by the bone flap or subcutaneous tunnel. If an issue with the graft is detected in the immediate postoperative period, it is usually revised. If complete graft occlusion occurs in a more delayed manner and the patient is asymptomatic, no intervention is performed. If partial graft occlusion occurs, tissue plasminogen activator is administered into the graft after obtaining endovascular access. Despite pressure distention, graft vasospasm may still occur rarely and can be treated by endovascular angioplasty with a high-pressure balloon such as the Gateway® balloon.[20,21] The patient is administered dual antiplatelet therapy and heparinized during the endovascular procedure. Stenosis of the graft near the proximal or distal end has been noted occasionally during follow-up. Short segment (<1 cm) stenosis can be repaired with segmental resection and re-anastomosis. Longer segment stenosis can be treated with segmental resection and replacement with new donor interposition graft or by creating a Y-shaped construct with a new donor graft connecting an area of the existing bypass graft that is proximal to the stenosis to a new distal site on the intracranial vessel.[20]

5.8 Outcomes and Complications

In our experience, 17 out of 221 bypasses performed from 2005 to 2018 were for skull base tumors (▶ Table 5.1). The distribution of those 17 tumors were as follows: Meningioma (n = 7; 41%), osteosarcoma (n = 3; 17%), chordoma (n = 3; 17%), chondrosarcoma (n = 1; 6%), schwannoma (n = 1; 6%), giant cell tumor (n = 1; 6%), and B-cell lymphoma (n = 1; 6%). The bypasses were performed in 14 patients for surgical vascular occlusion of a large artery: cavernous ICA in 12 patients, VA (V3 segment) in one patient, and combined VA and PICA sacrifice in another patient. Three patients underwent bypasses for intraoperative vascular injury of the petrous ICA, cavernous ICA, and AICA.

The bypass was patent at last follow-up in all patients (▶ Table 5.2). However, one patient had delayed graft stenosis that required revision and has been patent thereafter. None of the patients developed new symptomatic stroke postoperatively. Gross total resection of the tumor was achieved in 14 patients and near-total excision was performed in 3 patients. One patient who underwent near-total excision had tumor recurrence and required reoperation for additional resection. Five patients had died by last follow-up: two from medical illnesses, two from progression of their primary disease/metastasis, and one from stroke and subarachnoid hemorrhage sustained from ICA injury during trans-sphenoidal resection of sellar/parasellar tumor that had necessitated the bypass procedure.

Table 5.1 Our bypass experience for skull base tumors—indications

Total cases	17
Tumors	
• Meningioma	7 (41%)
• Osteosarcoma	3 (17%)
• Chordoma	3 (17%)
• Chondrosarcoma	1 (6%)
• Schwannoma	1 (6%)
• Giant cell tumor	1 (6%)
• B-cell lymphoma	1 (6%)
Bypass indications	
• Surgical vascular occlusion	14
– ICA (cavernous)	12 (85%)
– VA (V3 segment)	1 (7%)
– VA + PICA	1 (7%)
• Intraoperative vascular injury	3
– ICA (petrous or cavernous)	2 (66%)
– AICA	1 (33%)

Abbreviations: AICA, anterior inferior cerebellar artery; ICA, internal carotid artery; PICA, posterior inferior cerebellar artery; VA, vertebral artery.

5.9 Case Examples

Case 1: A 19-year-old male was incidentally found to have a large skull base tumor after a motor vehicle accident. In retrospect, he had a history of headaches, occasional double vision, and had experienced one transient episode of right arm weakness. On examination, he was found to have a partial sixth nerve palsy. Imaging demonstrated a heavily calcified spheno-petroclival tumor (see ▶ Fig. 5.1). He initially underwent a left frontotemporal craniotomy with orbitozygomatic osteotomy for resection of the tumor (chondrosarcoma). Intraoperatively, brisk arterial bleeding was encountered during tumor resection in the cavernous sinus. Further examination revealed tumor invasion of the ICA which could not be primarily repaired. The ICA was occluded by clips in the cervical and supraclinoid segments and an emergent RAG bypass from cervical ECA to an M2 division was performed (▶ Fig. 5.2). The patient then underwent two further surgeries including additional tumor resection via the prior craniotomy (▶ Fig. 5.3), followed by an extended bilateral subfrontal approach to achieve near-total tumor resection. This was followed by proton beam radiation to the resection bed. He had persistent left cranial nerve VI palsy which was later corrected with eye muscle surgery. On last follow-up 5 years postoperatively, he had no tumor recurrence (▶ Fig. 5.4), had completed college, and was working full time.

Case 2: A 62-year-old male with left cavernous sinus meningioma post treatment with gamma knife radiation presented with worsening left trigeminal neuralgia which was debilitating despite medical therapy. Clinical examination showed decreased sensation in left V1 and abnormal sensation in left V2 and V3 dermatomes, and partial left CN VI palsy. MRI of brain showed compression of the left trigeminal nerve by the left cavernous sinus tumor (▶ Fig. 5.5a–c). Angiography demonstrated severe stenosis of the left cavernous ICA (preocclusive state: Sekhar-Hirsch grade 3)[22] with presence of collateral flow (▶ Fig. 5.5d–f). However, CT perfusion demonstrated slightly decreased perfusion and cerebrovascular reserve on the left compared to right and neuropsychological testing was

Table 5.2 Our bypass experience for skull base tumors—outcomes and complications

Bypass outcome	
• Patent	17 (100%)
• Delayed stenosis	1 (Patent after graft revision)
• Postoperative stroke	None
• Tumor resection	
• Gross total excision	14 (82%)
• Near-total excision	3 (18%)
• Recurrence requiring reoperation	1
• Death	5 (31%)
• Medical complications	2
• Disease progression/metastatic disease	2
• Stroke and SAH from ICA injury	1

Abbreviations: ICA, internal carotid artery; SAH, subarachnoid hemorrhage.

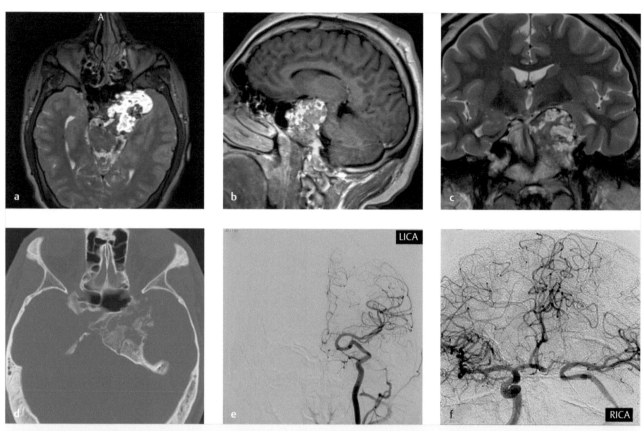

Fig. 5.1 Case 1: Preoperative axial T2-weighted magnetic resonance imaging (MRI) **(a)**, sagittal post-gadolinium T1-weighted MRI **(b)**, coronal T2-weighted MRI **(c)**, and axial noncontrast head computed tomography (CT) bone window **(d)** images demonstrating a large, heavily calcified spheno-petroclival tumor. Preoperative angiogram with anteroposterior views of left internal carotid artery (ICA) injection **(e)** demonstrating ICA encasement and displacement by the tumor, and right ICA injection **(f)** with cross compression of left ICA demonstrating limitation in collateral flow due to narrow left A1 segment.

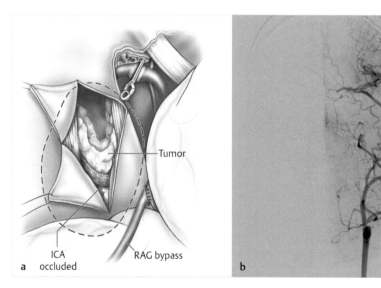

Fig. 5.2 Case 1: **(a)** Illustration demonstrating surgical view of the tumor, intracranial clip location in the clinoidal segment of left internal carotid artery (ICA), and distal anastomosis of the bypass graft to an M2 segment. **(b)** Angiogram with anteroposterior view of left common carotid artery injection demonstrating a patent left external carotid artery (ECA) to M2 segment radial artery graft (RAG) bypass, after the first surgery.

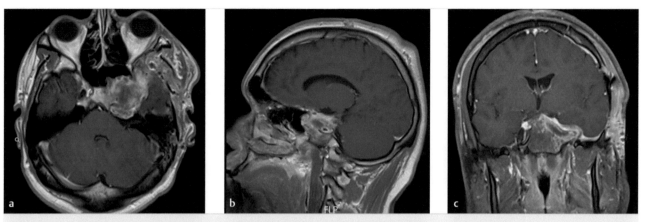

Fig. 5.3 Case 1: Axial **(a)**, sagittal **(b)**, and coronal **(c)** post-gadolinium T1-weighted magnetic resonance imaging (MRI) images demonstrating residual tumor in the sphenoid sinus and petroclival region after the second surgery.

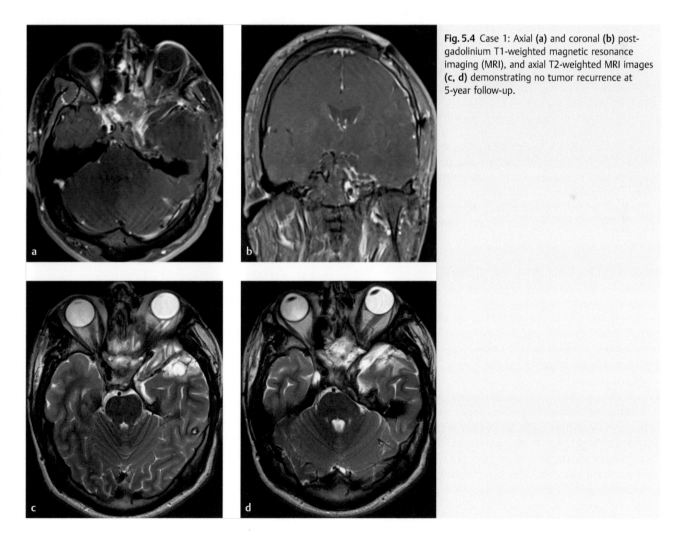

Fig. 5.4 Case 1: Axial **(a)** and coronal **(b)** post-gadolinium T1-weighted magnetic resonance imaging (MRI), and axial T2-weighted MRI images **(c, d)** demonstrating no tumor recurrence at 5-year follow-up.

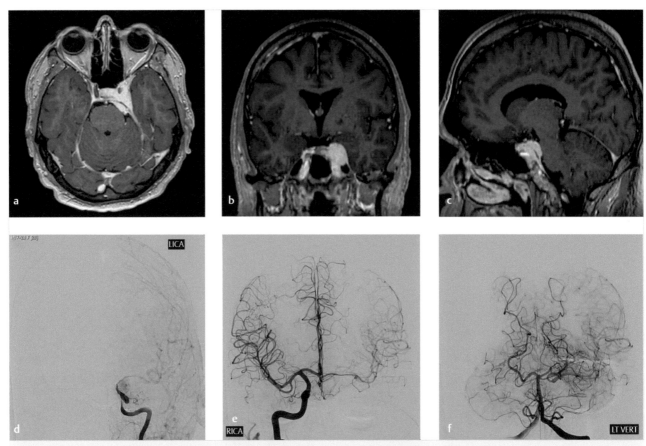

Fig. 5.5 Case 2: Preoperative axial (**a**), coronal (**b**), and sagittal (**c**) post-gadolinium T1-weighted magnetic resonance imaging (MRI) images demonstrating an enhancing tumor in the left cavernous sinus with internal carotid artery (ICA) stenosis. Preoperative angiogram with anteroposterior views of left ICA injection (**d**) demonstrating severe stenosis (Sekhar-Hirsch grade 3) of the left cavernous ICA with collateral flow from the right ICA (**e**) and vertebrobasilar circulation (**f**).

suggestive of vascular origin cognitive impairment. Given these findings, we recommended staged surgeries. In the first stage, the patient underwent a left frontotemporal craniotomy, zygomatic osteotomy, and complete posterolateral orbitectomy with partial tumor excision and decompression of cranial nerves in cavernous sinus. This was followed by the second-stage high-flow bypass surgery from left ECA to M2 segment with anterior tibial artery graft. The flow across the graft was confirmed intraoperatively with micro-Doppler and ICG angiography. Postoperative angiography was performed to confirm graft patency (▶ Fig. 5.6a–c). The immediate postoperative course was complicated by gram-negative wound infection and meningitis requiring wound washout and prolonged intravenous antibiotics. He also developed hydrocephalus necessitating a ventriculoperitoneal shunt placement. The patient had mild ophthalmoparesis postoperatively which recovered completely by 6-week follow-up, with the exception of baseline mild CN VI palsy which persisted. He had excellent relief of facial pain with only occasional episodes postoperatively. Postoperative MRI demonstrated expected residual tumor within the cavernous sinus (▶ Fig. 5.6d–f). His mRS was 1 at 6 months postoperatively.

5.10 Alternative Strategies

In recent years, a few groups have reported endovascular CCA or ICA stent placement followed by delayed tumor resection for benign skull base tumors,[23,24] and malignant head and neck tumors.[25] The underlying premise is that once neointimalization has occurred on the luminal surface of the stent, tumor resection from the vessel wall and adventitia outside the stent is safe. A limitation of stenting is that patients require dual antiplatelet therapy for at least 3 months following the procedure. However, stents are being developed which do not need prolonged dual antiplatelet therapy and this may be a reasonable alternative to bypass in the future.

5.11 Conclusion

High-flow bypass for flow replacement is a viable surgical option with good long-term outcomes for patients with benign or malignant skull base tumors requiring surgical resection of the ICA or VA, patients with ischemic symptoms due to large vessel occlusion by the tumor, or in situations of intraoperative injury to the ICA or VA. Intraluminal ICA stenting may be a potential option in the future for benign skull base tumors without ICA stenosis.

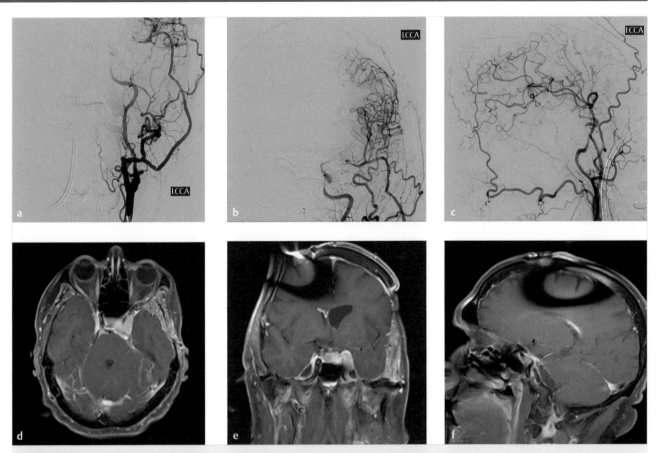

Fig. 5.6 Case 2: Postoperative angiogram with anteroposterior **(a, b)** and lateral **(c)** views of left CCA injection demonstrating a patent left ECA to M2 segment anterior tibial artery bypass graft with good filling of the left MCA territory. Postoperative axial **(d)**, coronal **(e)**, and sagittal **(f)** post-Gadolinium T1-weighted MRI images demonstrating expected decrease in tumor burden within the left cavernous sinus.

References

[1] Yasargil MG. Anastomosis between superficial temporal artery and a branch of the middle cerebral artery. Stuttgart: George Thieme Verlag; 1969

[2] Lougheed WM, Marshall BM, Hunter M, Michel ER, Sandwith-Smyth H. Common carotid to intracranial internal carotid bypass venous graft. Technical note. J Neurosurg. 1971; 34(1):114–118

[3] Group EIBS, EC/IC Bypass Study Group. Failure of extracranial-intracranial arterial bypass to reduce the risk of ischemic stroke. Results of an international randomized trial. N Engl J Med. 1985; 313(19):1191–1200

[4] Powers WJ, Clarke WR, Grubb RL, Jr, Videen TO, Adams HP, Jr, Derdeyn CP, COSS Investigators. Extracranial-intracranial bypass surgery for stroke prevention in hemodynamic cerebral ischemia: the Carotid Occlusion Surgery Study randomized trial. JAMA. 2011; 306(18):1983–1992

[5] Straus DC, Brito da Silva H, McGrath L, et al. Cerebral revascularization for aneurysms in the flow-diverter era. Neurosurgery. 2017; 80(5):759–768

[6] Sekhar LN, Cheng CY, Da Silva HB, Qazi Z. What is the current role of bypass surgery in the management of cerebral aneurysms? Neurol India. 2018; 66 (3):661–663

[7] Yang T, Tariq F, Chabot J, Madhok R, Sekhar LN. Cerebral revascularization for difficult skull base tumors: a contemporary series of 18 patients. World Neurosurg. 2014; 82(5):660–671

[8] Kim LJ, Tariq F, Sekhar LN. Pediatric bypasses for aneurysms and skull base tumors: short- and long-term outcomes. J Neurosurg Pediatr. 2013; 11(5):533–542

[9] Mohit AA, Sekhar LN, Natarajan SK, Britz GW, Ghodke B. High-flow bypass grafts in the management of complex intracranial aneurysms. Neurosurgery. 2007; 60(2) Suppl 1:ONS105–ONS122, discussion ONS122–ONS123

[10] Sekhar LN, Kalavakonda C. Cerebral revascularization for aneurysms and tumors. Neurosurgery. 2002; 50(2):321–331

[11] Sekhar LN, Tzortzidis FN, Bejjani GK, Schessel DA. Saphenous vein graft bypass of the sigmoid sinus and jugular bulb during the removal of glomus jugulare tumors. Report of two cases. J Neurosurg. 1997; 86(6):1036–1041

[12] Morita A, Sekhar LN. Reconstruction of the vein of Labbé by using a short saphenous vein bypass graft. Technical note. J Neurosurg. 1998; 89(4):671–675

[13] Sekhar LN, Patel SJ. Permanent occlusion of the internal carotid artery during skull-base and vascular surgery: is it really safe? Am J Otol. 1993; 14(5):421–422

[14] Ramanathan D, Hegazy A, Mukherjee SK, Sekhar LN. Intracranial in situ side-to-side microvascular anastomosis: principles, operative technique, and applications. World Neurosurg. 2010; 73(4):317–325

[15] Sekhar LN, Duff JM, Kalavakonda C, Olding M. Cerebral revascularization using radial artery grafts for the treatment of complex intracranial aneurysms: techniques and outcomes for 17 patients. Neurosurgery. 2001; 49(3):646–658, discussion 658–659

[16] Ramanathan D, Starnes B, Hatsukami T, Kim LJ, Di Maio S, Sekhar L. Tibial artery autografts: alternative conduits for high flow cerebral revascularizations. World Neurosurg. 2013; 80(3–4):322–327

[17] Sekhar LN, Bucur SD, Bank WO, Wright DC. Venous and arterial bypass grafts for difficult tumors, aneurysms, and occlusive vascular lesions: evolution of surgical treatment and improved graft results. Neurosurgery. 1999; 44(6):1207–1223, discussion 1223–1224

[18] Morton RP, Moore AE, Barber J, et al. Monitoring flow in extracranial-intracranial bypass grafts using duplex ultrasonography: a single-center experience in 80 grafts over 8 years. Neurosurgery. 2014; 74(1):62–70

[19] Morton RP, Abecassis IJ, Moore AE, et al. The use of ultrasound for postoperative monitoring of cerebral bypass grafts: a technical report. J Clin Neurosci. 2017; 40:169–174

[20] Ramanathan D, Temkin N, Kim LJ, Ghodke B, Sekhar LN. Cerebral bypasses for complex aneurysms and tumors: long-term results and graft management strategies. Neurosurgery. 2012; 70(6):1442–1457, discussion 1457

[21] Ramanathan D, Ghodke B, Kim LJ, Hallam D, Herbes-Rocha M, Sekhar LN. Endovascular management of cerebral bypass graft problems: an analysis of technique and results. AJNR Am J Neuroradiol. 2011; 32(8):1415–1419

[22] Hirsch WL, Sekhar LN, Lanzino G, Pomonis S, Sen CN. Meningiomas involving the cavernous sinus: value of imaging for predicting surgical complications. AJR Am J Roentgenol. 1993; 160(5):1083–1088

[23] Sanna M, Piazza P, De Donato G, Menozzi R, Falcioni M. Combined endovascular-surgical management of the internal carotid artery in complex tympanojugular paragangliomas. Skull Base. 2009; 19(1):26–42

[24] Konishi M, Piazza P, Shin SH, Sivalingam S, Sanna M. The use of internal carotid artery stenting in management of bilateral carotid body tumors. Eur Arch Otorhinolaryngol. 2011; 268(10):1535–1539

[25] Markiewicz MR, Pirgousis P, Bryant C, et al. Preoperative protective endovascular covered stent placement followed by surgery for management of the cervical common and internal carotid arteries with tumor encasement. J Neurol Surg B Skull Base. 2017; 78(1):52–58

6 Alternatives to Standard Bypass Techniques for Skull Base Tumors (Including Direct IMax Bypass)

Kevin Kwan, Julia R. Schneider, Ivo Peto, and Amir R. Dehdashti

Summary

The intimate involvement of major cerebral vessels by skull base tumors is often a barrier to gross total resection. If a multimodality evaluation by an interdisciplinary team determines that complete surgical resection is necessary, cerebral revascularization through the internal or external circulation might be deemed necessary. Although cerebral bypass may be utilized emergently for flow augmentation due to hypoperfused brain states secondary to vaso-occlusive disease, bypass for flow preservation for treating tumors remains mainly elective in nature and require planning for staged resections. This chapter will focus on the indications, operative technique, and alternative techniques to traditional bypass in the context of skull base tumor surgery. A novel method utilizing the internal maxillary artery as the donor vessel will be highlighted with reference to its indications, operative method, graft choices, and potential problems.

Keywords: Skull base tumor, carotid occlusion, revascularization, saphenous vein bypass graft, radial artery bypass graft, IMax bypass

6.1 Key Learning Points

- The IMax bypass is a safe and effective method to provide an extracranial-intracranial anastomosis without the need for a long conduit.
- The IMax bypass may be utilized to provide a mid- to high-flow alternative donor vessel if superficial temporal artery is not available.
- Detailed study of the IMax anatomy on the preoperative imaging, in particular its relationship with both heads of the lateral pterygoid muscle, is necessary.
- To obtain a longer segment of the IMax, initial localization can be based on the pterygomaxillary fissure as a landmark and drilling performed more posteriorly in the middle fossa toward foramen spinosum.
- Other alternative bypass techniques including intracranial-intracranial and bonnet bypass may also be considered based on surgeon's preference.

6.2 Indications

Invasive skull base tumors often become closely involved with the cerebral vasculature. In particular, in scenarios where gross total resection of the tumor is deemed to be clinically necessary, but the encasement of major vessels precludes its complete resection, arterial bypass may be required.

Tissue biopsy of the offending neoplasm may be necessary prior to the decision for an extensive skull base surgery, as certain tumors may be treated appropriately with aggressive chemoradiation therapy. Neoplasms that have demonstrated poor response to chemoradiation and have involvement of the vessel adventitia should be considered for aggressive resection to improve prognosis.[1] However, many tumors, when noninvasive and soft in consistency, may be dissected away and taken out microsurgically despite close proximity to the carotid artery.[2,3]

Careful consideration of the patient's overall functional status, disease burden, as well as the ability to obtain gross total resection should be evaluated prior to committing a patient for surgery.[2,4,5] Preoperative neuroradiologic imaging should be carefully evaluated to delineate the extent of neoplasm involvement of the skull base and cerebral vasculature. Noninvasive modalities such as computed tomography (CT) angiography or magnetic resonance (MR) angiography (MRA) may be useful in demonstrating spatial relationships, but definitive delineation of the vasculature by digital subtraction angiography (DSA) is recommended to understand the dynamic relationship between the tumor, surrounding cerebral vasculature, and collateral flow. Furthermore, understanding the anatomy of the internal maxillary artery is vital.

6.3 Determination of Cerebrovascular Reserve

Given the significantly increased risk of developing ischemia following carotid or middle cerebral artery (MCA) ligation, it is necessary to clearly delineate the presence of collateral flow from the posterior and contralateral circulation. MRI/MRA and most importantly a noninvasive optimal vessel analysis (NOVA) MRA can be utilized for this purpose and followed by formal angiography.[6] The NOVA MRA gives accurate quantitative measurement of flow inside cranial vessels, which could be helpful for planning of a cerebral revascularization.

More invasive procedures can be utilized to assess patient's tolerance to carotid occlusion, such as the temporary balloon test occlusion (BTO) (see Chapter 2). During this test, the carotid is temporarily occluded using an inflatable balloon positioned via endovascular access. Mean arterial pressure is then decreased by about 20%. The patient is then assessed clinically to see if there is a change in the neurologic examination. A single photon emission computed tomography (SPECT) scan, computed tomography perfusion (CTP), or transcranial Doppler (TCD) may be performed in conjunction with a BTO to further evaluate blood flow. However, the team must be prudent in interpreting the results from a normal BTO, as the risk of future cerebrovascular event may still be possible due to complications arising from thromboembolic events or revascularization injury.[7,8,9,10] In addition, skull base resections can often remove external carotid collateral supply.

6.4 Traditional High-Flow Cerebral Revascularization Methodology and Limitations

Standard high-flow bypass techniques were addressed in the previous chapter (see Chapter 5) and will only be described briefly here. In essence, the common carotid or external carotid artery in the neck is utilized as donor vessels and anastomosed via an autologous graft to the intracranial internal carotid or MCA. Typically, this graft is harvested from the saphenous vein or radial artery.[11,12,13] Complications may arise, however, when utilizing long grafts (approximately 20 cm), as they can be occluded along their course.[14,15,16] Three separate operative exposures must be created, including the intracranial exposure of the internal cerebral artery or MCA, the exposure in the neck of the common or external carotid, and the graft site (i.e., radial or saphenous), which requires constant change in surgical view. Often, an approximately 20 cm long graft must be tunneled in the neck to access the recipient site. These can contribute to patient morbidity and increased operative time.[1,4,12,17]

6.5 Advantages of the Internal Maxillary (IMax) External Carotid–Internal Carotid (EC-IC) Bypass

First described in cadaveric study over two decades ago, the IMax artery was noted to be feasible as a donor graft for EC-IC bypass.[18] Subsequent to its described initial use, the technique has been continuously refined with emphasis on the safe utilization of the IMax artery as an intermediate/high-flow (20–120 mL/minute) bypass source.

The IMax EC-IC bypass may be favored over traditional methods due to its ability to utilize a solitary surgical field, shortening surgical time, the ability to use a shorter graft (7–10 cm), decreasing the risk of occlusion, the capacity to see the entire graft length in the surgical field, and its utility for use as a salvage procedure in patients with prior cervical procedures.[4,19,20,21] A careful evaluation of required flow replacement is necessary prior to utilizing the IMax as the donor site.

6.6 IMax Artery—Importance of Preoperative Angiography

Prior to surgery, it is prudent to assess for differences in the course of the IMax artery to maximize the operative outcome and identify any abnormalities in the angiographic route of the IMax artery.[5] Furthermore, the possible anastomoses with intracranial circulation need to be identified. Attention should be paid to possible ophthalmic artery collaterals through the IMax and make sure the distal ligation of the IMax in its pterygoid segment does not interfere with intraocular blood supply if it is the solitary supply to the retina.

The utilization of noninvasive modalities like CT angiography and MR angiography are recommended initially and also very helpful as intraoperative imaging for IMax localization.

Specifically, CT or MR angiography will help delineate the availability, size, and course of the donor segments of the IMax artery, including the mandibular, pterygoid, and pterygopalatine segments,[22] in particular with regard to relationship to the lateral pterygoid muscle. To best delineate the availability, size, collaterals, and location of the donor vessel, an invasive, formal, four-vessel DSA should be performed to aid in appropriate patient selection and check availability of IMax vessel donors.[23,24,25] Specifically, the distal pterygoid segment, which allows for the easiest anastomosis due to its more superficial location and its cross-sectional diameter of 2.3 to 3.2 mm, is a suitable donor for most revascularization purposes. The preoperative decision-making process should include collaboration and discussion with endovascular colleagues to delineate which patients may be selected for the IMax EC-IC bypass.

6.7 IMax Artery Anatomical Considerations

Following its bifurcation from the common carotid artery, the external carotid artery divides into the superficial temporal artery and IMax artery distally. The IMax arises deep to the mandibular neck where it courses anteriorly and trifurcates into three segments: (1) mandibular, (2) pterygoid, and (3) pterygopalatine.[22] The mandibular division continues dorsal to the mandible. The pterygoid division continues to the pterygomaxillary fissure, while the pterygopalatine division continues where it runs inferior to V2.[26] Initially, the pterygopalatine division of the IMax was used as a intermediate- to high-flow bypass donor vessel. However, more recently, the pterygoid segment has been favored due to its wider operative exposure and more maneuverability, lower number of arterial side branches, and closer adjacent course to the floor of the middle fossa. The use of the pterygoid segment favors an end-to-end anastomosis to the graft as opposed to an end to side to the pterygopalatine segment.[27,28,29] Although there are variations in the diameter of the IMax, the average diameter of the pterygoid and pterygopalatine segments are similar (2.4–3.46 mm vs. 2.3–3.2 mm) which may theoretically translate into similar flow rates.[30] This matches closely with the diameter of the M2 segment of the MCA, making adequate anastomosis technically feasible.[31]

6.8 Autograft Selection for High-Flow Bypass

Suitable graft determination must consider the hemodynamic outflow necessary to maintain the cerebrovasculature of the target areas supplied by the artery that is being subjected to bypass. The diameter of the donor and recipient arteries, the usability of graft locations and the maximum span of the graft must also be taken into account.[15,32]

Typically, the graft types that are considered for high-flow carotid bypass (80–200 mL/minute) include the lower extremity saphenous, brachiocephalic veins, and radial artery.[33,34] Flow rates between venous grafts (70–140 mL/minute) and arterial grafts (40–150 mL/minute) are relatively comparable.[4,15,35] Radial artery grafts are initially preferred as vascular dissection is relatively uncomplicated due to its superficial course. The radial artery diameter matches well with the donor and recipient sites making anastomosis easier. Rates of vessel occlusion have been reported to be low when utilizing radial artery grafts, with documented better graft patency rates than venous autografts.[16,24,29,36] The risk of graft spasm remains the major downside of the radial artery graft and therefore a pressure distention technique[4] needs to be applied during the graft harvest to decrease the risk of spasm postoperatively. The pressure distention technique involves injecting saline into the vessel from either end (with the other end occluded) to forcibly inflate the vessel.[4] Other arterial graft options are anterior tibial artery, posterior tibial artery, lateral circumflex femoral artery, and

internal mammary artery. In the event an arterial graft cannot be acquired, or it is not preferred due to risk of spasm, saphenous venous grafts may also be utilized. However, close postoperative monitoring is required as venous grafts have been shown to be susceptible to the formation of accelerated atherosclerosis following the procedure.[37,38] Heparinization for a goal partial thromboplastin time (PTT) of 45 to 50 for vein grafts for up to 72 hours after surgery is recommended. Patients are routinely placed on ASA 81 mg on the morning of the surgery and subsequently kept on it indefinitely.

6.9 IMax Bypass Operative Technique

A frontotemporal skin flap is incised and reflected to anticipate the generous exposure of the sylvian fissure required for successful IMax bypass. We prefer the utilization of an interfascial dissection of the temporal muscle, with exposure of the frontal process of zygomatic bone.

Pterional craniotomy with addition of zygomatic or orbitozygomatic osteotomy are subsequently performed, allowing for access to the infratemporal fossa and inferior reflection of the temporalis muscle[39] (▶ Fig. 6.1). The pterygomaxillary fissure is identified by palpating the posterior wall of the maxilla and following it inferiorly. If the IMax is not immediately visible, then the superior head of lateral pterygoid muscle is partially detached from its insertion at the infratemporal crest for better visualization of infratemporal fossa contents. The IMax is identified between the lateral and medial pterygoid muscle entering the pterygo-maxillary fissure (PMF). A sufficient length of the vessel is dissected in a retrograde fashion in its pterygoid segment to increase the mobility of arterial stump. Deep temporal branches are identified, and usually a distal bifurcation in which the IMax size remains similar to the proximal segment is the limit of distal dissection and ligation of the IMax pterygoid segment. Following distal ligation (with hemoclips) and temporary occlusion of the proximal portion, the vessel is transected and mobilized superiorly for end-to-end anastomosis.[39]

Stereotactic navigation, with intraoperative merging of the preoperative CTA and MRI with contrast, is useful in all cases to help aid in determining the location of the IMax and confirming its position based on anatomical landmarks. With the use of navigation and Doppler, the IMax is identified medial (38%) or lateral (61.6%) to the lateral pterygoid muscle[40] (▶ Fig. 6.2).

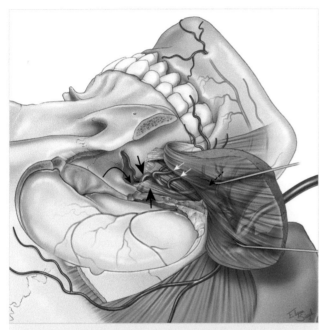

Fig. 6.1 Artistic illustration of a right pterional craniotomy with a zygomatic osteotomy demonstrating the relationship of the pterygo-maxillary fissure, superior head of the lateral pterygoid muscle, and the terminal portion of the pterygoid segment of the IMax. *Arrow*, distal pterygoid segment of the IMax; *arrowhead*, superior head of the lateral pterygoid muscle; *curved arrow*, pterygomaxillary fissure; *dashed arrow*, mandibular segment of IMax behind the reflected temporal muscle; *white arrows*, deep temporal arteries. (Reproduced with permission from Peto et al.[39])

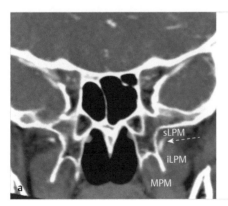
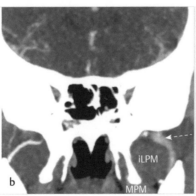

Fig. 6.2 Computed tomography (CT) angiography showing **(a)** medial position of the IMax in relation to the LPM. **(b)** Showing position of the IMax lateral to the LPM. Medial position often requires transection of the superior head of the LPM (sLPM). *Dash arrows*, pterygoid segment of the IMax; iLPM, inferior head of the lateral pterygoid muscle; LPM, lateral pterygoid muscle; MPM, medial pterygoid muscle; sLPM, superior head of the lateral pterygoid muscle.

The dural opening is centered around the sylvian fissure with the dural flap reflected anteriorly. The sylvian fissure is split and dissected in standard fashion, until appropriately sized MCA (M2 vessels) are visualized (▶ Fig. 6.3). We prefer to use the MCA as opposed to ICA for distal anastomoses.

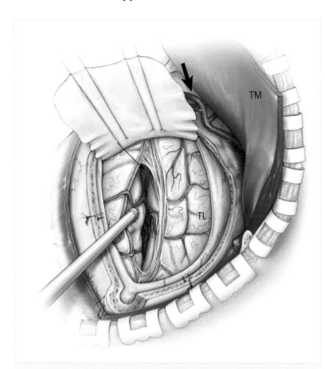

Fig. 6.3 Dissecting the right sylvian fissure with anterior reflection of dura to locate middle cerebral artery (MCA) vessels. *Arrow*, IMax; TL, temporal lobe; TM, temporal muscle. (Reproduced with permission from Nossek et al.[41])

The recipient vessel is dissected free of arachnoid and off the pia of the underlying cortex in a segment devoid of side branches to a length of approximately 1 to 2 cm. Patency of the recipient vessel is assessed by micro-Doppler probe. A colored plastic background is placed underneath the vessel to increase contrast between the vessel and underlying brain.

Analogous to the preparation of the recipient vessel, the IMax is dissected free of any soft tissue. After the patency is checked with micro-Doppler, a temporary clip is placed proximal to the intended implantation site for proximal anastomoses and the very distal segment is ligated. The IMax is subsequently liberated from its muscular attachments, transected, and mobilized superiorly up to the level of the middle fossa floor. The lumen of the proximal IMax stump distal to the temporary clip is flushed clear of blood using heparinized saline. The adventitia of both the IMax and the proximal part of the graft is meticulously dissected.

The harvested interposition graft is sewn onto the proximal end of the IMax in end-to-end fashion with an 8–0 suture/cutting needle[41] (▶ Fig. 6.4). The proximal temporary clip on the IMax is briefly opened to assess patency of the anastomosis. Once this is established, the proximal temporary clip on IMax is reapplied and the graft is flushed clear of blood with heparinized saline and is ready to be implanted onto the MCA vessel (▶ Fig. 6.5). The distal end of the graft is fish-mouthed (if necessary, to match recipient size) and implanted in an end-to-side fashion to the MCA vessel. Naturally, the recipient MCA vessel is temporarily clipped around the site of anastomosis. Using 9–0 or 10–0 sutures, the heel and toe are sewn first, followed by interrupted sutures on the back wall and running sutures on the front wall. This particular technique has worked very efficiently. Heparin saline is used to flush the anastomosis site during the suturing.

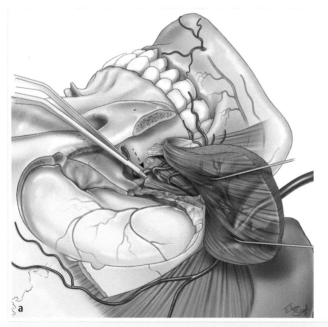
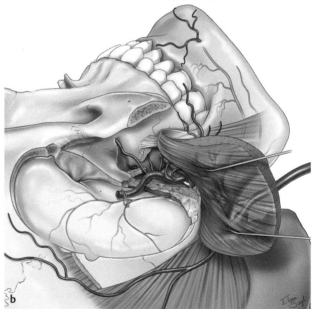

Fig. 6.4 **(a)** The right IMax is transected in its distal segment. The distal stump is ligated using hemoclips. **(b)** Proximal segment is mobilized superiorly into the middle fossa for the proximal anastomosis with the interposition graft. The *dash arrow* indicates the site of arteriotomy. (Reproduced with permission from Peto et al.[39])

Before tying the last stich, a temporary opening of clips on the IMax is conducted to observe flow across the implantation site. This helps to identify possible pitfalls with the anastomosis, including inadvertent suturing of both walls of MCA vessel together, occlusion of the recipient vessel resulting in thrombosis or the presence of an air leak. After this has been successfully accomplished, a temporary clip is placed back on IMax, the last knot of the anastomosis is tied, and all temporary clips removed. Clips are removed in sequence beginning first with distal MCA, then proximal MCA and last the IMax. Minor bleeding from the anastomosis site is expected and addressed by applying small Gelfoam pledgets to the suture line.

Intraoperative neuromonitoring should be utilized to monitor changes in motor or sensory evoked potentials, especially during occlusion time of the MCA. Papaverine may also be liberally used to prevent arterial vasospasm. Intraoperative indocyanine green, intraoperative flow assessment with Doppler flow probe as well as intraoperative angiography is advised to display adequate flow through the graft site.[42] If flow is maintained, subsequent ligation of the carotid artery or the relevant vessel may occur. In particular, dural, cranial, and skin closure should be completed with no compression or kinking of the graft. Patients typically receive 3,000 units of heparin during the temporary clipping and are placed on ASA 325 mg daily both pre- and postoperatively. For vein grafts, heparinization with a goal PTT of 45 to 50 for up to 72 hours after surgery is implemented.

6.10 Illustrative Case 1

A 64-year-old man presented with a large, 6-cm, left-sided parapharyngeal tumor extending proximally toward the skull base (▶ Fig. 6.6). The extracranial ICA was encased by the tumor and was resected along with the tumor based on the stability of neuromonitoring during ICA clamping time. The patient presented with recurrent transient ischemic attack (TIA) and eventually evidence of watershed infarct on diffusion-weighted imaging (DWI) sequence MRI in the frontal lobe, specifically in the centrum semiovale and operculum a few days after surgery (▶ Fig. 6.7). This presentation confirmed the need for cerebral revascularization. An IMax–MCA bypass was performed with robust filling through the graft evident on postoperative angiography (▶ Fig. 6.8). The patient had significant improvement of his right-sided weakness at short-term follow-up.

6.11 Illustrative Case 2

A 43-year-old female was diagnosed with an incidental 19-mm anterior choroidal artery segment fusiform aneurysm (▶ Fig. 6.9). An endovascular approach was limited as coiling alone was unfavorable while covered stents could compromise the patency of the choroidal artery. Clipping the aneurysm was not an option due to the fusiform aspect of the aneurysm, so a flow reversal strategy was decided upon that included: an IMax–MCA bypass with the brachiocephalic vein, partial trapping of the aneurysm with right ICA clipping (proximal to the PcomA), and right A1 clipping. The choroidal artery and the PcomA remained patent during retrograde flow of the bypass and the aneurysm thrombosis was confirmed at follow-up imaging at 3 months (▶ Fig. 6.10; **Video 6.1**).

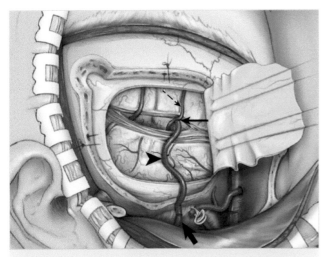

Fig. 6.5 Donor graft has been sewn onto right IMax and recipient middle cerebral artery (MCA) vessel. *Arrowhead*, radial interposition graft; *dashed arrow*, recipient MCA branch; *thick arrow*, proximal anastomosis site; *thin arrow*, distal anastomosis site. (Reproduced with permission from Nossek et al.[41])

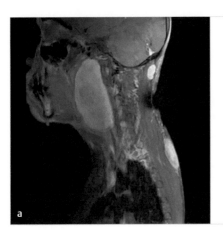
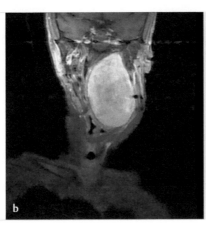

Fig. 6.6 Magnetic resonance imaging (MRI) demonstrating sagittal **(a)** and coronal **(b)** view of a large left-sided parapharyngeal tumor extending toward the skull base with encasement of extracranial internal carotid artery (not shown).

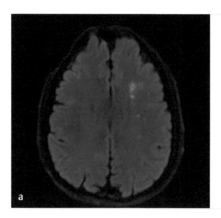
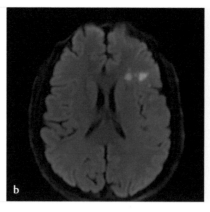

Fig. 6.7 Diffusion-weighted imaging (DWI) sequence demonstrating diffusion restriction—widespread cortical/subcortical foci of ischemia in centrum semiovale of frontal lobe (a) and left frontal operculum (b).

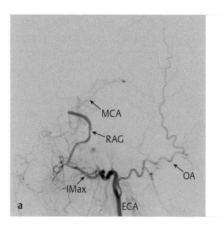
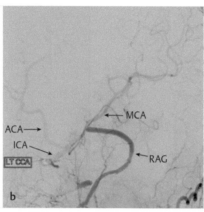

Fig. 6.8 Lateral (a) and zoomed in lateral and later phase of (b) CCA injection in arterial phase showing patent IMax to middle cerebral artery (MCA) bypass with filling of distal MCA branches and retrograde filling of ACA and terminal ICA (right). ACA, anterior cerebral artery; CCA, common carotid artery; ECA, external carotid artery; ICA, internal cerebral artery; IMax, internal maxillary artery; MCA, middle cerebral artery; RAG, radial artery graft.

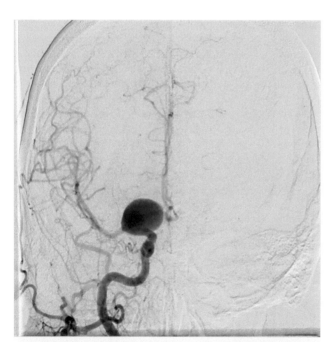

Fig. 6.9 Anteroposterior (AP) projection of right common carotid artery (CCA) injection demonstrating giant internal cerebral artery (ICA) C7 segment aneurysm.

6.12 Limitations of the IMax Bypass

Critics of the IMax bypass have mentioned the technical difficulty in comparison to the external carotid as the donor vessel, due the initial dissection of the IMax artery. The original techniques of the IMax exposure utilizing drilling of the middle fossa floor can be laborious. The smaller operative window may also make anastomosis of the IMax and vessel graft more limited; however, the use of the pterygoid segment of the IMax compared to the pterygopalatine segment has been very helpful to address this concern.[42] Furthermore, a surgical pearl to obtain a longer segment of the IMax includes drilling more posteriorly in the middle fossa toward foramen spinosum, allowing the exposure of an average of 17.6 mm of IMax.[27] Localizing the IMax based on the pterygomaxillary fissure as a landmark provides a longer segment, which is located more superficially due to the natural ascending course of the IMax. This allows more donor artery to be mobilized into the intracranial space for easier anastomosis. Also, when the distal IMax in its pterygoid segment is identified posterolateral to the maxillary sinus, it gives ample length of the IMax to be available for mobilization and bypass and avoids drilling of the middle fossa floor. Collaboration with colleagues from otolaryngology to aid in operative exposure may be helpful at the beginning of the surgeon's

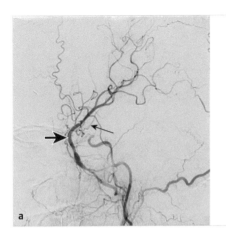 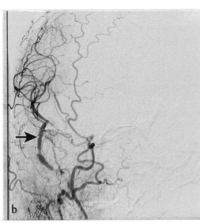

Fig. 6.10 Lateral **(a)** and anteroposterior (AP) **(b)** projection of common carotid artery (CCA) injection. Internal cerebral artery (ICA) is occluded at the C5 segment. *Large arrows,* bypass; *thin arrow,* anterior choroidal artery.

learning curve but becomes unnecessary when experience with the surgical technique is obtained. Detailed study of the IMax anatomy on the preoperative imaging, in particular its relationship with both heads of the lateral pterygoid muscle, is necessary. Image guidance or use of micro-Doppler probe provides additional safety to this procedure.

In our practice and with the technique described above, the IMax can be identified consistently and with a very little additional exposure. However, the IMax flow might not be enough to replace the whole carotid circulation and careful assessment of the flow requirement should be done preoperatively. Typically, the IMax can provide up to 100 mL/minute of flow which requires careful evaluation of flow replacement when the entire carotid circulation needs to be replaced. There should be little hesitation to use traditional techniques including the use of the external carotid artery as a donor for full carotid circulation replacement when the diameter of the IMax is less than usual (<2.6 mm).

Although rare, the superior thyroid artery and occipital artery have been reported in the literature for their use in the revascularization for skull base neoplasms. The former had limited success and occipital artery dissection can be tedious and the vessel lumen is small compared to the IMax so it cannot serve as an ideal alternative.[43,44]

6.13 Advantages of IC-IC Bypass

In the event of a lack of extracranial donor arteries, novel methods utilizing intracranial artery to intracranial artery (IC-IC) bypass have been developed. IC-IC bypasses, as compared to EC-IC bypasses, allow shorter connecting grafts, obviate the need for extracranial supply, and use recipient/donor sites of equal caliber. Surgical techniques for IC-IC bypass include *in situ* bypass, re-implantation, re-anastomosis, and intracranial bypass with grafts. Although there is seemingly a higher learning curve and degree of difficulty with IC-IC bypass, as well as potential impact on two intracranial vascular territories, this technique may be utilized in the hands of experienced bypass surgeons to provide favorable patient outcomes.[45]

6.14 Advantages of the "Bonnet" Bypass

In the event of an absence of an ipsilateral donor vessel, there is also an option to graft the contralateral superficial temporal artery with an interposition graft to the contralateral branch of the MCA. This technique has been called the "bonnet" bypass and has proven to be efficacious and safe in cases requiring a contralateral donor vessel. An advantage of this technique is the fact that the graft lies in close proximity to the skull during its trajectory, thus allowing the graft to remain motionless at its proximal and distal tip with head motion.[46]

6.15 Conclusion

The IMax artery is a valuable inclusion in the neurosurgeon's cerebrovascular armamentarium for use in EC-IC bypass providing a flow replacement of up to 100 mL/minute. It is our preferred choice when technically feasible and especially in cases where traditional methods of EC-IC bypass are not possible. The IMax EC-IC bypass is a clinically achievable route to provide intermediate to relatively high flow to the recipient arteries following carotid or MCA ligation. Careful flow assessment needs to be done preoperatively to confirm the adequacy of IMax flow for the flow replacement. Continued clinical evaluation is necessary to ascertain long-term efficacy of the IMax bypass in comparison to conventional methods of high-flow EC-IC bypass.

References

[1] Muhm M, Grasl MCh, Burian M, Exadaktylos A, Staudacher M, Polterauer P. Carotid resection and reconstruction for locally advanced head and neck tumors. Acta Otolaryngol. 2002; 122(5):561–564

[2] Lawton MT, Hamilton MG, Beals SP, Joganic EF, Spetzler RF. Radical resection of anterior skull base tumors. Clin Neurosurg. 1995; 42:43–70

[3] Meredith SD, Shores CG, Carrasco VN, Pillsbury HC. Management of the carotid artery at the skull base. Am J Otolaryngol. 2001; 22(5): 336–342

[4] Sekhar LN, Duff JM, Kalavakonda C, Olding M. Cerebral revascularization using radial artery grafts for the treatment of complex intracranial aneurysms: techniques and outcomes for 17 patients. Neurosurgery. 2001; 49(3):646–658, discussion 658–659

[5] Wright JG, Nicholson R, Schuller DE, Smead WL. Resection of the internal carotid artery and replacement with greater saphenous vein: a safe procedure for en bloc cancer resections with carotid involvement. J Vasc Surg. 1996; 23(5):775–780, discussion 781–782

[6] Bae YJ, Jung C, Kim JH, Choi BS, Kim E. Quantitative magnetic resonance angiography in internal carotid artery occlusion with primary collateral pathway. J Stroke. 2015; 17(3):320–326

[7] Drake CG, Peerless SJ, Ferguson GG. Hunterian proximal arterial occlusion for giant aneurysms of the carotid circulation. J Neurosurg. 1994; 81(5):656–665

[8] Origitano TC, al-Mefty O, Leonetti JP, DeMonte F, Reichman OH. Vascular considerations and complications in cranial base surgery. Neurosurgery. 1994; 35(3):351–362, discussion 362–363

[9] Gonzalez CF, Moret J. Balloon occlusion of the carotid artery prior to surgery for neck tumors. AJNR Am J Neuroradiol. 1990; 11(4):649–652

[10] Sekhar LN, Patel SJ. Permanent occlusion of the internal carotid artery during skull-base and vascular surgery: is it really safe? Am J Otol. 1993; 14(5):421–422

[11] Lougheed WM, Marshall BM, Hunter M, Michel ER, Sandwith-Smyth H. Common carotid to intracranial internal carotid bypass venous graft. Technical note. J Neurosurg. 1971; 34(1):114–118

[12] Sia SF, Morgan MK. High flow extracranial-to-intracranial brain bypass surgery. J Clin Neurosci. 2013; 20(1):1–5

[13] Amin-Hanjani S, Charbel FT. Flow-assisted surgical technique in cerebrovascular surgery. Surg Neurol. 2007; 68 Suppl 1:S4–S11

[14] Kalavakonda C, Sekhar LN. Cerebral revascularization in cranial base tumors. Neurosurg Clin N Am. 2001; 12(3):557–574, viii–ix

[15] Sekhar LN, Bucur SD, Bank WO, Wright DC. Venous and arterial bypass grafts for difficult tumors, aneurysms, and occlusive vascular lesions: evolution of surgical treatment and improved graft results. Neurosurgery. 1999; 44(6): 1207–1223, discussion 1223–1224

[16] Sekhar LN, Kalavakonda C. Cerebral revascularization for aneurysms and tumors. Neurosurgery. 2002; 50(2):321–331

[17] Ashley WW, Amin-Hanjani S, Alaraj A, Shin JH, Charbel FT. Flow-assisted surgical cerebral revascularization. Neurosurg Focus. 2008; 24(2):E20

[18] Vrionis FD, Cano WG, Heilman CB. Microsurgical anatomy of the infratemporal fossa as viewed laterally and superiorly. Neurosurgery. 1996; 39(4):777–785, discussion 785–786

[19] Ustun ME, Buyukmumcu M, Ulku CH, Cicekcibasi AE, Arbag H. Radial artery graft for bypass of the maxillary to proximal middle cerebral artery: an anatomic and technical study. Neurosurgery. 2004; 54(3):667–670, discussion 670–671

[20] Arbağ H, Ustun ME, Buyukmumcu M, Cicekcibasi AE, Ulku CH. A modified technique to bypass the maxillary artery to supraclinoid internal carotid artery by using radial artery graft: an anatomical study. J Laryngol Otol. 2005; 119(7):519–523

[21] Büyükmumcu M, Ustün ME, Seker M, Karabulut AK, Uysal YY. Maxillary-to-petrous internal carotid artery bypass: an anatomical feasibility study. Surg Radiol Anat. 2003; 25(5–6):368–371

[22] Allen WE, III, Kier EL, Rothman SL. The maxillary artery in craniofacial pathology. Am J Roentgenol Radium Ther Nucl Med. 1974; 121(1):124–138

[23] Arimoto S, Hasegawa T, Okamoto N, et al. Determining the location of the internal maxillary artery on ultrasonography and unenhanced magnetic resonance imaging before orthognathic surgery. Int J Oral Maxillofac Surg. 2015; 44(8):977–983

[24] Akiyama O, Güngör A, Middlebrooks EH, Kondo A, Arai H. Microsurgical anatomy of the maxillary artery for extracranial-intracranial bypass in the pterygopalatine segment of the maxillary artery. Clin Anat. 2018; 31(5): 724–733

[25] Gulses A, Oren C, Altug HA, Ilica T, Sencimen M. Radiologic assessment of the relationship between the maxillary artery and the lateral pterygoid muscle. J Craniofac Surg. 2012; 23(5):1465–1467

[26] Osborn AG. The external carotid vasculature. Philadelphia: Lippincott Williams & Wilkins; 1999:31–55

[27] Feng X, Meybodi AT, Rincon-Torroella J, El-Sayed IH, Lawton MT, Benet A. Surgical technique for high-flow internal maxillary artery to middle cerebral artery bypass using a superficial temporal artery interposition graft. Oper Neurosurg (Hagerstown). 2017; 13(2):246–257

[28] Uysal II, Buyukmumcu M, Dogan NU, Seker M, Ziylan T. Clinical significance of maxillary artery and its branches: a cadaver study and review of the literature. Int J Morphol. 2011; 29(4):1274–1281

[29] Eller JL, Sasaki-Adams D, Sweeney JM, Abdulrauf SI. Localization of the internal maxillary artery for extracranial-to-intracranial bypass through the middle cranial fossa: a cadaveric study. J Neurol Surg B Skull Base. 2012; 73 (1):48–53

[30] Wang L, Cai L, Lu S, Qian H, Lawton MT, Shi X. The history and evolution of internal maxillary artery bypass. World Neurosurg. 2018; 113:320–332

[31] Ma L, Ren HC, Huang Y. Bypass of the maxillary artery to proximal middle cerebral artery. J Craniofac Surg. 2015; 26(2):544–547

[32] Ban SP, Cho WS, Kim JE, et al. Bypass surgery for complex intracranial aneurysms: 15 years of experience at a single institution and review of pertinent literature. Oper Neurosurg (Hagerstown). 2017; 13(6):679–688

[33] Roberts B, Hardesty WH, Holling HE, Reivich M, Toole JF. Studies on extracranial cerebral blood flow. Surgery. 1964; 56:826–833

[34] Nossek E, Costantino PD, Chalif DJ, Ortiz RA, Dehdashti AR, Langer DJ. Forearm cephalic vein graft for short, "middle"-flow, internal maxillary artery to middle cerebral artery bypass. Oper Neurosurg (Hagerstown). 2016; 12(2):99–105

[35] Drake CG. Giant intracranial aneurysms: experience with surgical treatment in 174 patients. Clin Neurosurg. 1979; 26:12–95

[36] Ulku CH, Ustun ME, Buyukmumcu M, Cicekcibasi AE, Ziylan T. Radial artery graft for bypass of the maxillary to proximal posterior cerebral artery: an anatomical and technical study. Acta Otolaryngol. 2004; 124(7): 858–862

[37] Kocaeli H, Andaluz N, Choutka O, Zuccarello M. Use of radial artery grafts in extracranial-intracranial revascularization procedures. Neurosurg Focus. 2008; 24(2):E5

[38] Purohit M, Dunning J. Do coronary artery bypass grafts using cephalic veins have a satisfactory patency? Interact Cardiovasc Thorac Surg. 2007; 6(2): 251–254

[39] Peto I, Nouri M, Agazzi S, Langer D, Dehdashti AR. Pterygo-maxillary fissure as a landmark for localization of internal maxillary artery for use in extracranial-intracranial bypass. Oper Neurosurg (Hagerstown). 2020; 19 (5):E480–E486

[40] Maeda S, Aizawa Y, Kumaki K, Kageyama I. Variations in the course of the maxillary artery in Japanese adults. Anat Sci Int. 2012; 87(4):187–194

[41] Nossek E, Costantino PD, Eisenberg M, et al. Internal maxillary artery-middle cerebral artery bypass: infratemporal approach for subcranial-intracranial (SC-IC) bypass. Neurosurgery. 2014; 75(1):87–95

[42] Abdulrauf SI, Sweeney JM, Mohan YS, Palejwala SK. Short segment internal maxillary artery to middle cerebral artery bypass: a novel technique for extracranial-to-intracranial bypass. Neurosurgery. 2011; 68(3):804–808, discussion 808–809

[43] Hanakita S, Lenck S, Labidi M, Watanabe K, Bresson D, Froelich S. The occipital artery as an alternative donor for low-flow bypass to anterior circulation after internal carotid artery occlusion failure prior to exenteration for an atypical cavernous sinus meningioma. World Neurosurg. 2018; 109: 10–17

[44] Mura J, Cuevas JL, Riquelme F, Torche E, Julio R, Isolan GR. Use of superior thyroid artery as a donor vessel in extracranial-intracranial revascularization procedures: a novel technique. J Neurol Surg B Skull Base. 2014; 75(6):421–426

[45] Sanai N, Zador Z, Lawton MT. Bypass surgery for complex brain aneurysms: an assessment of intracranial-intracranial bypass. Neurosurgery. 2009; 65(4): 670–683, discussion 683

[46] Spetzler RF, Roski RA, Rhodes RS, Modic MT. The "bonnet bypass". Case report. J Neurosurg. 1980; 53(5):707–709

7 Skull Base Approaches for Aneurysm

Rokuya Tanikawa and Kosumo Noda

Summary

Skull base approaches can be used to augment all standard cranial approaches to aneurysms. Anterior petrosectomy and posterior petrosectomy with mastoidectomy, condylar fossa, sphenoid, or temporal bone drilling all help reduce or avoid brain retraction when accessing deep-seated aneurysms. Even removal or disconnection of the zygomatic arch, when added to frontotemporal craniotomy, enables the visualization and treatment of high-riding lesions. In this chapter, the application of skull base approaches to intracranial aneurysm surgery will be described.

Keywords: Frontotemporal craniotomy, orbitozygomatic approach, transzygomatic approach, anterior clinoid process, cavernous sinus, petrous bone, suboccipital muscles, condylar fossa

7.1 Key Learning Points

- Frontotemporal craniotomy:
  - It can be used for distal basilar aneurysms and all anterior circulation aneurysms except distal anterior cerebral artery aneurysm.
  - Frontal and temporal lobes should be exposed evenly to place the sylvian fissure in the middle of the craniotomy window.
  - Resecting the lateral sphenoid ridge to flatten the base of the craniotomy provides maximal exposure of the supraclinoid carotid artery.
  - Drilling and skeletonizing the posterolateral wall of orbit extend the basal operative space.
- Transzygomatic approach:
  - It can be used for high-positioned aneurysms like basilar tip aneurysms, carotid bifurcation aneurysms, and superiorly projecting M1 aneurysms.
  - Further inferior retraction of the temporalis muscle by removing the zygomatic arch extends the basal operative field at the pterion compared to standard frontotemporal craniotomy.
- Lateral cavernous wall dissection:
  - Increases the anterior temporal space without sacrificing tributaries of superficial sylvian veins crossing the sylvian fissure by retracting the temporal lobe epidurally.
  - Reduces mechanical injury to the oculomotor nerve by opening the oculomotor foramen and releasing the cavernous segment of the nerve by incising the connective tissue between it and the cavernous sinus.
- Anterior petrosectomy:
  - The operative field obtained via anterior petrosectomy is the space between the trigeminal foramen and internal auditory canal (IAC).
  - Midbasilar aneurysms between the IAC and trigeminal foramen can be exposed through this approach.
  - Important landmarks, like superior orbital fissure, foramen rotundum, spinosum, ovale, posterior border of V3, greater superficial petrosal nerve (GSPN), C6 segment of internal

carotid artery (ICA), petrosal edge, superior petrosal sinus (SPS), arcuate eminence, geniculate ganglion, inner petrosal dura, IAC, and cochlea must all be identified during middle fossa dissection.
  - It is key to identify Glasscock's and Kawase's triangles and the rhomboid of middle fossa.
- Posterior petrosectomy:
  - It can be used to access distal vertebral or lower basilar aneurysms located between the jugular foramen and IAC.
  - The space between superior semicircular canal and sinodural angle is opened via a mastoidectomy with removal of the petrous edge.
- Mastoidectomy:
  - Mastoidectomy is necessary to perform a posterior petrosectomy.
  - Important anatomical landmarks for mastoidectomy are the root of zygoma, supramastoid crest, parietomastoid suture, lambdoid suture, occipitomastoid suture, asterion, spine of Henle, mastoid tip, outer mastoid triangle, sinodural angle, SPS, sigmoid sinus, transverse sinus, digastric ridge, jugular bulb, mastoid antrum, incus, lateral semicircular canal, Fallopian canal, posterior semicircular canal, superior semicircular canal, endolymphatic sac, presigmoid dura, stylomastoid foramen, chorda tympani, facial recess, and the outer rim of the tympanic membrane.
- Suboccipital muscular layer-by-layer dissection:
  - This technique provides a shallow operative field without a bulky suboccipital muscle mass and enables use of shorter instruments (e.g., during occipital artery–posterior inferior cerebellar artery [OA-PICA] bypass).
  - The layers of muscle are divided with suboccipital muscles, occipital muscle, sternocleidomastoid, and trapezius in the first layer; splenius capitis, longissimus capitis, semispinalis capitis, and digastric muscle in the second layer; and superior oblique, rectus capitis major and minor, and inferior oblique muscles in the third layer.
  - All muscles except the sternocleidomastoid, trapezius, and occipital muscles are innervated by a posterior branch of the C2 spinal nerve. The sternocleidomastoid and trapezius muscles are innervated by the accessory nerve, and the occipital muscle is innervated by the facial nerve.
- Lateral suboccipital craniotomy:
  - The intracranial vertebral artery can be exposed by this approach if the aneurysm is located lower than the eighth nerve.
  - If the vertebral aneurysm is shifted ipsilaterally this approach alone is adequate.
- Transcondylar fossa approach:
  - Aneurysms involving the entire intracranial vertebral artery to the lower basilar artery (BA) can be exposed using this approach.
  - This provides the extended view necessary for distal vertebral or lower BA shifted contralaterally.
  - Important landmarks are the hip of sigmoid sinus where the sigmoid sinus curves anteromedially toward the jugular bulb, occipital condyle, C1 condylar facet where it faces the occipital

condylar facet, posterior condylar emissary vein and canal, marginal sinus, vertebral venous plexus covering the V3 segment of vertebral artery, and the hypoglossal canal.

7.2 Introduction

The concept of a skull base approach is the removal of bone to reduce brain retraction and neurovascular manipulation when approaching various deep-seated lesions.

An accurate knowledge of osseous, vascular, and neural anatomy is critical. Their relationships are relatively simple because every important neural and vascular structure is surrounded by compact bone which works as a protector and potential conduit for these vital structures.

7.3 Transzygomatic Approach

Removal of the zygomatic arch provides wide subtemporal exposure with added inferior retraction of the temporalis muscle. As a result, the retracted temporalis muscle bulk does not encroach on the middle fossa floor and pterion enabling a bright and wide operative field. Although the orbitozygomatic approach may be necessary if the main operative corridor is a subfrontal or transcavernous route, a transzygomatic approach is sufficient when a distal transsylvian with anterior temporal approach is the main corridor to the target lesion. For example, basilar tip superior cerebellar artery aneurysms are a good indication for a transzygomatic approach.

The patient should be supine with the head rotated 30 degrees toward the contralateral side and the head of bed elevated 15 to 20 degrees (Low-Fowler's position).

The skin incision is designed as a curved line which starts in front of the tragus just posterior to the trunk of the superficial temporal artery, in order to avoid its injury, then curving up toward the midline hairline (▶ Fig. 7.1).

The skin flap is elevated just above the temporalis fascia in a two-layer/differential fashion until exposing the orbitozygomatic process with frontozygomatic suture which is covered by the periosteum and connective tissue connecting to the deep temporal fascia. The fat pad of the superficial temporal fascia is elevated with a semicircular arc incision in order to expose the zygomatic arch between the root of zygoma and temporal zygomatic process (▶ Fig. 7.2).

The exposed zygomatic arch is cut obliquely at just anterior to the root of the zygoma and just anterior to the temporal zygomatic process with a bone saw or reciprocating saw as a T-bone shape. The masseter muscle, which attaches to the inferior border of zygomatic arch, and temporalis muscle, which connects to the inner surface of the zygomatic arch, must be detached to remove the zygomatic arch (▶ Fig. 7.3).

The temporalis muscle can be incised in line with the posterior vertical part of skin incision down to the root of the zygoma, then detached from the superior temporal line and dissected and retracted inferiorly (▶ Fig. 7.4).

Next, a frontotemporal craniotomy can be performed. After the bone flap is removed, the remaining lateral sphenoid ridge is drilled away until the meningo-orbital band is exposed (▶ Fig. 7.5). Drilling the remaining bone lateral to the meningo-orbital band extends the basal operative field and ensures no disturbance of microscope illumination regardless of zygoma retraction

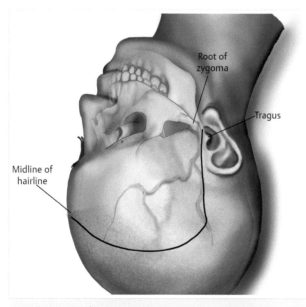

Fig. 7.1 L- or reverse L-shaped skin flap for frontotemporal craniotomy is designed with preservation of the superficial temporal artery. The skin incision is started just in front of the tragus and extends superiorly before turning toward the midline hairline in order to not cut the trunk of the superficial temporal artery.

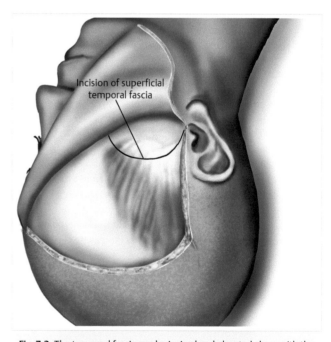

Fig. 7.2 The temporal fascia can be incised and elevated along with the fat pad deep to it as a semicircular curve between orbital zygomatic process and root of zygoma in order to expose the zygomatic arch.

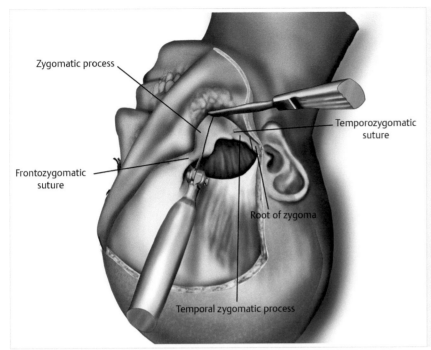

Fig. 7.3 L-shaped zygoma removal can be performed using a sagittal saw for two osteotomies. The frontal zygomatic process is cut vertically, and the temporal zygomatic process is cut obliquely just anterior to the root of the zygoma.

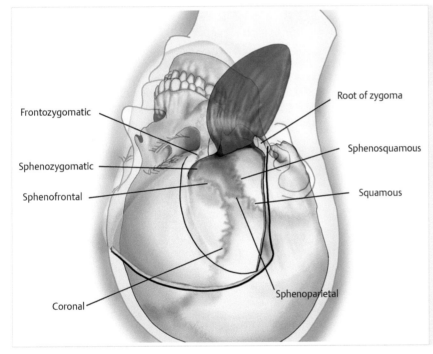

Fig. 7.4 Coronal, squamous, sphenoparietal, sphenofrontal, sphenozygomatic, and sphenosquamous sutures are exposed by elevation of temporalis muscle after it is incised posteriorly in line with the vertical skin incision.

7.4 Transpetrosal Approach (Includes Posterior Petrosectomy and Anterior Petrosectomy)

7.4.1 Posterior Petrosectomy

A posterior petrosectomy can be done via mastoidectomy which involves bone removal posterolateral to the superior semicircular canal, whereby the semicircular canals and Fallopian canal are skeletonized, exposing the sigmoid sinus, SPS, endolymphatic sac, presigmoid dura, and digastric ridge. This is used to access distal vertebral or lower basilar aneurysms located between the jugular foramen and IAC.

Mastoidectomy[1] with preservation of the labyrinth is not easy; it requires not only careful training with a high-speed drill, but also a thorough comprehension of the anatomy. The landmarks to begin a mastoidectomy are the root of the zygoma, external ear canal, spine of Henle, supramastoid crest, mastoid tip, digastric groove, and asterion. The outer mastoid triangle can be defined by the root of zygoma, spine of Henle, mastoid tip, and asterion (▶ Fig. 7.6).

The rough drilling of superficial compact bone along the outer mastoid triangle to expose the cancellous bone and mastoid air cells is the first step of a mastoidectomy. The superoposterior wall of the external ear canal must be preserved as a thin wall of 0.5 to 1.0 mm thickness[1] while preserving the spine of Henle which attaches to the posterior external ear canal in order to preserve the very thin skin layer of this canal (▶ Fig. 7.7).

The sigmoid sinus can be skeletonized as a blueish bulging along the posterior aspect of the outer mastoid triangle. The

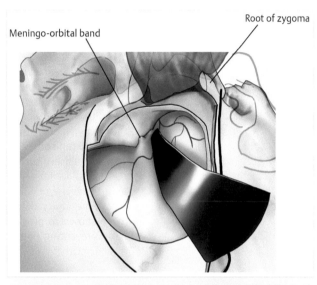

Fig. 7.5 Meningo-orbital band can be exposed by the skeletonization of orbit to reduce brain retraction.

wall of the sigmoid sinus should be protected by retaining an "eggshell" or "paper thin" compact bone on it to not disrupt the venous sinus wall. The presigmoid dura can be exposed gradually after skeletonization of the sigmoid sinus.

The temporal dura can be exposed by drilling the bone along the superior aspect of the outer mastoid triangle and the SPS can be exposed by the skeletonization of the temporal dura and sigmoid sinus at the sinodural angle.

The mastoid antrum will be opened in the depth posterior to the root of the zygoma and a yellow compact bone can be found beside the mastoid antrum which is the lateral semicircular canal. The lateral semicircular canal is generally 15 mm from the surface of the mastoid bone.[1] It is important to find the mastoid antrum first, not to try to find the lateral semicircular canal directly. As the lateral semicircular canal is in the posterior part of the antrum, it can then be exposed just after opening the mastoid antrum (▶ Fig. 7.8).

The tympanic segment of the facial nerve lies just anterolateral to the lateral semicircular canal and the corner between the tympanic segment and the Fallopian segment is called the genu of the facial nerve.

As the semicircular canals are surrounded by cancellous bone in the mastoid air cells, their yellow, hard, compact bone can be recognized easily under microscope. Each plane of the semicircular canals crosses at right angles: the posterior semicircular canal is posterior to the lateral semicircular, and the superior semicircular canal is superior to the lateral semicircular canal (▶ Fig. 7.9).

The jugular bulb can be skeletonized by taking cancellous bone inferior to the posterior semicircular canal and posterior to the Fallopian canal, which overhangs the anterior half of the jugular bulb. In order to remove the bone over the jugular bulb, accurate skeletonization of the Fallopian canal and eggshell

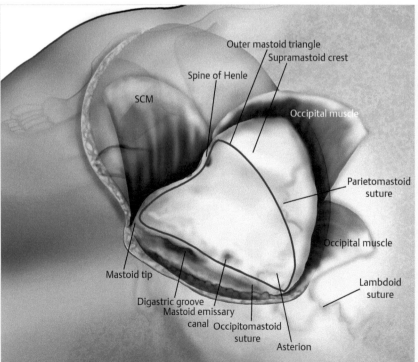

Fig. 7.6 The outer mastoid triangle (left side), which is defined by the root of the zygoma, the spine of Henle, mastoid tip, and asterion, is exposed by elevating the sternocleidomastoid muscle anteriorly, detaching the splenius capitis from the posterior border of the mastoid body, and elevating the occipital muscle.

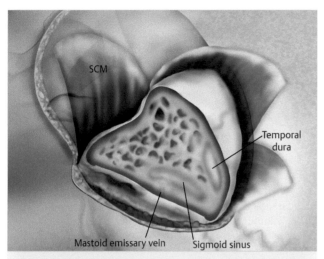

Fig. 7.7 Drilling of surface cortical bone of the left mastoid process should be done in a flat drilling manner, not going deeper locally to maintain the thin compact bone on important dural, vascular, or neural structures.

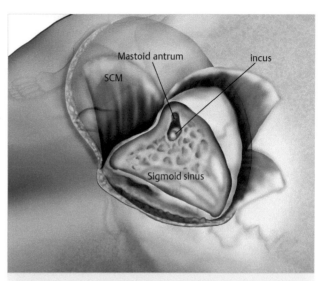

Fig. 7.8 The first landmark to find the labyrinth is the antrum of the middle ear. The incus, one of the ear ossicles, can be found in the antrum and the yellow compact bone which is the lateral semicircular canal will be recognized just posterior to the incus.

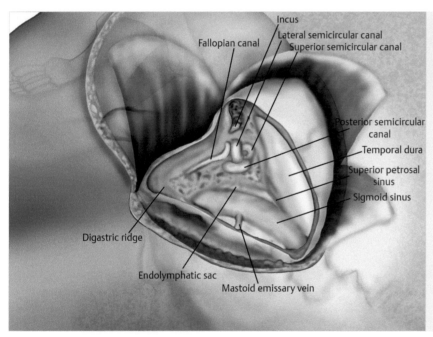

Fig. 7.9 The genu of the facial nerve can be found at the same depth as the lateral semicircular canal. The lateral, posterior, and superior semicircular canals cross at 90 degrees to each other.

exposure of the facial nerve for its protection is necessary. The digastric ridge is found by the drilling cancellous bone lateral to the digastric groove where the posterior belly of the digastric muscle attaches. The Fallopian canal connects to the stylomastoid foramen at the anterior part of digastric ridge (▶ Fig. 7.10).

The purpose of this approach is to obtain a sufficient operative field between the labyrinth and cerebellum to approach the ventral brainstem and the distal vertebral and lower BA. Complete drilling of the petrous edge posterior to the superior semicircular canal maximizes the operative field because the posterior edge of the petrous bone remaining after mastoidectomy blocks the corridor to the ventral pons.

7.4.2 Anterior Petrosectomy

Midbasilar aneurysms between the IAC and trigeminal foramen can be exposed through the anterior transpetrosal approach. The boundary between the posterior and anterior petrosectomy is the superior semicircular canal which is localized by the arcuate eminence. The temporal rhomboid is defined by the posterior border of the mandibular branch of the trigeminal nerve (V3), the petrous edge, arcuate eminence, and GSPN and can be exposed by the elevation of the middle fossa dura after ligating the middle meningeal artery at foramen spinosum and incision of the dura propria to expose V3 at foramen ovale. Care is taken to preserve GSPN to avoid

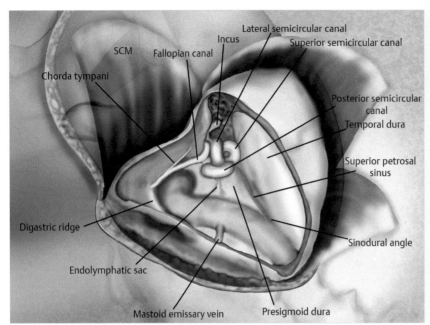

Fig. 7.10 The posterior petrous bone surrounding the labyrinth can be drilled away to maximize the presigmoid operative space. The superior petrosal sinus between sinodural angle and superior semicircular canal can be exposed by removing the petrous ridge.

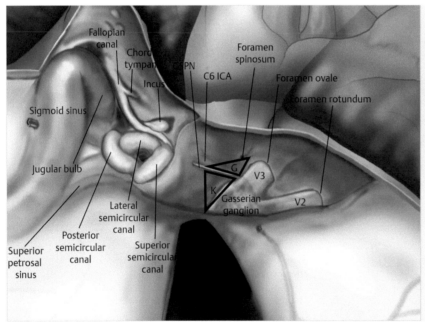

Fig. 7.11 Left side. Glasscock's triangle (G) is defined by the posterior edge of foramen ovale, the cochlea, and the intersection of greater superficial petrosal nerve (GSPN) and V3; Kawase's triangle (K) is defined by the junction of GSPN and V3, the cochlea, and the posterior edge of trigeminal foramen. Both are important triangles to localize the C6 segment of the internal carotid artery (ICA), tensor tympani, and the transition of the C6 and C7 segments of ICA.

damage to the facial nerve via retraction injury to the geniculate ganglion.[1] GSPN must be identified in the bony hiatus between the geniculate ganglion and V3. GSPN continues into the vidian canal under the mandibular nerve (V3) as the vidian nerve which connects to the pterygopalatine ganglion which innervates secreting glands in the head and neck including the lacrimal glands.

Glasscock's triangle (G) and Kawase's triangle (K) are important triangles to locate the petrous (C6) portion of ICA just beneath GSPN (▶ Fig. 7.11).

Drilling the temporal rhomboid begins at the anteromedial corner of the rhomboid and proceeds toward the posteromedial corner at the crossing point of the petrous edge and arcuate eminence. The bone along the petrous edge is a safe area to drill and the superior wall of the IAC is covered by thick bone (▶ Fig. 7.12).

On the other hand, drilling near GSPN must be done carefully because the C6 segment of ICA is just below GSPN and the cochlea is just medial to the corner of C6–C7 segment of ICA (▶ Fig. 7.13).

The petrous apex can be drilled by elevating the trigeminal root after releasing the fibrous ring of the trigeminal foramen. Exposure and drilling of the petrous apex is only necessary to approach midbasilar to lower basilar lesions. Upper basilar lesions can be exposed in the space anterior to the trigeminal nerve root by opening the porus trigeminus.

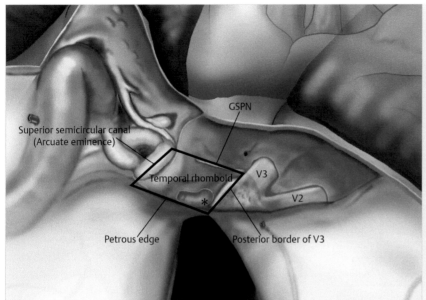

Fig. 7.12 Temporal rhomboid which is defined by posterior border of V3, greater superficial petrosal nerve (GSPN), arcuate eminence, and petrous edge is an important anatomy to perform safe drilling in the anterior petrosal approach. The anteromedial corner of the temporal rhomboid is a safe point to begin drilling in the temporal rhomboid (*).

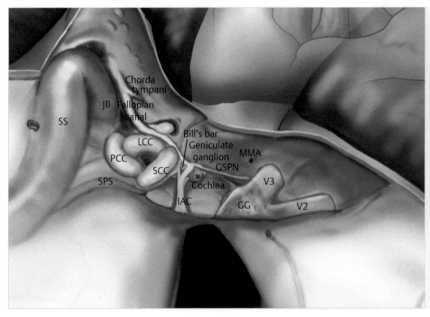

Fig. 7.13 Temporal rhomboidectomy provides the skeletonization of the C6 internal carotid artery, the cochlea at the posterior genu of the C6 carotid, the internal auditory canal (IAC), and the inner petrosal dura. The vestibular nerve and facial nerve can be skeletonized at the distal end of IAC between Bill's bar which indicates the beginning of the tympanic segment of the facial nerve. GG, gasserian ganglion; IAC, internal auditory canal; JB, jugular bulb; LCC, lateral semicircular canal; MMA, middle meningeal artery at foramen spinosum; PCC, posterior semicircular canal; SCC, superior semicircular canal; SPS, superior petrosal sinus; SS, sigmoid sinus; *, cochlea.

The IAC is skeletonized by drilling the posterior part of the temporal rhomboid. The axis of the IAC divides the angle between GSPN and the superior semicircular canal at 60-degree angles between the cochlea and superior semicircular canal.[1]

7.5 Far Lateral Suboccipital Approach

A far lateral, suboccipital approach can reduce cerebellar retraction and provide more anterior and inferior access to the cerebellopontine (CP) angle and lateral brainstem. The intracranial vertebral artery can be exposed by this approach if an aneurysm is located lower than the eighth nerve.

Space is obtained by skeletonizing the posterior half of the sigmoid sinus between the transverse–sigmoid junction and turn toward the jugular bulb. One must pay careful attention to the mastoid emissary vein which connects the occipital venous plexus to the lateral surface of the sigmoid sinus.[2] Eggshell drilling is used to expose the wall of the sigmoid sinus (► Fig. 7.14).

7.5.1 Suboccipital Layer-by-Layer Muscular Dissection

Initial dissection for a far lateral approach can be done in a layer-by-layer fashion to dissect out the suboccipital muscles.[3] The sternocleidomastoid, trapezius, and occipital muscles are the first layer; splenius, longissimus, and semispinalis capitis

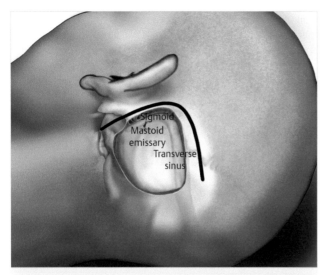

Fig. 7.14 A standard lateral suboccipital craniotomy is demonstrated with exposure of the posterior half of the sigmoid sinus without exposing the condylar fossa. Occipital bony exposure for a standard suboccipital craniotomy should expose the asterion, superior nuchal line, and inferior nuchal line by detaching superior oblique, capitis, and posterior major/minor rectus capitis muscles. This reverse "L"-shaped incision may not be common but is preferred by the author.

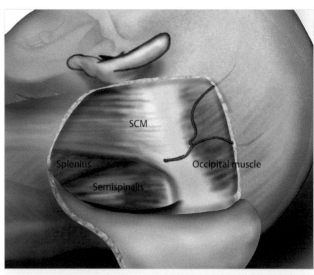

Fig. 7.15 The occipital artery is superficial to the occipital muscle and galea aponeurosis superior to the superior nuchal line. Occipital muscle, sternocleidomastoid muscle, and trapezius muscle all gather at the superior nuchal line and the occipital artery usually penetrates the sternocleidomastoid tendon at this insertion. The incision used is not typical but used extensively by the senior author.

muscle are the second layer; and superior oblique, posterior major and minor rectus, and inferior oblique capitis muscles are the third layer of suboccipital muscles[2,3,4] (▶ Fig. 7.15).

The sternocleidomastoid muscle can be detached at the superior nuchal line as a triangular flap, elevated and retracted anteriorly. The origin of the occipital muscle can also be detached from the superior nuchal line and reflected superiorly so that the asterion can be identified as a gathering point of three bony sutures (parietomastoid, occipitomastoid, and lambdoid suture). The splenius capitis muscle attaches on the mastoid body and mastoid tip and it can be elevated inferoposteriorly (▶ Fig. 7.16).

The intermuscular occipital artery runs between the splenius capitis muscle and inferior nuchal line. It runs medially to longissimus capitis in 70% and laterally in 30%.[2,3,4] When harvesting the occipital artery is necessary as a donor graft (e.g., for fusiform posterior inferior cerebellar artery [PICA] aneurysms) a careful observation and recognition of the occipital artery whether it runs at medial or lateral to the longissimus capitis muscle is important during elevation of the splenius capitis and longissimus capitis muscles. The intermuscular occipital artery can be fully skeletonized by the elevation of longissimus capitis muscle.

The third layer of occipital muscles is exposed at the inferior nuchal line and makes up the suboccipital triangle with its associated fat pad. The suboccipital triangle covers the extradural (V3 segment) vertebral artery and is comprised of the superior oblique, posterior rectus capitis major, and inferior oblique capitis muscles (▶ Fig. 7.17).

The V3 segment of the vertebral artery is surrounded by a venous plexus in the "J groove" at the superior aspect of the lamina of the atlas and lies in the suboccipital triangle. The

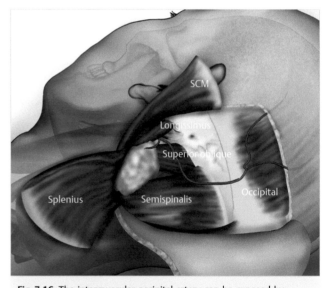

Fig. 7.16 The intermuscular occipital artery can be exposed by elevation of the splenius capitis muscle. The occipital artery has a course medial (deep) to the longissimus capitis muscle in 70% and lateral (superficial) to it in 30% of patients.

superior oblique muscle crosses over the posterior rectus capitis major muscle and the superior oblique muscle should be detached from inferior nuchal line. The (posterior) rectus capitis major muscle can be detached next which opens the upper suboccipital triangle. The extracranial V3 segment with associated vertebral venous plexus can then be identified with its fat pad in the opened suboccipital triangle (▶ Fig. 7.18).

7.6 Transcondylar (Fossa) Approach

When an approach to aneurysms involving the PICA, vertebrobasilar junction, or lower BA is required, the bulging of

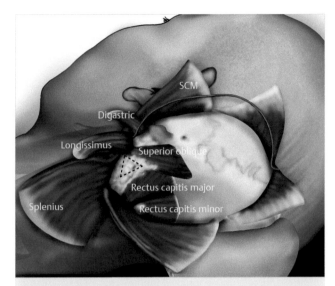

Fig. 7.17 The third layer of muscles is exposed by detaching the longissimus and semispinalis capitis muscles. The suboccipital triangle (*dotted triangle*) is defined by the medial edge of the superior oblique, the superior margin of the inferior oblique, and the medial edge of the rectus capitis major muscle.

the jugular tubercle obscures the deep field which is superomedial to the tubercle. A transcondylar (fossa) approach exposes the lower basilar area by the removal of the jugular tubercle in the epidural space. In order to drill the jugular tubercle, which is medial to the jugular bulb, exposure of the condylar fossa is necessary after managing the posterior condylar emissary vein which connects the vertebral venous plexus that surrounds the extracranial vertebral artery (V3 portion) to the jugular bulb[3,5] (▶ Fig. 7.19).

The posterior condylar emissary vein can be cauterized and cut after it is exposed by removing the adipose tissue around it. Then the condylar fossa can be exposed and identified.

The bone of the condylar fossa is a bone between the occipital condylar facet and the bottom of the sigmoid sinus which includes the hypoglossal canal.

The hypoglossal canal can be skeletonized by drilling the condyle bone after a retrosigmoid suboccipital craniotomy with skeletonization of the sigmoid sinus and posterolateral surface of the foramen magnum has been performed. The marginal sinus at the foramen magnum can be skeletonized using the eggshell technique. Because the plexus surrounding the hypoglossal nerve connects with the marginal sinus, skeletonization of the marginal sinus creates a good landmark to identify the hypoglossal canal.[1,5,6]

Since the jugular tubercle is medial to the jugular bulb, superior to the hypoglossal canal, and anteromedial to the turn of the sigmoid sinus, identification and skeletonization of these anatomical landmarks are necessary to safely drill the jugular tubercle (▶ Fig. 7.20).

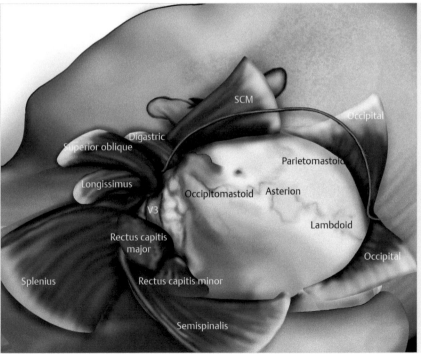

Fig. 7.18 The V3 segment of the vertebral artery can be exposed by opening the suboccipital triangle. The V3 segment is surrounded by the vertebral venous plexus. SCM, sternocleidomastoid muscle; V3, mandibular nerve.

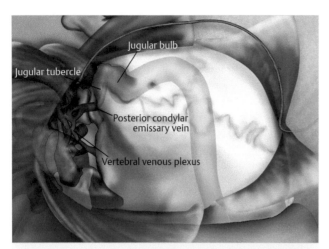

Fig. 7.19 The posterior condylar emissary vein connects the vertebral venous plexus and jugular bulb. The condylar fossa can be exposed after cauterizing and cutting the posterior condylar emissary vein.

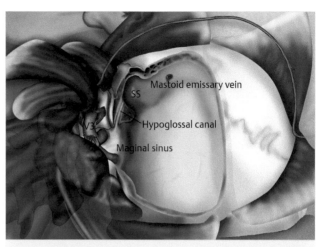

Fig. 7.20 Skeletonization of the foramen magnum followed by condylar fossa drilling will provide transcondylar fossa approach with skeletonization of the hypoglossal canal. The jugular tubercle superior to the hypoglossal canal can be drilled away as necessary. SS, sigmoid sinus.

7.7 Vascular Challenges

7.7.1 High-Riding Distal Basilar Aneurysm (Basilar Tip and Basilar-Superior Cerebellar Artery [SCA] Aneurysm)

For surgery of distal basilar aneurysms through a transsylvian or anterior temporal route, where the neck is 15 mm above the clinoid line, zygomatic arch resection is effective to visualize not only the aneurysm neck, but also important perforators like the posterior thalamoperforating arteries.

7.7.2 P2p or P2-P3 Junction Aneurysm

A combined supra- and infratentorial (transtentorial) approach via mastoidectomy with preservation of the labyrinth enables access to a superiorly located P2p or P2-P3 junction aneurysm while minimizing retraction of the temporal lobe.

7.7.3 VA-PICA Aneurysm

For Vertebral artery-posterior inferior cerebellar artery (VA-PICA) aneurysms which exist medial to the jugular tubercle or immediately distal to the dural ring of the vertebral artery, a far lateral or even transcondylar approach is an effective addition to ensure complete distal or proximal control, respectively.

7.7.4 VA-AICA Aneurysm (Midbasilar Aneurysm)

The midbasilar region can be the most challenging to access. An anterior petrosectomy with release of the fibrous dural ring of the trigeminal foramen and opening of the IAC can secure the operative field in between the fifth nerve and seventh/eighth complex to expose the midbasilar artery and basilar–AICA aneurysms.

7.8 Injury Avoidance

All of the approaches described in this chapter require significant dissection for bone removal but help to avoid vascular injury or inadequate treatment by dramatically improving access to difficult to access aneurysms. In addition, they can be critical for proximal and/or distal control for these aneurysms, which is a basic vascular tenet critical in treatment of any aneurysm.

7.8.1 Prevention of Frontalis Nerve and Temporomandibular Joint (TMJ) Injury

Exposure of the zygomatic arch can be performed by elevating the temporal fascial flap from superior to inferior between the frontal zygomatic process and root of the zygoma (▶ Fig. 7.3). Next, the temporalis muscle can be elevated by detaching it from the frontotemporosphenoidal bone. The exposure of the root of the zygoma should be carefully performed to avoid injury to the temporomandibular joint (TMJ) by accidentally incising the articular capsule due to excessive exposure or disorientation, as the TMJ is just under the root of the zygoma.

Facial nerve frontalis branches cross the zygomatic arch around the midpoint in the subcutaneous tissue of the temporal scalp. Elevating a superficial temporal fascial flap subperiosteally from the surface of zygomatic arch protects these facial branches.

7.8.2 Preservation of Orbital Fascia

The removal of the sphenoid ridge is effective to widen the basal operative field below the pterion in order to visualize deep and high-positioned basilar apex aneurysms. Removal of the posterior orbital bone helps create a wide corridor to approach deep midline structures, because the wall of the posterior orbit is a limitation to the anteromedial border of the operative corridor to the basilar bifurcation. Since the inner cortical bone of the posterior wall of the orbit is very thin, orbital skeletonization must be performed carefully to avoid injury to periorbita. If the periorbita is injured, orbital fat and any bleeding must be carefully cauterized and opened fascia covered with gelfoam soaked with fibrinogen to avoid the protrusion of fat.

Orbital rim resection as an orbitozygomatic approach should be performed for limited cases. When performed, to avoid overzealous exposure of orbital tissue, especially orbital fat tissue, an eggshell orbital roof skeletonization can help the neurosurgeon perform orbital rim resection without disruption of orbital fascia and the resulting fat extrusion which reduces the operative visual field in spite of more invasive orbital resection.

7.8.3 Avoiding Optic Nerve and Internal Carotid Artery (ICA) Injury

Optic canal skeletonization during anterior clinoidectomy must be performed with "eggshell" technique to avoid injury to the optic nerve. The proximal roof of the optic canal (closer to the orbit) usually has thinner bone than the distal optic canal.

By drilling inside of the anterior clinoid process, at the so-called "Anteromedial Triangle (Dolenc)," the C3 segment of the ICA, which is surrounded by thin compact bone, can be skeletonized. This thin cortical bone must be shaved smoothly with a diamond burr until "eggshell" thin to skeletonize the C3 portion of the ICA. The same technique can be applied to the C6 segment of the ICA during drilling of the petrous rhomboid for anterior petrosectomy after confirmation of the precise location of the C6 portion of the ICA. This can be localized using Glasscock's (posteromedial) triangle with its boundaries of foramen spinosum, arcuate eminence, GSPN, and mandibular nerve.

7.9 Related Pathologies

In addition to aneurysms, these approaches can be used to address pituitary macroadenomas with suprasellar extension;

clinoid meningiomas; sphenoid ridge, cavernous, and Meckel's cave meningiomas; trigeminal schwannomas; petrous apex or petroclival meningiomas; jugular foramen dumbbell shape schwannomas and meningiomas; and hypoglossal schwannomas.

7.10 Case Examples

7.10.1 Case 1

A 69-year-old woman presented with an incidentally discovered, asymptomatic BA apex aneurysm (▶ Fig. 7.21).

Family History: Mother Died Due to Subarachnoid Hemorrhage (SAH)

The aneurysm was 19.4 mm above the clinoid line (▶ Fig. 7.22). A previous endovascular surgeon referred the patient to us because the aneurysm was wide-based and low-height shape which has relatively high recurrence rate after the coiling even with adjuvant assist techniques. Clipping of this basilar tip aneurysm was performed via a left transzygomatic frontotemporal craniotomy anterior temporal approach. All the perforators around the aneurysm could be confirmed through the anterior temporal route and were preserved during the neck clipping (▶ Fig. 7.23). The aneurysm could be clipped using two fenestrated straight clips. The left posterior thalamo-perforating artery was preserved by using a fenestrated clip (▶ Fig. 7.24) and all other important perforators were safely preserved. The patient was discharged on postoperative day 14 without any assistance.

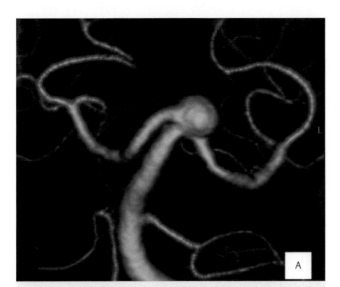

Fig. 7.21 Three-dimensional computed tomography (CT) angiogram reconstruction showing a wide neck basilar bifurcation aneurysm projecting superolaterally to the left.

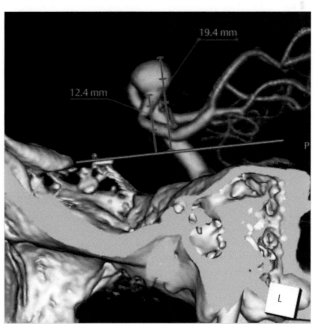

Fig. 7.22 Three-dimensional computed tomography (CT) angiogram reconstruction showing that the aneurysm is located in a high position, 19.4 mm above the clinoid line (between the apex of the anterior clinoid process and tip of the posterior clinoid process).

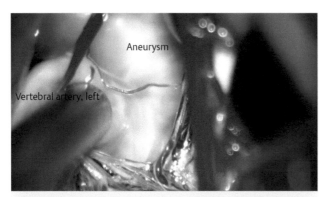

Fig. 7.23 The aneurysm and the vital perforating arteries could be exposed by a left transzygomatic anterior temporal approach.

7.10.2 Case 2

A 27-year-old woman presented with an asymptomatic giant vertebrobasilar junction aneurysm (▶ Fig. 7.25) discovered because of headaches.

A left, combined posterior and anterior petrosectomy was performed in order to secure a sufficient operative field to manipulate and observe the aneurysm in the operative field between not only seventh and nineth nerves but also between the fifth nerve and seventh/eighth nerve complex. A posterior petrosectomy with mastoidectomy was performed to remove the petrous edge lateral to the superior semicircular canal and afterward the anterior petrosectomy was performed (▶ Fig. 7.26). The aneurysm could be exposed directly between the seventh/eighth complexes and fifth nerve (▶ Fig. 7.27). The aneurysm was deflated by the temporary trapping by bilateral vertebral and proximal BA. The aneurysm could be trapped safely between ipsilateral vertebral artery proximal to the aneurysm and the distal vertebral artery proximal to the union (▶ Fig. 7.28). Patient recovered immediately without any deficits and was discharged on postoperative day 21.

7.10.3 Case 3

A 60-year-old man presented with asymptomatic, bilateral vertebral artery fusiform aneurysms found during screening for headache (▶ Fig. 7.29). The patient insisted on treatment due to significant anxiety of aneurysm rupture. A right transcondylar (fossa) approach (▶ Fig. 7.29) was performed in order to bypass the right vertebral artery after trapping the aneurysm. A direct reconstruction was performed using a radial artery interposition graft between the extracranial V3 segment proximal and the intracranial V4 segment distal to the aneurysm[4] (▶ Fig. 7.30, ▶ Fig. 7.31, and ▶ Fig. 7.32). After surgery, the patient recovered well; he had no new neurological deficit and was discharged on postoperative day 30 without any assistance. The contralateral aneurysm was treated 1 year later by proximal clip occlusion preserving the perforator to the medulla oblongata with an uneventful clinical course.

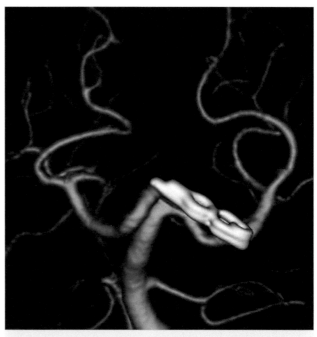

Fig. 7.24 The aneurysm was occluded with multiple clipping technique across the neck using fenestrated clips to preserve the posterior thalamoperforating artery which was adherent to the aneurysm neck.

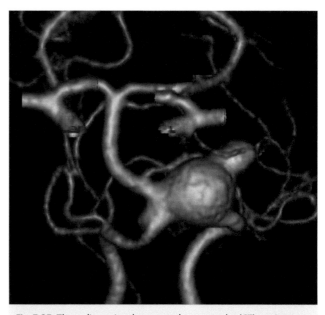

Fig. 7.25 Three-dimensional computed tomography (CT) angiogram shows a giant fusiform aneurysm at the vertebral basilar junction.

7.11 Management Strategy

7.11.1 Preoperative Management

The general fitness of the patient is important to safely undergo extensive skull base approaches. A patient with vascular lesions like aneurysm often has diabetes mellitus or glucose

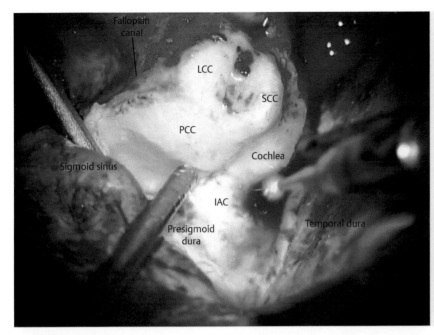

Fig. 7.26 Intraoperative view showing full skeletonization of the anterior petrous and posterior petrous bone with mastoidectomy and anterior petrosectomy in a left combined petrosal approach. IAC, internal auditory canal; LCC, lateral semicircular canal; PCC, posterior semicircular canal; SCC, superior semicircular canal.

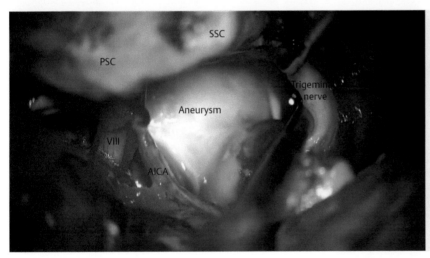

Fig. 7.27 Intraoperative view showing that the aneurysm could be manipulated in between the trigeminal and seventh/eighth complexes by the combined petrosal approach.

intolerance, and the poor control of glucose metabolism is an important cause of postoperative delay of wound healing and/or an infection. Strict control of diabetes mellitus is necessary before surgery and because chronic diabetes mellitus induces dehydration, appropriate perioperative hydration should be considered if the patient does not have cardiac or pulmonary congestion. Steroid administration before the surgery is important to protect the patient from surgical trauma and a short period (approximately 3 days) of prednisolone or dexamethasone is useful in perioperative management. The authors do not use lumbar drainage routinely, but lumbar or ventricular drainage should be used as needed.

7.12 Potential Complications

Early visual disturbance: Caused by optic nerve injury due to mechanical damage during optic canal drilling. Any disruption of periorbita will cause early postoperative periorbital ecchymosis and swelling. Rarely, there can be delayed enophthalmos due to significant disruption of the periorbita with complete orbital roof removal.

Delayed visual disturbance after 12 hours: May be caused by intraorbital venous congestion due to the obstruction of superior ophthalmic vein at its outlet into the anterior cavernous sinus just inferior to the proximal ring of the ICA.[7,8,9] All patients who experienced delayed monocular blindness had ipsilateral conjunctival edema immediately after surgery. Vasospasm or hematoma should be ruled out as reversible causes of vision loss.

Oculomotor palsy: Caused by mechanical damage to the oculomotor nerve in the lateral cavernous wall when the temporal lobe dura propria is elevated from the superior orbital fissure and lateral wall of the cavernous sinus.

Facial numbness: Caused by mechanical damage to the trigeminal nerve during dissection of the dura propria.

Dry eye: Caused by the loss of lacrimation due to injury or sacrifice of GSPN.

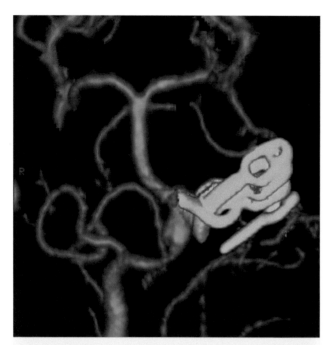

Fig. 7.28 Postoperative three-dimensional computed tomography (CT) angiogram shows the main part of the aneurysm obliterated and right distal vertebral artery fusiform dilation remaining.

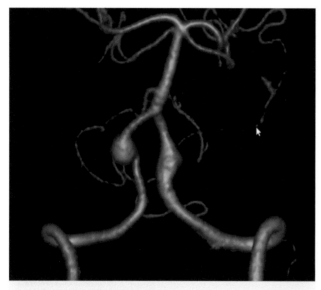

Fig. 7.29 Computed tomography (CT) angiography showing bilateral fusiform vertebral artery aneurysms.

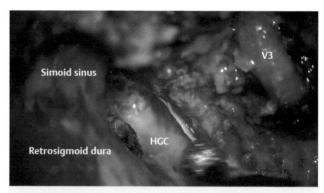

Fig. 7.30 Intraoperative view after a right transcondylar fossa approach was performed. HGC, hypoglossal canal.

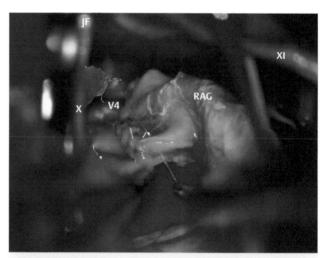

Fig. 7.31 Intraoperative, intradural view after the right vertebral artery was reconstructed directly using an interposition radial arterial graft (RAG) between the V3 and intracranial V4 segments. JF, jugular foramen.

Facial nerve palsy: The facial nerve and its branches can be injured in several locations. Injury can be caused by traction on the geniculate ganglion and facial nerve during elevation of dura propria from GSPN. It can also be caused by direct injury to the facial nerve in the Fallopian canal during mastoidectomy. Finally, injury to the frontal branch can occur during dissection of the superficial temporal fascia during frontotemporal craniotomy or zygomatic osteotomy.

Carotid injury: Can occur at the C6 segment by careless drilling of the temporal rhomboid bone under GSPN or at the C3 segment during anterior clinoidectomy.

Auditory disturbance: Caused by opening the labyrinth during skeletonization of the semicircular canals during mastoidectomy or the cochlea during temporal rhomboidectomy.

Injury to the sigmoid sinus: Caused by inappropriate skeletonization of the sigmoid sinus without eggshell technique.

7.13 Conclusion

Understanding vital structures within the skull base is critical to perform safe skull base approaches for challenging aneurysms.

These approaches play a critical role in providing adequate vascular control for many challenging posterior circulation and some anterior circulation aneurysms and should be applied carefully and with full understanding of the access they provide. These include distal basilar aneurysms such as basilar tip and superior cerebellar through an epi- and/or sub-dural anterior temporal approach, midbasilar aneurysms through an anterior transpetrosal approach, distal vertebral and lower basilar aneurysms through a combined petrosal approach, and

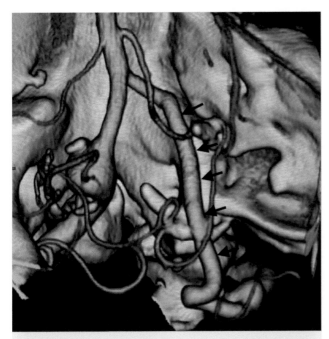

Fig. 7.32 Postoperative three-dimensional computed tomography (CT) angiogram shows a well-reconstructed, right vertebral artery by radial artery graft (*black arrows*) and disappearance of the aneurysm.

intradural juxta-dural ring vertebral aneurysms and contralaterally shifted aneurysms and distal vertebral aneurysms through a transcondylar fossa approach.

Surgeons should practice as much as possible in cadaver dissection courses to fully understand skull base anatomy prior to attempting these approaches.

References

[1] Fukushima T, Nonaka Y. Fukushima manual of skull base dissection. 3rd ed. Raleigh: AF-Neuro Video Inc.; 2010

[2] Hatano Y, Ota N, Noda K, et al. Surgical microanatomy of the occipital artery for suboccipital muscle dissection and intracranial artery reconstruction. Surg Neurol Int. 2019; 10:127

[3] Katsuno M, Tanikawa R, Uemori G, Kawasaki K, Izumi N, Hashimoto M. Occipital artery-to-posterior inferior cerebellar artery anastomosis with multiple-layer dissection of suboccipital muscles under a reverse C-shaped skin incision. Br J Neurosurg. 2015; 29(3):401–405

[4] Matano F, Tanikawa R, Kamiyama H, et al. Surgical treatment of 127 paraclinoid aneurysms with multifarious strategy: factors related with outcome. World Neurosurg. 2016; 85:169–176

[5] Matsukawa H, Tanikawa R, Kamiyama H, et al. Risk factors for visual impairments in patients with unruptured intradural paraclinoid aneurysms treated by neck clipping without bypass surgery. World Neurosurg. 2016; 91:183–189

[6] Ota N, Tanikawa R, Miyazaki T, et al. Surgical microanatomy of the anterior clinoid process for paraclinoid aneurysm surgery and efficient modification of extradural anterior clinoidectomy.World Neurosurg. 2015; 83(4):635–643

[7] Ota N, Tanikawa R, Yoshikane T, et al. Surgical microanatomy of the posterior condylar emissary vein and its anatomical variations for the transcondylar fossa approach. Oper Neurosurg (Hagerstown). 2017; 13(3):382–391

[8] Ota N, Tanikawa R, Eda H, et al. Radical treatment for bilateral vertebral artery dissecting aneurysms by reconstruction of the vertebral artery. J Neurosurg. 2016; 125(4):953–963

[9] Tanikawa R, Sugimura T, Seki T, et al. Basic surgical techniques and pitfalls in vascular reconstruction in the posterior fossa: surgical anatomy for OA-PICA anastomosis (Japanese). Jpn J Neurosurg. 2008; 17:587–595

8 Endoscopic Endonasal Aneurysm Treatment

Aneek Patel, Hussam Abou-Al-Shaar, Michael M. McDowell, Georgios A. Zenonos, Eric W. Wang, Carl H. Snyderman, and Paul A. Gardner

Summary

This chapter reviews the current application of endoscopic endonasal surgery for intracranial aneurysms. Although all aneurysms can be managed endovascularly or through microscopic open surgery, there is a specific subset of aneurysms for which an endonasal approach can be considered to minimize the need to work across critical neurovascular structures and to maximize exposure and vascular control. We review the optimal selection of these aneurysms and the technical nuances associated with managing these aneurysms.

Keywords: Endoscopic endonasal approach, aneurysm clipping, microneurosurgery, nasoseptal flap, cerebrovascular, learning curve, multidisciplinary approach, indocyanine green

8.1 Key Learning Points

- The utilization of the endoscopic endonasal approach for properly and comprehensively selected aneurysms can minimize the amount of manipulation of neurovascular structures, provide superior proximal vascular control and visualization, and minimize complications in comparison to traditional microscopic approaches.
- The established principles of microsurgical and microvascular techniques should be employed during endoscopic endonasal surgery.
- Complications can be avoided through interdisciplinary collaboration to overcome the steep learning curve, prepare for possible vessel injury, and provide contingency planning.
- Detailed knowledge of the anatomy and practicing endoscopic techniques can mitigate complications, along with the adjuvant utilization of intraoperative endoscopic indocyanine green (ICG) videoangiography/Doppler ultrasound/intraoperative angiography and multilayered, vascularized flap reconstruction that takes clip protrusion into account.
- There are two specific locations which have the strongest anatomic basis for endonasal aneurysm treatment: (1) medial/inferior pointing paraclinoidal aneurysms (superior hypophyseal artery/carotid cave); (2) low-lying basilar apex or basilar trunk and branches.
- The steep learning curve associated with endoscopic endonasal surgery must be considered when evaluating vascular indications. Only teams with significant experience with both simple and advanced cases should contemplate these Level 5 approaches.

8.2 Introduction

The endoscopic endonasal approach (EEA) has seen an increase in the breadth of its applications in neurosurgery in recent years. Although the EEA may reduce certain components of invasiveness, such as the area of exposed tissue and external incisions, it should not be seen merely as a minimally invasive alternative to transcranial approaches to the ventral skull base.

Rather, as part of an overarching approach selection paradigm in surgery, particularly when dealing with regions with a high density of critical structures, the EEA provides a corridor with the potential to minimize the exposure and manipulation of major vessels and neural elements. By providing direct access to lesions which are midline or medial to key structures (e.g., optic nerve), these corridors can reduce the likelihood and severity of complications.

Favorable aneurysms may be selected generally based on (1) the location and (2) the projection of the aneurysm relative to the parent vessel and neighboring nerves. This is a small proportion of aneurysms generally near the central skull base. Additionally, this approach presents a steep surgical learning curve for a team of neurosurgeons and otolaryngologists. However, the approach mitigates a substantial number of risks and challenges in certain cases, and therefore slowly continues to enter discussions of intracranial aneurysm management. Hopefully, this framework will help determine which aneurysms may be best treated with EEA, but each aneurysm is unique and calls for a tailored and thorough consideration of endoscopic, microscopic, and endovascular modalities.

8.3 Vascular Challenge

Although endovascular intervention has revolutionized the management of intracranial aneurysms, there remains a set of aneurysms that are best addressed using clipping based on criteria including morphology, neck anatomy, location, as well as the demographic of the patient.[1] For younger patients, clipping (open or EEA) provides a strong option that avoids the long-term, dual antiplatelet therapy needed after endovascular management without requiring a craniotomy. Clipping may also be a safer option for patients with a history of bleeding complications or poor response to oral antiplatelet or anticoagulant therapy. Additionally, endovascular intervention may not be indicated for aneurysms with wide necks at major branch points, saccular aneurysms with multiple arterial outputs, multilobed aneurysms, or large aneurysms exerting mass effects on surrounding structures.[2] For some of these patients for which clipping is indicated, EEA offers a microsurgical clipping option via a potentially superior corridor compared to "open" craniotomy.

The primary argument against EEA for appropriate aneurysms is one of expertise and experience. Currently, microsurgical clipping is vastly more well-studied and has proven excellent long-term outcomes and cure rates. Beyond the literature, the approach is more comfortable and familiar to a majority of surgeons. EEAs require a steep learning curve to master the techniques. Snyderman et al developed a training program for EEA that stratifies the type of EEA surgery into levels of difficulty; use of the approach for intracranial aneurysms was placed at the highest level of difficulty.[3,4] Importantly, Lavigne et al found that certain surgical complications, including blood loss, cranial nerve injury, and cerebrospinal fluid (CSF) leaks, rose as the level of EEA difficulty escalated to that of an intracranial aneurysm. This highlights the need for substantial training in this approach by the endonasal team both inside and outside of operating room in order to minimize avoidable adverse outcomes.[4] Once sufficiently experienced, an advanced endonasal team can begin to explore aneurysm treatment safely.

Certain aneurysms present a challenge and/or drawback when managed through a traditional craniotomy. In the anterior circulation, transcranial access to inferomedial-pointing paraclinoid aneurysms arising from the internal carotid artery (ICA) provides poor visualization requiring manipulation of the optic nerve. It also poses a significant challenge for proximal ICA control, requiring at least anterior clinoidectomy (which still may be subpar even with division of the dural rings), transcavernous dissection (with cranial nerve manipulation), or cervical ICA exposure (which does not account for intervening collaterals). In addition to the optic nerve exposure and mobilization required to visualize and access the aneurysm neck, the superior hypophyseal artery is also poorly visualized. This has the potential for increased risk of visual loss and even hypopituitarism postoperatively. Similarly, aneurysms arising from the medial aspect of the ophthalmic artery also present anatomical challenges due to their intracranial depth, which may require substantial optic retraction and avoidance of critical and often anatomically variable vessels.[5,6] In the posterior circulation, the relationship of basilar trunk and distal vertebral aneurysms to cranial nerves, brainstem, and varying perforating vasculature that must be identified and dissected imposes significant challenges to transcranial approaches, which present an inherently lateral to medial corridor. This is especially true for aneurysms that arise close to the midline (for retrosigmoid or far-lateral approaches) or for low-lying basilar apex or trunk aneurysms (for orbitozygomatic or subtemporal approaches).[7]

The ventral pons and medulla and associated vasculature are not well accessed through traditional, "open" posterolateral or anterolateral approaches. Low-lying basilar, midbasilar/anterior inferior cerebellar artery (AICA), ventromedial posterior inferior cerebellar artery (PICA), and vertebrobasilar junction aneurysms all present challenges with simultaneous proximal and distal control and full visualization of aneurysm neck and associated perforators. An endonasal, transclival approach can provide direct access and visualization of all these regions.

Due to the direct view of the endoscope and somewhat narrow corridor relative to the parasellar contents, utilization of endoscopy-specific tools for aneurysm clipping is necessary in order to prevent obscuration of the target during clipping. An elongated, single-shaft applier, potentially with a malleable portion system, maximizes the ability to maintain *en face* visibility while placing aneurysm clips. In addition, some clip constructs require more creativity and clip variability given the lack of wide angles for application. Curved or angled clips may provide better visibility than straight clips depending on the location. These technical limitations can often be mitigated and accounted for in ways that will be discussed in the following sections, but they must always be considered when discussing microscopic versus endoscopic aneurysm surgery.

8.4 Injury Avoidance

The basic principle in complication avoidance is a robust understanding of anatomic landmarks from an endonasal perspective (▶ Fig. 8.1). Two-surgeon teams provide numerous advantages

including consensus verification of critical neurovascular structures. A more subtle benefit of having a second surgeon driving the endoscope versus an endoscope holder is that dynamic endoscopy helps to provide the ideal view constantly as well as some degree of depth perception despite the two-dimensional video screen.[7] Lastly, in the case of a vascular injury or aneurysm rupture, having a mobile endoscope ensures being able to clear the view from torrential bleeding so that the site of injury can be addressed expediently. Frequent repositioning of the endoscope on either side of instruments or even between instruments is necessary in order to continue to maintain a clear view of vessels and the aneurysm during the clipping process. A well-coordinated team learns to move together to ensure this can be performed quickly. This is one of the key reasons that these cases are considered Level 5 for any team to even consider.[5,6] The surgical team must be very far into their combined learning curve to attempt endonasal clipping.[3,4]

The most important way to avoid severe complications with endoscopic endonasal surgery is to be lucid about its indications and limitations. This includes strict selection criteria for aneurysms that are optimal for an endoscopic approach, interdisciplinary collaboration between neurosurgeons and otolaryngologists in planning and operation, optimization of distal and proximal control, and contingency planning.

Just as in open approaches, ICG angiography can improve the safety and efficacy of endoscopic endonasal aneurysm surgery. Endoscopic ICG angiography ensures lack of aneurysm filling without jeopardizing the parent artery or perforators (often angiographically occult) and allows for immediate intraoperative assessment of clip placement and adjustment, if needed. Likewise, utilization of intraoperative Doppler can be useful to ensure adequate flow within larger arteries after clipping as well as the absence of pulsations within the aneurysm dome. Finally, the use of intraoperative digital subtraction angiogram can be easily done utilizing the EEAs. With the patient being supine, access to the femoral or radial artery is easily established to assess complete aneurysm obliteration and patency of surrounding vessels.

Due to the EEA's ability to access the full ventral skull base, there is an inherent risk of injury to neurovascular structures and cranial nerves (CNs) III to XII. To proactively foresee and reduce the likelihood of postoperative neurological deficits, intraoperative neurophysiologic monitoring is commonly used in endoscopic endonasal surgery.[8] Somatosensory evoked potentials (SSEPs) allow for intraoperative detection of perfusion changes to the spinal dorsal columns, medial lemniscal pathways, and thalamic projections to the primary sensory cortex. Brainstem auditory evoked potentials (BAEPs) allow for active monitoring of hearing function. The multimodal use of SSEPs and BAEPs intraoperatively allows for real-time injury detection and active intervention that has been shown to provide value in endoscopic endonasal surgery by preventing potentially permanent and disabling neurological defecits.[9]

8.4.1 Case Selection

The location and direction of projection of an aneurysm are critical when determining the value and utility of an endoscopic approach. A particularly effective application of the EEA is for paraclinoid aneurysms that project toward the midline into the

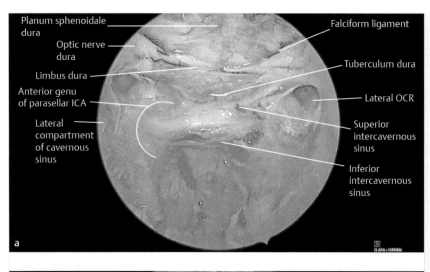

Planum sphenoidale dura
Optic nerve dura
Limbus dura
Anterior genu of parasellar ICA
Lateral compartment of cavernous sinus
Falciform ligament
Tuberculum dura
Lateral OCR
Superior intercavernous sinus
Inferior intercavernous sinus

a

Limbus
Medial OCR
Dehiscent anterior genu of ICA
Tuberculum sellae
Sellar floor
Clival recess
Planum sphenoidale
Optic canal
Lateral OCR
Middle clinoid
Drilled down septation
Dehiscent vertical segment/paraclival ICA

b

Fig. 8.1 (a,b) Anatomic landmarks for endoscopic endonasal surgery. ICA, internal carotid artery; OCR, opticocarotid recess.

suprasellar space. Current risks of microscopic clipping for paraclinoid aneurysms include optic nerve manipulation and the need to unroof the cavernous sinus, with or without division of the dural rings for subpar proximal vascular control.[10] For these reasons, management of paraclinoid aneurysms has largely shifted to endovascular coiling and/or flow diversion. However, endovascular options are particularly contraindicated in wide-necked aneurysms at major branch points, saccular aneurysms with multiple arterial outputs, certain multilobed aneurysms, and aneurysms exerting mass effect, such as compression of the optic nerve.[2] Additionally, consistent dual antiplatelet therapy is mandatory and flow diversion is a relatively novel technology that requires further study to understand long-term outcomes as well as the mechanisms that lead to its rare risk of subsequent intraparenchymal hemorrhage.[11] In such cases in which clipping is indicated, the endoscopic approach affords minimal manipulation of surrounding structures with good proximal and distal control. The trajectory of the endonasal corridor here provides an excellent view of the vasculature without the need for anterior clinoidectomy or manipulation of the optic nerve.[12] Additionally, direct proximal control can be established through the medial compartment of the cavernous sinus, which is associated with low rates of postoperative complications when compared to opening the roof of the cavernous sinus.[13] The medial cavernous sinus can be opened sharply medial to the carotid

and a hemostatic agent gently injected to obtain hemostasis. An upgoing knife such as a feather blade (Mizuho) can then be used to incise the dura laterally over the carotid genu.

The EEA is also used for select anterior communicating artery (AComm) aneurysms, largely depending on the angle of projection. In the case of a medial inferior projection that allows for aneurysm neck exposure from the endoscopic corridor, for instance, an endoscopic approach can be considered.[14] However, the endoscopic approach is often not favorable for AComm aneurysms because it frequently involves manipulation above the optic chiasm. For AComm aneurysms in which a midline corridor is indicated, for instance, an interhemispheric approach can provide similar exposure while avoiding the optic chiasm. Additionally, only select AComm aneurysms allow for sufficient proximal control to be established. Aneurysms in which the optic chiasm is post-fixed (overlying the dorsum sellae) and/or in which the AComm is more anterior relative to the chiasm allow for better proximal control; in most other cases, obtaining adequate proximal control in the event of an intraoperative rupture proves challenging. Although EEA is possible for many AComm aneurysms and has some cosmetic advantage, it is not an ideal choice unless the projection of that specific aneurysm, spatial relation to the optic chiasm, and plan for vascular control have been carefully considered (▶ Fig. 8.2).

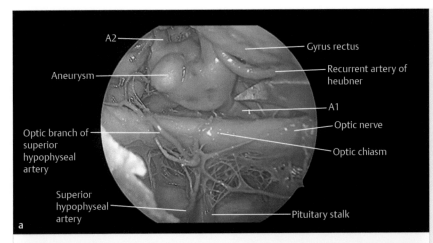

A2

Aneurysm

Gyrus rectus

Recurrent artery of heubner

A1

Optic nerve

Optic chiasm

Optic branch of superior hypophyseal artery

Superior hypophyseal artery

Pituitary stalk

a

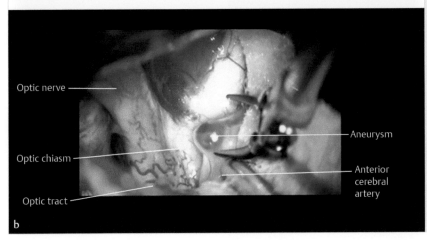

Optic nerve

Aneurysm

Optic chiasm

Anterior cerebral artery

Optic tract

b

Fig. 8.2 **(a)** Endoscopic endonasal view of an anterior communicating artery (AComm) aneurysm discovered during cadaver dissection. The neck is accessible with an angled clip, but the dome is facing the operator and proximal control (A1) requires passing the aneurysm dome and manipulation of the optic nerve/chiasm. **(b)** Similar, small aneurysm clipped via an eyebrow/supra-orbital craniotomy which allows more direct access to the aneurysm neck without passing the dome or optic nerve and early ipsilateral/dominant A1 (anterior cerebral artery) control.

As mentioned, EEA may also be indicated for low-riding basilar apex or basilar trunk aneurysms, along with superior cerebellar artery (SCA) and AICA aneurysms, which require complication-prone posterior clinoidectomy with or without a transcavernous corridor when approached microsurgically, while the subtemporal approach provides poor visibility and vascular control of the contralateral vessels.[13] The anterior trajectory of the endoscope provides excellent visualization of the basilar trunk, perforators, and distal arteries in many cases, particularly if the basilar apex arises low in the prepontine cistern. Nonetheless, in large superiorly pointing low-lying basilar tip aneurysms, especially those that are retroflexed, the limitations in visualization of the basilar perforators remain, as these vessels are draped on the back of the aneurysm, and a purely ventral approach may not be ideal. Unlike paraclinoid aneurysms, clipping trajectory is less predictable and may require more creativity; it is most feasible if the basilar aneurysms projects laterally.[7]

A general rule of thumb for posterior circulation aneurysms is that this approach provides good access to lesions that are ventral to the brainstem and at or below the sella (see Case II below), in which the approach offers more adequate proximal control and visualization when compared to transcranial approaches.[15]

8.4.2 Proximal and Distal Control

Preoperative planning should consider the level of vascular control that can be achieved endonasally. For larger paraclinoid aneurysms which block access to the supraclinoidal ICA distal to the aneurysm neck, this may indicate the addition of a transsylvian microsurgical approach for more adequate distal vascular control.[5] In fact, some surgeons may prefer preparing for a pterional craniotomy before the endonasal approach is undertaken for additional control in the event of a rupture.[16]

Both proximal and distal control should always be preplanned before the surgery. Gaining quick control is more critical in the case of an intraoperative rupture. Depending on the location of the aneurysm, a proximal region along the parasellar or paraclival ICA that can be quickly clipped should be identified and adequately exposed prior to aneurysm exposure. These considerations are particularly important in endoscopic surgery, where limited maneuverability within the endoscopic corridor should be accounted for when exposing a site of proximal control. Proximal control for basilar trunk or apex aneurysms is also often superior via an endonasal approach, given the ability for wide access from the vertebrobasilar junction to the basilar apex afforded by a wide clival resection ("far medial approach") or by pituitary transposition.[17,18,19]

Preoperative planning of distal control is equally important for aneurysms arising from large vessels, which can have significant retrograde bleeding from collateral circulation. After a proximal control point is identified and exposed, a region of the artery "downstream" from the aneurysm should also be adequately visualized and exposed, with equal consideration to clipping angle through the endoscopic corridor.[20] As referenced

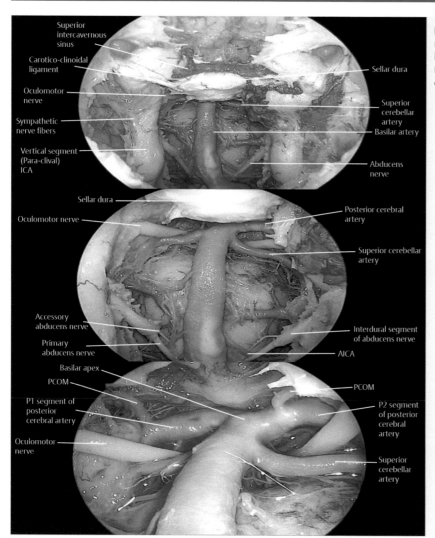

Fig. 8.3 Relationship between the sella, endonasal transclival approach, and posterior circulation. AICA, anterior inferior cerebellar artery; ICA, internal carotid artery; PCOM, posterior communicating artery.

above, distal control for some paraclinoidal aneurysms may be compromised endonasally. In these situations, a craniotomy or distal endovascular balloon should be considered to ensure distal control. Distal control of the basilar artery is relatively straightforward unless the artery is high riding. Understanding its relationship to the sella is critical in addition to understanding the collateral circulation provided by the posterior communicating arteries (▶ Fig. 8.3).

8.4.3 Contingency Planning

Due to all of the limitations of EEA discussed, particularly those of limited expertise, need for team surgery, a field of view that can be easily obscured in the event of bleeding, and the narrow access corridor, the level of contingency planning for aneurysms approached endonasally should extend beyond identification and exposure of proximal and distal control points. A microscope should always be immediately available in the operating room as well as a sheath in place for angiographic control in the event of complications that cannot be adequately managed endoscopically.[20] Endovascular access can be particularly useful in the surgical setting for gaining both proximal and distal control of the aneurysm through

balloon occlusion if control sites cannot be clearly visualized and/or accessed surgically. This has been well described for craniotomy to achieve proximal control, but this is relatively well-established endonasally and would be more helpful for distal control. Additionally, a balloon can be inflated across the aneurysm neck in some cases to improve control and increase clip placement accuracy.[21,22, 23]

8.4.4 Reconstruction

Endoscopic skull base surgery has a steep learning curve and requires extensive collaboration between neurosurgery and otolaryngology before, during, and after the surgery.[3] The position and angle of the clip have a significant potential impact on the subsequent reconstruction. If improperly angled, a protruding clip can tent the nasoseptal flap and prevent it from adhering directly to the defect, resulting in a higher likelihood of a CSF leak. In addition, aneurysm clips pulsing in direct contact with the flap can erode through the flap over time (▶ Fig. 8.4). CSF leak rates are high following these surgeries and the team must be prepared for a robust, multilayer reconstruction.[5] Although vascularized nasoseptal flaps have significantly decreased rates of CSF leaks in EEA surgeries, protrusion of the clip into the

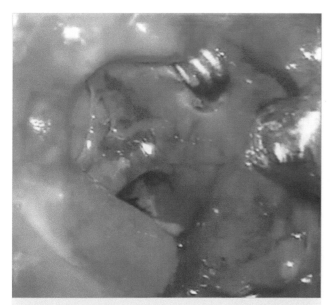

Fig. 8.4 Intraoperative endoscopic view demonstrating erosion of the proximal aneurysm clip through the necrotic vascularized nasoseptal flap.

sphenoid sinus requires greater coverage, and we prefer to place an inlay collagen graft around the clip, followed by fascia and/or fat with a nasoseptal flap covering the entire reconstruction. As a result, a full size or even extended flap is recommended even if the primary dural opening is small.

8.5 Related Pathologies

A number of other vascular pathologies can also be effectively approached endonasally. Several reports describe perichiasmatic and brainstem cavernomas that have been successfully removed with an endoscopic endonasal approach.[24] The approach allows for direct visualization of the inferior chiasm, infrachiasmatic space, and anterior circulation while minimizing dissection and manipulation of the neighboring neurovasculature.[25,26] EEA has also been utilized for arteriovenous malformations (AVMs) along the ventral skull base, as described by Kassam et al in 2007.[27] Interesting cases of its utilization in select cases of anterior dural arteriovenous fistulas supplied from ophthalmic artery branches have also been reported.[28] Although the approach should still be considered novel for these applications and should not be considered as a first-line approach for any cerebrovascular pathology, it demonstrates a growing avenue warranting further study and offers an alternative approach for lesions that are otherwise difficult to access using traditional open approaches.

8.6 Case Examples

8.6.1 Case 1

A 55-year-old female with history of hypertension and smoking and a positive family history of ruptured intracranial aneurysms was found to have a large left paraclinoidal aneurysm during the workup of longstanding headaches (▶ Fig. 8.5). The aneurysm neck was likely subarachnoid by crossing the diaphragma/distal

dural ring and was wide and deemed not ideal for endovascular intervention (prior to flow diversion era). The patient strongly wished to have the aneurysm treated and elected for clipping. Given the aneurysm's projection into the sellar compartment, endoscopic endonasal approach was chosen.

The patient was placed supine on the operating table in three-pin radiolucent head fixation. The vascularized nasoseptal flap was harvested and a wide sphenoidotomy and partial posterior ethmoidectomy was performed. A high-speed drill was used to reduce the sphenoid rostrum down to the clival recess and the sphenoid septations. The paraclival carotid artery was exposed for proximal control. The dural face of the sella was completely exposed followed by the planum sphenoidale, the parasellar carotid artery, and the left medial optic canal. A retractable blade, scissor, and hook blade were used to open the parasellar cavernous sinus and proximal dural ring, followed by the tuberculum and prechiasmatic dura extending to the proximal left optic canal. While opening the distal dural ring/diaphragma with a scissor at the distal aneurysm neck where it extended into the subarachnoid space, the aneurysm ruptured. Large bore suctions were utilized to control bleeding and maintain visualization and an attempt to coagulate the bleeding source was unsuccessful. A cottonoid patty was used to tamponade and localize the bleeding site and permanent clips were applied in successive manner to control bleeding. Once controlled, a proximal clip was placed, and the clips repositioned for final control using the "cotton clipping" technique.[29]

An intraoperative angiogram showed complete obliteration of the aneurysm and no stenosis of the parent vessel (▶ Fig. 8.6). Hemostasis and inspection of the surgical cavity were performed. Intraoperative Doppler was utilized to ensure patency of the ICA with absence of flow within the dome of the aneurysm. A piece of Duragen was placed as an inlay graft. Fat graft was placed around the clips and folded around to cover the entire field. The nasoseptal flap was then used to cover the entire fat graft as well as come up through the floor of the sphenoid and be in contact with the lateral recess of sphenoid as well as the planum. This was covered with Surgicel, DuraSeal, and gentle Merocel packing. Finally, the patient was taken out of three-pin Mayfield head fixation and a lumbar drain was subsequently placed. The patient tolerated the procedure well with no complications. She was monitored in the intensive care unit. Postoperative computed tomography (CT) angiogram showed complete obliteration of the aneurysm (▶ Fig. 8.6). The lumbar drain was removed on postoperative day 4 and she was discharged home on postoperative day 10.

8.6.2 Case 2

A 67-year-old man with history of diabetes and hyperlipidemia presented to our service with 3 months of progressive frontal headaches and double vision. On examination, he had a partial oculomotor nerve palsy. CT angiogram depicted a giant left-sided posterior cerebral artery aneurysm (▶ Fig. 8.7). Endovascular intervention was not feasible. Therefore, we recommended clipping through the EEA.

The patient was placed supine on the operating table and in three-pin Mayfield head fixation. The vascularized nasoseptal flap was harvested. After a wide sphenoidotomy was performed, the upper and midclivus were drilled and the dura

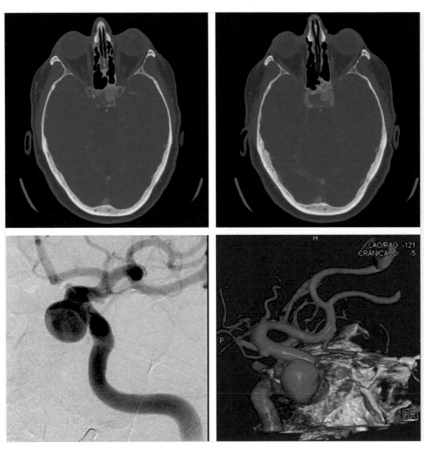

Fig. 8.5 Computed tomography (CT) angiography and digital subtraction angiogram showing a large left-sided paraclinoid aneurysm.

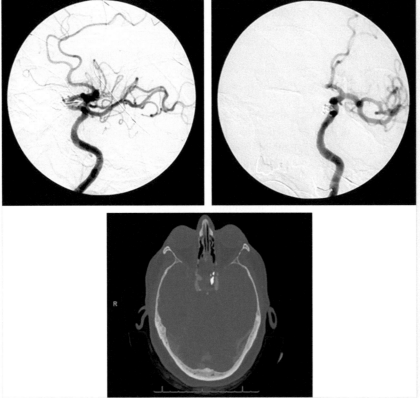

Fig. 8.6 Intraoperative angiogram and computed tomography (CT) angiogram demonstrating complete abolishment of the aneurysm and patency of the parent vessel.

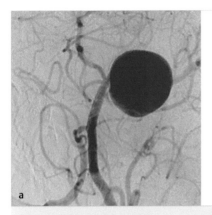
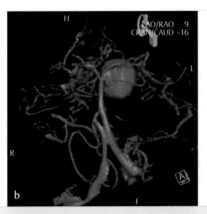
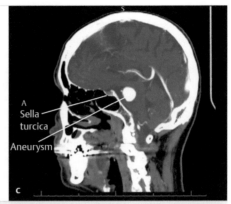

Fig. 8.7 **(a)** Anteroposterior (AP) view and **(b)** three-dimensional reconstruction of a digital subtraction angiogram depicting a giant left-sided posterior cerebral artery aneurysm. **(c)** Sagittal view of CT angiogram showing the relationship of this low-lying basilar apex and PCA aneurysm (at or below the sella) which allowed for endonasal clipping. PCA, posterior cerebral artery.

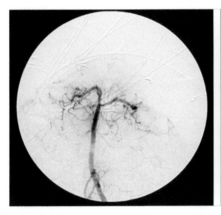
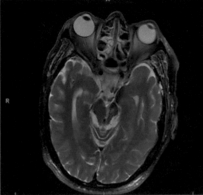

Fig. 8.8 Intraoperative angiogram showing complete abolishment of the aneurysm and patency of the parent vessel. Magnetic resonance imaging (MRI) demonstrating a small infarct due to occlusion/manipulation of a small perforator.

exposed. The dura was opened eccentric to the left side with a retractable blade. The basilar artery, superior cerebellar arteries, posterior cerebral arteries, and the large aneurysm were clearly visualized.

ICG Angiography was performed to confirm the anatomy. A temporary clip was applied over the basilar trunk. The aneurysm was inspected, and perforators were peeled away from its dome. Clips were placed in tandem. Intraoperative Doppler, ICG, and angiography confirmed obliteration of the aneurysm and patency of the parent vessel (▶ Fig. 8.8).

Warm water irrigation was utilized for meticulous hemostasis. The defect was covered with intradural DuraMatrix inlay followed by fat and Surgicel, DuraSeal, and gentle Merocel packing as previously described. A lumbar drain was placed at the completion of the procedure.

The patient tolerated the procedure well. He developed a small infarct secondary to manipulation of the small perforators as depicted on his postoperative magnetic resonance imaging (▶ Fig. 8.8). The lumbar drain was removed on postoperative day 3 and he was discharged home on postoperative day 4. Upon his last follow-up appointment, he had complete recovery of his oculomotor nerve palsy and resolution of his diplopia.

8.7 Management Strategy and Potential Complications

The risk of complication can be minimized by stringent selection criteria for aneurysms that may benefit from an endonasal approach as well as comprehensive contingency planning. The most feared complications of cerebrovascular surgery—endoscopic or transcranial—are arterial injury or aneurysm rupture. Planning and experience, both to avoid these complications and manage them, are critical.

8.7.1 Management of Intraoperative Rupture

In the event of intraoperative aneurysm rupture, it is important to first control bleeding and then ensure proximal and distal control. Visualization poses the initial challenge, as active bleeding can easily obscure the field of view. When operating an endoscope in the event of a significant hemorrhage, visualization can be re-established by pulling back the endoscope slightly to avoid being within the bleed itself; at this point, the endoscope can provide equal if not potentially superior visualization for hemorrhage management when compared to a microscope. There may be a psychological component of dealing with such a complication through an endonasal corridor, but most difficult aneurysms are accessed via deep corridors. The two-surgeon, four-hand technique with an experienced endoscopist is key. Control can be reestablished by surgical packing, which is safe but temporary.[30] The first-line packing is a small cottonoid, which often can be pressed against the site of bleeding in order to suppress blood and improve visibility. Suctioning up the active bleeding as the cottonoid is being placed is key. For long-term packing or occlusion, muscle may be harvested, or cotton applied. Small tears in an artery may be amenable to closure via careful bipolar cauterization. If the rent is too large, clipping off the defect may be possible. For ruptured aneurysms, ultimately, the bleed can be immediately addressed with suction and cottonoid tamponade and then either initial clip placement across the aneurysm dome (if it is the source of bleeding) or temporary clips placed proximally and distally.[14,20,31] Once control has been established, the aneurysm can be more aggressively manipulated and neck definitively clipped (or at least the site of bleeding if temporary trapping is used, to reduce the duration of ischemia). During temporary trapping, mean arterial blood pressure should be kept moderately elevated (approximately 80–90 mm Hg) to promote collateral perfusion before the temporary proximal and distal clips are removed.[20] Transient adenosine-induced flow arrest can also be safely used for rapid clipping and can help establish control temporarily in the event that temporary trapping is not immediately feasible.[32]

8.7.2 ICA Sacrifice

Given the nasal starting point and trajectory of the endonasal approach, it follows that the majority of EEA surgeries are along the ventral skull base and in close proximity to the ICA, if not directly dealing with ICA itself. For this reason, acute management of vessel injury with vessel sacrifice must always be considered, although as a method of last resort when hemostasis cannot be otherwise achieved. For high-risk aneurysms (giant/sessile/ICA pseudoaneurysm, etc.), balloon test occlusion (BTO) of the ICA may be done preoperatively to ensure that an ICA sacrifice could be tolerated, if needed.[33] Aneurysms associated with other skull base lesions should be considered as particularly fragile and may represent a consequence of tumor invasion. Approximately 70% of patients are able to tolerate ICA sacrifice without an ischemic event, but this is heavily

dependent on both the patient's age and comorbidities, but more importantly on the individualized vascular anatomy.[34,35] For this reason, careful examination of preoperative vascular studies, and understanding the potential collaterals, may help predict to some extent whether the patient would tolerate the vascular sacrifice. Neurophysiologic monitoring, with somatosensory and motor evoked potentials, as well as continuous EEG, is extremely important and help guide management intraoperatively.

8.7.3 Minimizing Postoperative Complications

Ensuring complete clipping and optimal flap reconstruction intraoperatively are critical for minimizing the likelihood of postoperative complications, which include recurrence and/or rupture of the clipped aneurysm and postoperative CSF leakage through an incomplete flap or graft.

Complete occlusion of the aneurysm as well as adequate perfusion of neighboring vasculature can be assessed intraoperatively by near-infrared, endoscopic ICG videoangiography, microvascular Doppler sonography, and/or formal digital subtraction angiography.

Endoscopic ICG videoangiography is available (Karl Storz) and can confirm aneurysm occlusion, assess the aneurysm neck post-clipping, and can ensure flow in the parent vessels (▶ Fig. 8.9).[36] Ensuring that these core metrics of clipping success have been achieved intraoperatively can reduce the rate of aneurysm recurrence and the need to reoperate at that site. A study of 232 patients found a 13.5% incidence of ICG videoangiography findings that indicated either clip replacement or additional clipping, preventing aneurysm recurrence and/or follow-up surgery in approximately one-sixth of patients.[37]

As with other EEA surgeries, CSF fistula can also occur following aneurysm surgery due to inadequate coverage of a protuberant clip, leading to incomplete dural and skull base reconstruction,[5] or posthemorrhagic hydrocephalus. The potential clip construct should always be considered in preoperative reconstructive planning. The use of pedicled vascularized nasoseptal flaps has been shown to significantly decrease CSF leak rates following EEA.[38,39] Additionally, optimal coverage or fat packing around the clip prior to laying the flap on top of it is of paramount importance in order to decrease direct pressure from the clip on the flap and lower the likelihood of subsequent flap necrosis or erosion of a pulsatile clip.

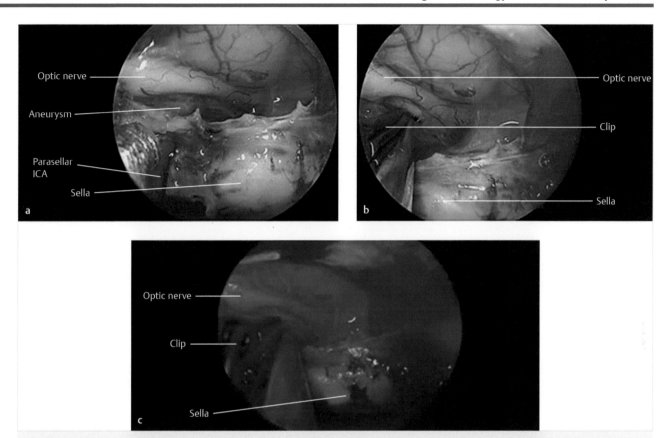

Fig. 8.9 Intraoperative endoscopic (**a, b**) and indocyanine green videoangiography (**c**) demonstrating aneurysm occlusion and patency of parent vessels following ophthalmic artery aneurysm clipping. ICA, internal carotid artery.

Poor Case Selection	EEA for aneurysm surgery is still a relatively novel approach and is only indicated for a specific subset of aneurysms. Selection of aneurysms that may benefit from this approach rather than a conventional and well-studied transcranial approach and endovascular interventions should be comprehensive, conservative, and should consider the aneurysm characteristics, anatomy, the patient, and the surgical team's experience.
Inadequate Exposure	Incomplete preoperative planning can result in partial exposure of the lesion that may not allow for full visualization of the parent vessel or budding point of the neck. Additional consideration should be given to the narrow corridor that endoscopy provides, which can limit clipping angle and instrumental mobility depending on the direction of projection of the aneurysm. Inadequate exposure can lead to failure to identify and preserve critical neural and vascular structures, restriction of movement, inadequate clip constructs, a failure to achieve adequate proximal or distal control, or the need for additional exposure after dural opening or aneurysm rupture.
Variation in Anatomy	Due to the two-dimensional visual field of the endoscope and lack of depth perception along with a steep learning curve required to master endoscopic techniques for vascular pathologies, it may be difficult to appreciate variations in anatomy that can make it difficult to navigate to the lesion or preserve sensitive structures, both during the approach and during clipping. Calcification of the carotid-clinoidal ligament or dural ring may make exposure of the parent vessel and aneurysm higher risk. In addition, complete connection between the middle and anterior clinoid (carotico-clinoidal ring) poses additional challenges for exposure and, if not appropriately disconnected and removed, may result in carotid injury.[40]
Intraoperative Rupture	As with any cerebrovascular surgery, the risk of aneurysm rupture must always be considered. Preoperative contingencies and acute management planning should be done to promptly reestablish vascular control and to stabilize the patient. Standard neurovascular concepts such as avoidance of the dome and early proximal and distal control are key.
Inadequate Visualization	A lack of dynamic or experienced endoscopy may lead to an inability to maintain an adequate view. Two-surgeon, four-hand technique is critical for these surgeries. Careful examination of the entire aneurysm can help avoid inadvertent rupture (see Rupture Case above).
Inadequate Instrumentation	Key instruments for advanced endoscopic surgery include: Single shaft bipolar cautery, single shaft microscissors, and single shaft aneurysm clip appliers. Backup endoscopes and cameras as well as adjuncts such as fluorescence endoscopy can add a level of confidence.
Flap Failure and Necrosis	Failure to account for clip size and direction can lead to incomplete dural and skull flap closure that can moreover lead to CSF leak. Poor perfusion of the flap from inadequate pedicle can lead to its necrosis. Direct pressure of the clip on the flap can lead to erosion. Leak and erosion can both be prevented by using multilayer reconstruction.

8.8 Management Algorithm

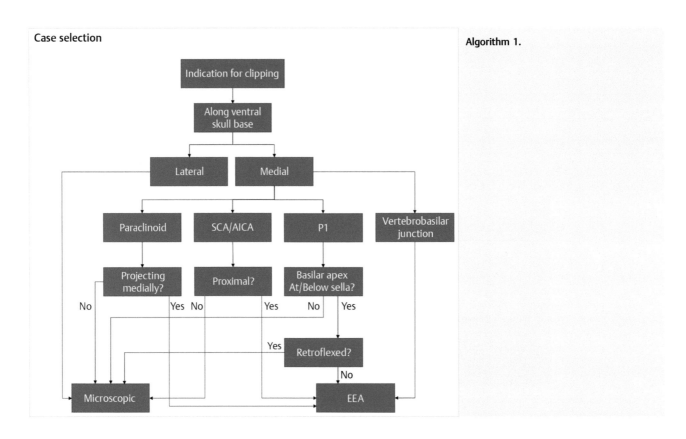

Algorithm 1.

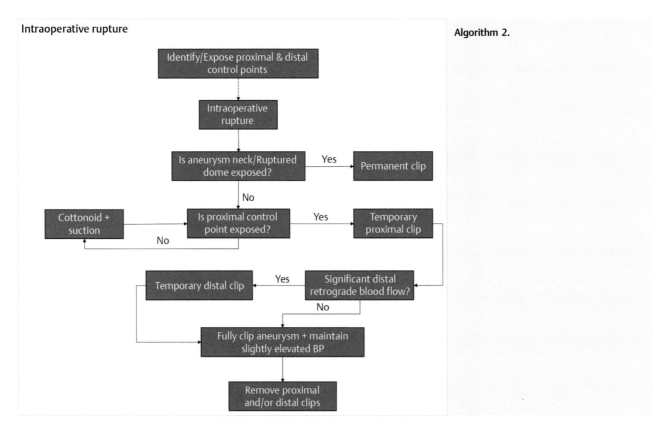

Algorithm 2.

8.9 Root Cause Analysis

Due to the technical complexity and team surgical approach in EEA for aneurysm surgery, it is important to categorize the potential causes of complications with this approach so that each cause can be systematically considered and accounted for to minimize error.

8.10 Conclusion

The EEA for aneurysm surgery remains a novel approach that has powerful applications in the management of a specific subset of intracranial aneurysms. Although promising, the approach still plays a limited role in aneurysm surgery as part of a comprehensive armamentarium for aspiring skull base and cerebrovascular neurosurgeons. A particular limitation is the steep learning curve, requiring practiced cooperation of a multidisciplinary team of a neurosurgeon and an otolaryngologist along with all other members of the surgical team. However, with careful case selection and contingency planning, EEA can be highly effective for aneurysms of certain positions and projections along the skull base. Given the novelty of this approach, large multicentric and long-term studies are warranted to determine more definitively its role and efficacy in cerebrovascular surgery.

References

[1] Raja PV, Huang J, Germanwala AV, Gailloud P, Murphy KP, Tamargo RJ. Microsurgical clipping and endovascular coiling of intracranial aneurysms: a critical review of the literature. Neurosurgery. 2008; 62(6):1187–1202, discussion 1202–1203

[2] Mazur MD, Taussky P, Park MS, Couldwell WT. Contemporary endovascular and open aneurysm treatment in the era of flow diversion. J Neurol Neurosurg Psychiatry. 2018; 89(3):277–286

[3] Snyderman C, Kassam A, Carrau R, Mintz A, Gardner P, Prevedello DM. Acquisition of surgical skills for endonasal skull base surgery: a training program. Laryngoscope. 2007; 117(4):699–705

[4] Lavigne P, Faden D, Gardner PA, Fernandez-Miranda JC, Wang EW, Snyderman CH. Validation of training levels in endoscopic endonasal surgery of the skull base. Laryngoscope. 2019; 129(10):2253–2257

[5] Gardner PA, Vaz-Guimaraes F, Jankowitz B, et al. Endoscopic endonasal clipping of intracranial aneurysms: surgical technique and results. World Neurosurg. 2015; 84(5):1380–1393

[6] Szentirmai O, Hong Y, Mascarenhas L, et al. Endoscopic endonasal clip ligation of cerebral aneurysms: an anatomical feasibility study and future directions. J Neurosurg. 2016; 124(2):463–468

[7] Montaser AS, Prevedello DM, Gomez M, et al. Extended endoscopic endonasal clipping of intracranial aneurysms: an anatomic feasibility study. World Neurosurg. 2020; 133:e356–e368

[8] Thirumala PD, Kassasm AB, Habeych M, et al. Somatosensory evoked potential monitoring during endoscopic endonasal approach to skull base surgery: analysis of observed changes. Neurosurgery. 2011; 69(1) Suppl Operative:ons64–ons76, discussion ons76

[9] Thirumala PD, Kodavatiganti HS, Habeych M, et al. Value of multimodality monitoring using brainstem auditory evoked potentials and somatosensory evoked potentials in endoscopic endonasal surgery. Neurol Res. 2013; 35(6):622–630

[10] Khan N, Yoshimura S, Roth P, et al. Conventional microsurgical treatment of paraclinoid aneurysms: state of the art with the use of the selective extradural anterior clinoidectomy SEAC. Acta Neurochir Suppl (Wien). 2005; 94:23–29

[11] Walcott BP, Stapleton CJ, Choudhri O, Patel AB. Flow diversion for the treatment of intracranial aneurysms. JAMA Neurol. 2016; 73(8):1002–1008

[12] Germanwala AV, Zanation AM. Endoscopic endonasal approach for clipping of ruptured and unruptured paraclinoid cerebral aneurysms: case report. Neurosurgery. 2011; 68(1) Suppl Operative:234–239, discussion 240

[13] Koutourousiou M, Vaz Guimaraes Filho F, Fernandez-Miranda JC, et al. Endoscopic endonasal surgery for tumors of the cavernous sinus: a series of 234 patients. World Neurosurg. 2017; 103:713–732

[14] Xiao LM, Tang B, Xie SH, et al. Endoscopic endonasal clipping of anterior circulation aneurysm: surgical techniques and results. World Neurosurg. 2018; 115:e33–e44

[15] Sanai N, Tarapore P, Lee AC, Lawton MT. The current role of microsurgery for posterior circulation aneurysms: a selective approach in the endovascular era. Neurosurgery. 2008; 62(6):1236–1249, discussion 1249–1253

[16] Kassam AB, Gardner PA, Mintz A, Snyderman CH, Carrau RL, Horowitz M. Endoscopic endonasal clipping of an unsecured superior hypophyseal artery aneurysm. Technical note. J Neurosurg. 2007; 107(5):1047–1052

[17] Morera VA, Fernandez-Miranda JC, Prevedello DM, et al. "Far-medial" expanded endonasal approach to the inferior third of the clivus: the transcondylar and transjugular tubercle approaches. Neurosurgery. 2010; 66(6) Suppl Operative:211–219, discussion 219–220

[18] Filho FVG, Wang EW, Snyderman CH, Gardner PA, Fernandez-Miranda JC. Endoscopic endonasal "far-medial" transclival approach: surgical anatomy and technique. Oper Tech Otolaryngol–Head Neck Surg. 2013; 24(4):222–228

[19] Fernandez-Miranda JC, Gardner PA, Rastelli MM, Jr, et al. Endoscopic endonasal transcavernous posterior clinoidectomy with interdural pituitary transposition. J Neurosurg. 2014; 121(1):91–99

[20] Lawton MT. Seven Aneurysms: Tenets and Techniques for Clipping. New York: Thieme; 2011

[21] Mizoi K, Yoshimoto T, Takahashi A, Ogawa A. Direct clipping of basilar trunk aneurysms using temporary balloon occlusion. J Neurosurg. 1994; 80(2):230–236

[22] Steiger HJ, Lins F, Mayer T, Schmid-Elsaesser R, Stummer W, Turowski B. Temporary aneurysm orifice balloon occlusion as an alternative to retrograde suction decompression for giant paraclinoid internal carotid artery aneurysms: technical note. Neurosurgery. 2005; 56(2) Suppl:E442–, discussion E442

[23] Thorell W, Rasmussen P, Perl J, Masaryk T, Mayberg M. Balloon-assisted microvascular clipping of paraclinoid aneurysms. Technical note. J Neurosurg. 2004; 100(4):713–716

[24] Ezequiel G, Andrew SV, Maximiliano N, Eric W, Carl S, Paul G. Endoscopic endonasal approach for brainstem cavernous malformation. Neurosurgical Focus: Video FOCVID.. 2019; 1(2):V2. https://thejns.org/video/view/journals/neurosurg-focus-video/1/2/article-pV2.xml

[25] Zoia C, Bongetta D, Dorelli G, Luzzi S, Maestro MD, Galzio RJ. Transnasal endoscopic removal of a retrochiasmatic cavernoma: a case report and review of literature. Surg Neurol Int. 2019; 10:76

[26] Meng X, Feng X, Wan J. Endoscopic endonasal transsphenoidal approach for the removal of optochiasmatic cavernoma: case report and literature review. World Neurosurg. 2017; 106:1053.e11–1053.e14

[27] Kassam AB, Thomas AJ, Zimmer LA, et al. Expanded endonasal approach: a fully endoscopic completely transnasal resection of a skull base arteriovenous malformation. Childs Nerv Syst. 2007; 23(5):491–498

[28] Jankowitz BGP, McDowell MM, Zhu X, Friedlander RM. Anterior fossa, superior sagittal sinus, and convexity dural arteriovenous malformations. In: Macdonald RL, ed. Neurosurgical Operative Atlas: Vascular Neurosurgery, 3rd ed. New York, NY: Thieme Medical Publishers; 2019

[29] Safavi-Abbasi S, Moron F, Sun H, et al. Techniques and long-term outcomes of cotton-clipping and cotton-augmentation strategies for management of cerebral aneurysms. J Neurosurg. 2016; 125(3):720–729

[30] Safaee M, Young JS, El-Sayed IH, Theodosopoulos PV. Management of noncatastrophic internal carotid artery injury in endoscopic skull base surgery. Cureus. 2019; 11(8):e5537

[31] Goldschmidt E, Lavigne P, Snyderman C, Gardner PA. Endoscopic endonasal approach for clipping of a PICA aneurysm. Neurosurgical Focus: Video FOCVID.. 2020; 2(2):V14

[32] Powers CJ, Wright DR, McDonagh DL, Borel CO, Zomorodi AR, Britz GW. Transient adenosine-induced asystole during the surgical treatment of anterior circulation cerebral aneurysms: technical note. Neurosurgery. 2010; 67(2) Suppl Operative:461–470

[33] Kikuchi K, Yoshiura T, Hiwatashi A, Togao O, Yamashita K, Honda H. Balloon test occlusion of internal carotid artery: angiographic findings predictive of results. World J Radiol. 2014; 6(8):619–624

[34] Tan TW, Garcia-Toca M, Marcaccio EJ, Jr, Carney WI, Jr, Machan JT, Slaiby JM. Predictors of shunt during carotid endarterectomy with routine electroencephalography monitoring. J Vasc Surg. 2009; 49(6):1374–1378

[35] Plestis KA, Loubser P, Mizrahi EM, Kantis G, Jiang ZD, Howell JF. Continuous electroencephalographic monitoring and selective shunting

reduces neurologic morbidity rates in carotid endarterectomy. J Vasc Surg. 1997; 25(4):620–628

[36] Fischer G, Rediker J, Oertel J. Endoscope- versus microscope-integrated near-infrared indocyanine green videoangiography in aneurysm surgery. J Neurosurg. 2018:1–10.–Online ahead of print

[37] Roessler K, Krawagna M, Dörfler A, Buchfelder M, Ganslandt O. Essentials in intraoperative indocyanine green videoangiography assessment for intracranial aneurysm surgery: conclusions from 295 consecutively clipped aneurysms and review of the literature. Neurosurg Focus. 2014; 36 (2):E7

[38] Patel MR, Stadler ME, Snyderman CH, et al. How to choose? Endoscopic skull base reconstructive options and limitations. Skull Base. 2010; 20(6): 397–404

[39] Heiferman DM, Somasundaram A, Alvarado AJ, Zanation AM, Pittman AL, Germanwala AV. The endonasal approach for treatment of cerebral aneurysms: a critical review of the literature. Clin Neurol Neurosurg. 2015; 134:91–97

[40] Fernandez-Miranda JC, Tormenti M, Latorre F, Gardner P, Snyderman C. Endoscopic endonasal middle clinoidectomy: anatomic, radiological, and technical note. Neurosurgery. 2012; 71(2) Suppl Operative:ons233–ons239, discussion ons239

9 Dealing with Major Intraoperative Vascular Injury During Endonasal Approaches to the Anterior Skull Base

Vincent Dodson, Neil Majmundar, Gurkirat Kohli, Wayne D. Hsueh, Jean Anderson Eloy, and James K. Liu

Summary

Development of advanced endoscopic endonasal approaches have equipped skull base surgeons with additional routes for treating a wide variety of pathologies at the skull base. However, the proximity of critical vascular structures to the endoscopic surgical corridors and to the pathologies being treated makes these surgical approaches particularly susceptible to potentially fatal vascular complications. This chapter reviews the relevant anatomy of endoscopic endonasal approaches to the anterior skull base, the common vascular complications encountered, and methods to minimize and deal with these complications.

Keywords: Endonasal, endoscopic, vascular complications internal carotid artery, anterior cerebral artery

9.1 Key Learning Points

- It is critical to check preoperative labs prior to any surgical procedure to assess for thrombocytopenia or any coagulopathy.
- A patient's past medical history which may include bleeding disorders or use of antiplatelet agents or anticoagulation must be considered. Patients should hold all antiplatelet medications for at least 5 to 7 days prior to the procedure, and all anticoagulation at least 3 days prior to the procedure. The indications for the patient's antiplatelet/anticoagulant use must be discussed with the patient's primary provider to limit risk of potential thromboembolic complications while the medication is held.
- Preoperative imaging should be extensively studied for any vascular involvement by the pathology being treated. Bilateral internal carotid arteries (ICAs) and all its terminal branches must be evaluated. Specifically, thorough evaluation of anterior cerebral arteries (ACAs), A1, A2, anterior communicating artery (AComA), and its branches must be evaluated for encasement.
- If the pathology involves the ICAs extensively, preoperative balloon test occlusion (BTO) is recommended to evaluate collateral flow in case the ICA is injured and needs to be sacrificed intraoperatively or postoperatively. The BTO will also guide the total extent of resection the surgeon may pursue.
- Preoperative planning of resection of tumors encasing anterior cerebral vasculature should include evaluation of a potential "cortical cuff." This layer of protective noneloquent brain matter separating tumor and vasculature is best visualized with magnetic resonance imaging (MRI), and the presence of a cortical cuff makes resection by endoscopic approach more feasible. However, the absence of a cortical cuff, as in the case of almost all tuberculum sellae meningiomas, does not eliminate the feasibility of an endoscopic endonasal approach.
- Intraoperative image guidance with merged MRI and computed tomography angiography (CTA) modalities is a useful tool during the treatment of complex skull base pathologies.
- Prior to starting the procedure, the availability of all surgical instruments and tools which may be required in case of vascular injury should be confirmed. In addition, cross matching the patient and having blood available is recommended.
- An experienced team with a two-surgeon, four-handed approach is recommended for complex pathologies in which vascular injuries may be encountered.
- We also recommend that more complex pathologies during which vascular injury may be encountered are performed at an institution where both a multidisciplinary team experienced with handling complex pathologies with neurovascular considerations as well as an endovascular team with neurointerventional capabilities are available.

9.2 Introduction

Over the past two decades, expanded endoscopic endonasal approaches (EEAs) have enabled alternate access to anterior skull base pathologies from a route through the paranasal sinuses.[1,2] The EEAs via transcribriform or transplanum/transtuberculum corridors have allowed treatment of various lesions such as meningiomas, schwannomas, craniopharyngiomas, esthesioneuroblastomas, and other sinonasal malignancies.[2] Despite offering a minimal access approach to anterior skull base pathologies, EEAs have the potential for a variety of complications including postoperative cerebrospinal fluid (CSF) leak, impaired olfaction, infection, and vascular injury. Major vascular injury to neighboring structures such as the internal carotid artery (ICA) and anterior cerebral arteries (ACAs) and their branches can result in major morbidity and even mortality. In general, tumors encasing vessels or in the absence of a protective cortical cuff may be better suited for treatment via open transcranial approach. In addition, in the event of a major vascular injury, such as an arterial vessel tear or transection, the ability to perform safe vascular control with temporary clips and direct suture repair, anastomosis, or bypass is more feasible with an open transcranial approach than it is with a narrow endonasal corridor. However, if the tumor is demonstrated on preoperative imaging to be adequately separate from crucial vasculature, the EEAs can be considered as these approaches allow for improved visualization and reduced brain retraction, and a possible lower risk of vascular injury (as opposed to tumors that have vessel encasement). Despite allowing for improved visualization and minimal retraction, whether the EEAs reduce vascular complication rates when compared to open approaches is disputed. In either approach, the occurrence of major vascular injury is rare and EEAs have been repeatedly demonstrated to achieve vascular complication rates that are comparable to those seen in open surgery.[3,4] Endonasal approaches for pituitary tumor resection have a reported incidence of ICA injury ranging from 0.5 to 1.1%, while more extended approaches have a higher incidence of 4 to 9%.[5,6,7,8,9] Injuries do occur in both types of procedures but one could argue that it is easier to deal with complications in the open case because of better visualization and a larger working corridor to quickly apply temporary clips and perform direct vessel repair with microanastomosis techniques. In this chapter, we focus on the vascular challenges encountered during EEAs to pathologies affecting the anterior skull base, techniques and strategies which can be employed to reduce vascular complications, and the management of vascular complications intra- and postoperatively.

9.3 Relevant Anatomy

Knowledge of the relevant vascular anatomy is essential to avoid major vascular complications (▶ Fig. 9.1). One of the risk factors for vascular injury is lack of familiarity of the neurovascular anatomy of the skull base and the variations which can be encountered, especially with existing pathologic conditions. The rate of injury to the ICA in transsphenoidal surgery is inversely related to the surgeon's experience.[10] This can be supplemented by careful study of the relationships between major blood vessels and surgical landmarks seen on preoperative imaging in conjunction with the use of image guidance; this is crucial due to anatomical variations. The vasculature at risk depends on the pathology and approach utilized. In particular, the vasculature at risk of injury during an EEA to the anterior fossa includes the ICAs, ACAs, and the ethmoidal arteries.

In this chapter we will refer to the Bouthillier et al classification of the segments of the ICA: C1 cervical, C2 petrous, C3

lacerum, C4 cavernous, C5 clinoid, C6 ophthalmic, and C7 communicating (▶ Fig. 9.2).[11,12] The C3, C4, and C5 segments of the ICA can be injured during a variety of EEA. The C3 segment runs from the end of the carotid canal, passes above the cartilage-filled foramen lacerum, and extends to the anterior portion of the petrolingual ligament.[11,13] The C4 segment starts from the superior margin of the petrolingual ligament and ends as it exits the cavernous sinus at the proximal dural ring. The cavernous portion of the ICA is divided into three segments—posterior ascending, horizontal, and anterior vertical segments.[11] The C5 segment, also known as the clinoid segment, starts its course at the proximal dural ring and ends at the distal dural ring where the ICA enters the subarachnoid space.[11] In 71% of patients the ICA bulges into the sphenoid sinus but is covered by bone.[14] Dehiscence of the ICA is seen when the ICA is exposed to the sphenoid sinus due to the absence of the bony wall. The incidence of this variant is not well studied, but its range is estimated from 5 to 30%.[15,16] This anatomic variant can be dangerous to encounter during EEAs as the bony layer normally serves as a useful protective barrier from injury to the ICA. Additionally, the ICAs may have a smaller inter-artery distance and compress the pituitary gland. In these cases, the vessels may be injured if the dura is opened more laterally without caution.[4] Furthermore, the anatomic protection of the cavernous portion of the ICA is limited, as the bony wall covering the ICA is variable and usually thin and insufficient for protection especially during drilling.[17]

Although it is uncommon, there is increased risk of injury to the ACA, especially the orbitofrontal and frontopolar branches due to the proximity of the frontal lobe during transcribriform approaches.[18,19,20] The orbitofrontal artery, usually the first branch of the A2 segment of the ACA, resides in the olfactory sulcus on the frontobasal surface, and it provides the vascular supply to the gyrus rectus.[21] The frontopolar artery, usually the second branch of the A2 segment of the ACA, resides superior and medial to the orbitofrontal artery, and it provides the vascular supply to the medial portions of the frontal lobe.[21] Both the A1 and A2 segments can be displaced or encased by tumors affecting the anterior skull base and suprasellar region, such as tuberculum sellae meningiomas and craniopharyngiomas. Careful review of the imaging, including MRI, CT angiogram, and sometimes cerebral angiogram, must be performed prior to attempting an EEA.

In the endonasal transcribriform approach, the anterior and posterior ethmoidal arteries, branches of the ophthalmic artery, are typically ligated and divided to devascularize cribriform tumors.[22] The anterior ethmoidal artery enters the nasal cavity and courses between the second and third lamellae. The posterior ethmoidal artery resides along the roof of the ethmoid, anterior to the sphenoid sinus, approximately 5 mm anterior to the optic canal, and it supplies the posterior ethmoid air cells and the nasal septum.[22,23] The superior portion of the lamina papyracea is removed to expose the posterior or anterior ethmoidal artery. At this point, the ethmoidal arteries may be ligated. The posterior ethmoidal artery is usually larger than the anterior ethmoidal artery and runs more closely to the skull base.[24] Identification of these ethmoidal vessels allows accurate cauterization and division to devascularize the anterior skull base tumor in preparation for

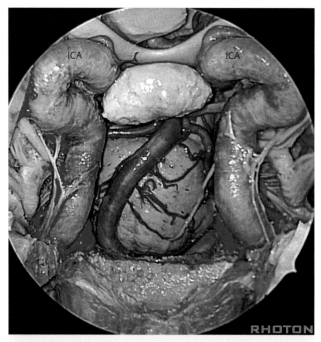

Fig. 9.1 Cadaveric dissection revealing the sphenoid sinus. The cavernous segment of the right and left internal carotid arteries (ICAs) can be seen bilaterally. (Courtesy of the Rhoton collection.)

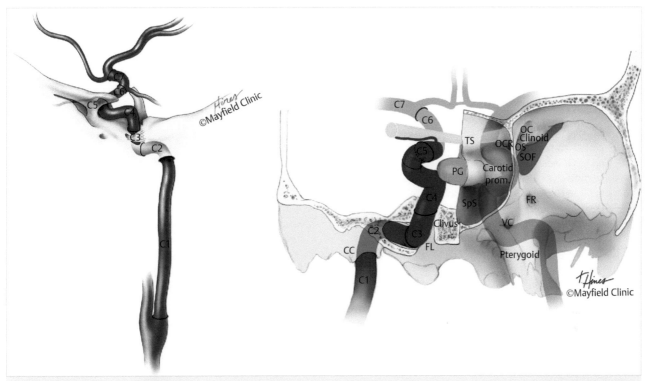

Fig. 9.2 Segments of the internal carotid artery: C1 (cervical), C2 (petrous), C3 (lacerum), C4 (cavernous), C5 (clinoid), C6 (ophthalmic), and C7 (communicating).[12]

cribriform plate resection. One must be cautious not to allow inadequate cauterization and retraction of the artery into the orbit resulting in retrobulbar hematoma, orbital compartment syndrome, and visual loss.

9.4 Vascular Challenges

One of the most significant challenges of endoscopic endonasal surgery (EES) is using instruments in narrow corridors without causing injury to nearby anatomical structures. The narrow nasal corridor and the distances at which instruments are used can present significant challenges during EES especially when vascular complications occur. This can happen at any point during the surgery: during bony exposure, resection of the lesion, and closure of the skull base defect.

The ICA is the most commonly injured vessel during EEAs. Romero et al performed a literature review of vascular injuries during endoscopic procedures that included 7,336 patients and found the arterial injury rate to be 0.34%, and of the 25 cases with an arterial injury, 19 were ICA injuries.[4] From these injuries to the ICA, four patients died and two developed neurological deficits.[4] Although the reported rates of vascular injury during endonasal endoscopic surgery may potentially be low due to the wider view offered by the endoscope and improved localization of the ICA, injury to the ICA is the most common vascular complication. These rates may increase as the procedure is more frequently used. Injuries to other arteries are less common but have been reported in various retrospective reviews.

Injury to the ACA and its branches is also possible. In a retrospective review done by Kassam et al on 800 cases of endoscopic endonasal skull base surgeries, they found only seven vascular injuries, one of which was an avulsion of the frontopolar (A2) artery which eventually resulted in permanent right hemiparesis. This patient required endovascular treatment to control the bleeding.[25] Romero et al described a case during which a perforator of A1 was torn during removal of a meningioma. The injured vessel was clipped but no new neurological deficit was identified.[4] Although injuries to these branches are relatively rare, they are possible during expanded EEAs. These branches can be injured directly or commonly avulsed during tumor removal. It is imperative to avoid removal of tumor until it has been thoroughly dissected off the surrounding tissue, especially when removing the most dorsal portions. When these small caliber arteries are injured, direct repair is nearly impossible from an EEA. Management will generally involve direct coagulation or clipping of the injured vessel. Postoperative angiogram can be performed if there is concern for a pseudoaneurysm or injury to a larger vessel.

9.5 Injury Avoidance

As with any other surgical complication, injury avoidance begins with knowledge of normal anatomy. A thorough knowledge of the sinonasal and intracranial vasculature is required prior to any surgical intervention. Furthermore, the patient's own preoperative imaging must be studied to examine any anatomical variance as well as any vascular involvement with the lesion itself.

In addition to the MRI to evaluate the lesion, a CTA should be obtained for all lesions involving the anterior skull base and parasellar regions. CTA can provide critical information regarding the location of the ICAs, the ACAs, and their branches. In addition, CTA provides the ability to view the vessels in relation to the bony anatomy of the skull base and the involved pathology. For example, in a case where a tumor is encasing the paraclival segment of the ICA seen on an MRI, it would be useful to know if the bony canal over the ICA is intact or dehiscent on a CTA. Dissecting the tumor off an intact bony carotid canal is much easier and has lower risk for ICA injury than a "naked" ICA without bony protection. We routinely use the preoperative MRI and merge it with the CTA for intraoperative image guidance. A blended hybrid view can help visualize tumor pathology in conjunction with the course of the vasculature (ICA) and the bony structures of the skull base.

If the pathology significantly involves the ICAs or any of the other major surrounding vessels or appears hypervascular with flow voids on the T2 MRI, a diagnostic cerebral angiogram may be helpful to further delineate the surrounding vasculature and blood supply to the tumor. Only a small portion of these skull base lesions will be amenable to preoperative embolization. If the arterial supply is from the ICA, the lesion is typically not amenable to embolization, as there is a considerable risk of causing a thromboembolic complication. In situations where the lesion encases the ICA or if an ICA appears to be at high risk of injury, a preoperative balloon test occlusion (BTO) with hypotensive challenge of the involved ICA can be performed to determine if there is adequate collateral circulation for carotid in the case of an intraoperative ICA injury. If the patient develops focal symptoms during the test, this is an indication that the patient may have an adverse outcome if carotid injury occurs intraoperatively. This test can guide the aggressiveness of resection or raise consideration of preparing for a bypass.[26] Nevertheless, it may be prudent to perform a more conservative resection leaving residual adherent tumor on the ICA in these cases. For more on BTO and evaluation of tumor vasculature, see Chapter 2.

Intraoperative Doppler ultrasound can also be useful to guide the bony exposure of the ICAs as well as tumor dissection off the ICAs. If visualization of the ICA protuberances and the normal bony landmarks (optical carotid recess, optic canal) is inadequate after the sphenoid sinus has been opened, the Doppler can be used in conjunction with image guidance to confirm location of the ICAs.[27] The Doppler also helps in identifying the location of the cavernous portion of the ICA before dural opening.

It is best to have a two-surgeon team with a four-handed approach during complex cases involving the anterior skull base.[28] Having two surgeons with experience in their respective fields improves decision-making and provides the ability for dynamic movement of the endoscope. Before the operation, it is important to review the angiographic imaging, determine the patient risk factors, extent of the tumor, and its relation to the nearby neurovascular structures. It is also important to be comfortable with the anatomy, specifically, the location of the arteries and their landmarks from the endoscopic viewpoint. There are well-established landmarks that can be used to determine the location of specific segments of the ICA (see Chapter 1).[29]

Intraoperatively, since the vessels can be pushed away from their normal course, the tumor should be debulked prior to performing extracapsular dissection. It is important to use sharp dissection to release adherent arachnoid that could be tethering the neighboring vessels to the tumor capsule, as in the case of some olfactory and tuberculum meningiomas. If there is tumor encasement or strict adherence, it may be safer to trim the tumor sharply to release the vessel from the tumor, leaving a small residual amount of tumor adherent to the vessel. This is a better alternative than vessel avulsion injury which can result in potential hemorrhage and ischemic stroke.[30]

The proper use of surgical equipment also can minimize the risk of arterial injury. Romero et al made some recommendations based on their experiences with arterial complications. They recommended to always keep surgical equipment in view with the endoscope and to only remove the tumor when it is adequately dissected from adjacent structures.[4] Angled endoscopes allow the surgeon greater access and generally a wider view. However, greater angulation may mean that there are additional structures which can be visualized but cannot be safely dissected or controlled. We therefore recommend the use of 30-degree angled endoscopes, and increasing angulation only as necessary, particularly in cases that involve the ACAs. In addition, avoiding the use of some equipment in certain locations can help to minimize risk of arterial injury. Romero et al demonstrated one case in which the use of an ultrasonic aspirator during the resection of a pituitary macroadenoma resulted in brisk arterial bleeding which needed to be controlled quickly. Based on their experience, they recommend avoiding the use of ultrasonic aspirators near the cavernous sinus.[4] In the event that there is tumor adherence to the ACAs, we recommend that it is better to leave a small remnant attached to the vessels than to risk avulsion or tear to the ACAs.

In the case of the ACAs (A1, A2, and anterior communicating artery) and their branches, tumors of the skull base can adhere to or encase these arteries rendering endoscopic approaches difficult to perform. In these cases, open transcranial approaches may be preferable as these approaches would allow for better control of vascular complications such as hemorrhage. Open approaches would allow the surgeon to repair any arterial injury via direct suture repair or bypass under temporary occlusion. Preoperative imaging with MRI with and without gadolinium and CTA is crucial for determining the extent of vascular involvement of the tumor. However, these studies are limited in their ability to differentiate between visualizing vessels encased by a tumor and a highly vascular tumor.

Also, in the context of ACA injury, the presence of a "cortical cuff" makes an endoscopic approach more favorable. A "cortical cuff" is defined as a protective layer of noneloquent brain tissue that provides a natural plane of separation between tumor and the anterior cerebral vessels. Koutourousiou et al demonstrated that the absence of a cortical cuff between the tumor and anterior cerebral vasculature limited the extent of resection performed endoscopically.[31] Therefore, open approaches should be considered when preoperative MRI demonstrates vascular encasement and a gross total resection is indicated.

9.6 Related Pathologies

The risk of vascular injury may be dependent on the characteristics of the pathology being operated. The size, location, and extension into the surrounding neurovasculature are all dependent

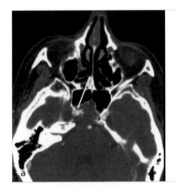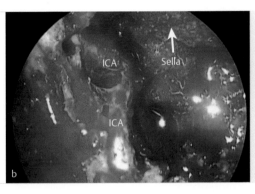

Fig. 9.3 **(a)** Computed tomography (CT) angiogram reveals dehiscence of the right paraclival carotid artery canal (*yellow arrow*). **(b)** Intraoperative image demonstrates dehiscence of the internal carotid artery (ICA) secondary to erosive skull base chondrosarcoma.

on the aggressiveness of the lesion. Prior to the operation, it is important to know how the pathology of the patient might alter the surrounding anatomy and change the course of the vasculature. Tumor consistency also plays an important role on how readily dissection away from vascular structures can be performed. Softer tumors (most adenomas and chordomas) can be aspirated with suctions away from vascular structures, whereas firm tumors require more microdissection. Tumors with a firmer, more fibrous consistency present a challenge for endoscopic endonasal removal. Not only do these tumors require more microdissection, but because of their firmer consistency, they may not descend into the sella as easily and may require additional bony removal of the planum sphenoidale.[32,33]

For suprasellar tumors, such as tuberculum sellae meningiomas and craniopharyngiomas, the ICAs and posterior communicating arteries laterally, the anterior communicating artery and ACAs superiorly, the basilar apex and P1 vessels posteriorly, are at risk. Tuberculum sellae meningiomas tend to occur inferiorly and anteriorly at the anterior wall of the sella turcica. As a result, they are more likely to involve the ACAs.[34] Although craniopharyngiomas can also extend anteriorly, according to the Kassam classification of craniopharyngiomas, types II and III can extend posteriorly, potentially involving the posterior communicating artery and posterior cerebral artery.[28] Again, these tumors should be debulked prior to performing extracapsular dissection to ensure safe vascular dissection. Internal debulking makes it easier to collapse the tumor capsule away from the neurovascular structures. It is important to keep the plane of dissection between the tumor capsule and the tumor arachnoid so that the arachnoid is mobilized toward the side of the vessel which offers a subtle extra barrier of protection. Sometimes the arachnoid needs to be incised sharply to free the adjacent vessel away from the tumor capsule. For both craniopharyngiomas and meningiomas, it is paramount to identify and preserve the superior hypophyseal vessel and perforators that supply the optic apparatus since inadvertent injury to this vessel could lead to postoperative visual loss. For tuberculum sellae meningiomas that invade the optic canal, it is important to identify and protect the ophthalmic artery coursing inferomedial in the optic canal when opening the optic dural sheath.

Chondroid tumors of the clivus are associated with a greater risk of injury compared to pituitary adenomas due to greater involvement of one or both paraclival ICAs (▶ Fig. 9.3 and ▶ Fig. 9.4). ▶ Fig. 9.3 and ▶ Fig. 9.4 demonstrate an illustrative case in which a skull base chondrosarcoma erodes the bony wall around the right paraclival ICA. When there is tumor adjacent or encasing vascular structures without intervening bony

protection, such as in the case of a clival chordoma or invasive pituitary adenoma eroding the paraclival carotid canals, a two-suction technique with strong 12 to 14 French Frazier suctions to initially aspirate the tumor followed by smaller size, controlled suctions is recommended. Ultrasonic and side-cutting aspirators should not be used next to the ICA. In addition, sharp ringed curettes should be avoided as these can cut the vessel wall. Blunt ringed/looped curettes can be used judiciously with extreme caution but has less of a vascular risk than sharp (Hardy) curettes. In pathologies that have eroded bone, such as chondrosarcomas, it is important to outfracture and mobilize the fragmented bone away from the ICA vessel wall in order to avoid the sharp edges from encroaching the artery (▶ Fig. 9.3 and ▶ Fig. 9.4).

Functional macroadenomas can also increase the risk of vascular injury as their respective hormonal changes can affect tissues and introduce unique difficulties during surgery. High levels of cortisol results in hypertension and connective tissue changes, which can lead to friable changes of the ICA, increasing risk of injury.[4,35] Growth hormone-secreting adenomas resulting in acromegaly cause anatomic changes such that intranasal anatomy is altered due to bony overgrowth and soft tissue hypertrophy, as well as arterial ectasia, potentially decreasing the intercarotid distance. Both of these anatomical alterations need to be considered and evaluated for with neuroimaging.[36]

Furthermore, pathologies including olfactory groove and tuberculum sellae meningiomas may be susceptible to bilateral ACA injury upon their resection. It is therefore important to assess for vascular encasement and for the presence of a cortical cuff between the tumor and arteries on preoperative MRI (T1 + gadolinium and T2 sequences). In olfactory groove meningiomas, the presence of a cortical cuff provides a protective layer of noneloquent brain tissue for the ACAs. This lessens the risk of a vascular injury and impacts the extent of resection.[31] However, in tuberculum sellae meningiomas, there is almost always no cortical cuff present because the superior portion of these tumors abut directly against the A1 or AComA (anterior communicating artery) vessels in the suprasellar cistern. Extension of this relationship can lead to encasement and it is important to assess for any tumor encasement of the ACAs and its branches.

9.7 Case Example

An endoscopic endonasal transplanum transtuberculum approach was used to remove a large tuberculum sellae meningioma in a 58-year-old female (▶ Fig. 9.5). During the tumor

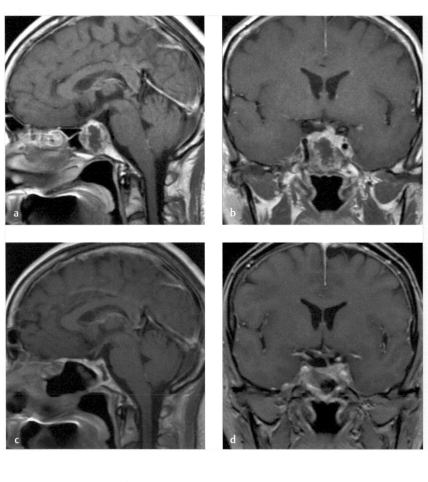

Fig. 9.4 Preoperative T1-weighted post-gadolinium magnetic resonance (MR) of the brain in (a) sagittal and (b) coronal images demonstrating chondrosarcoma of the skull base. (c) Sagittal and (d) coronal images of postoperative MR demonstrating resection of the chondrosarcoma.

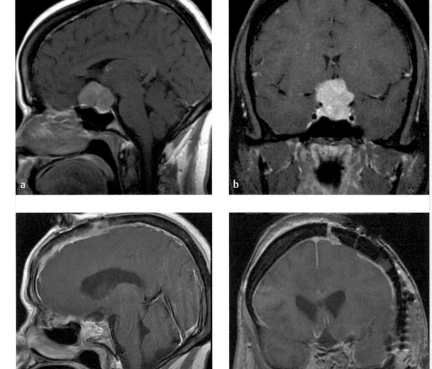

Fig. 9.5 Preoperative T1-weighted post-gadolinium magnetic resonance (MR) of the brain in (a) sagittal and (b) coronal planes demonstrating a tuberculum sellae meningioma. Postoperative T1-weighted post-gadolinium MR of the brain in (c) sagittal and (d) coronal planes demonstrating successful resection of the tumor. This postoperative MRI was taken after craniotomy for aneurysm clipping.

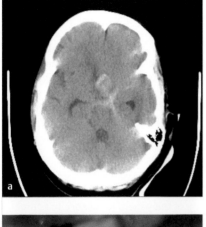
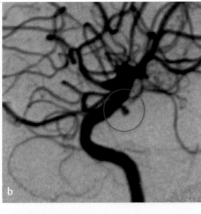
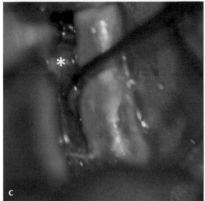
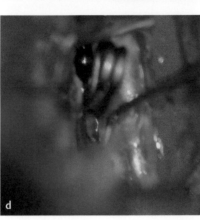

Fig. 9.6 Postoperative computed tomography (CT) demonstrated subarachnoid hemorrhage on postoperative day 10 after endoscopic endonasal resection of the meningioma (**a**). Digital subtraction angiography (**b**) of the internal carotid artery demonstrates a posterior communicating artery aneurysm (*red circle*). It was unclear whether this was a true aneurysm versus a traumatic pseudoaneurysm. Intraoperative images confirmed a true aneurysm with the neck arising from the posterior communicating artery (**c**) (*asterisk*) which was successfully clipped (**d**).

removal, a jet of bright arterial blood was encountered. The area of arterial bleeding was packed off with cottonoids. Once the bleeding was stabilized, the remainder of the tumor was removed. The cottonoids were then removed and there was no active bleeding and no obvious pseudoaneurysm. Postoperatively, the patient was neurologically intact. Immediate postoperative imaging which included a CTA was unremarkable. However, on postoperative day 10, the patient suffered a subarachnoid hemorrhage (▶ Fig. 9.6). A diagnostic cerebral angiogram demonstrated an aneurysm in the supraclinoid ICA region. The endovascular team did not believe they could treat this lesion through endovascular means; therefore, the aneurysm was clipped surgically. If there is a concern for cerebrovascular injury, it is imperative to obtain diagnostic cerebral angiography immediately, especially to identify potential sites of vascular injury (e.g., dissection, early pseudoaneurysm formation). Delayed cerebral diagnostic angiography (5–10 days) can demonstrate formation of a pseudoaneurysm as well as vasospasm.

Romero et al performed a retrospective review of 800 endoscopic endonasal skull base surgeries and found only four cases of arterial injuries.[4] Similar to the above, in one of their cases, a 67-year-old female with a diaphragma sella meningioma with bitemporal hemianopsia was removed via an EEA. While the tuberculum sella was being removed, high pressure bright red blood started to pool in the sphenoid sinus. To control the bleeding, the sella was packed off and a Foley balloon was deployed within the nasopharynx. An angiogram showed active bleeding from the cavernous segment of the right ICA. The patient demonstrated good collateral circulation,

so the right ICA was occluded with coils. The patient was discharged 6 days later and eventually had the tumor resected by craniotomy.

9.8 Management Strategy

9.8.1 Initial Steps

During any intraoperative vascular injury, prompt identification of the site of injury and obtaining hemostasis are the primary goals. One of the major challenges in endoscopic surgery is that the relatively small visual field will become quickly obscured by any brisk bleeding. The first step is adequate visualization of the injury. A two-surgeon, four-handed technique is best for management as one surgeon can drive the endoscope with one hand free to clear the view while the other uses a bimanual technique to attend to the vascular injury.

9.8.2 ICA Injury

Valentine et al demonstrated in a sheep model the high-flow nature of ICA injury. They demonstrated that the stream of blood from the injury generally flows into one nasal cavity; therefore, the endoscope can be placed in the nasal cavity shielded by the posterior septal edge from the blood stream.[37] In addition, a foot-controlled lens cleaning system is valuable for continuous visualization, as the endoscope does not have to be removed from the field.[37] At least two large suctions, 12 French or greater, should be placed in the nostril contralateral to the endoscope.[37]

After hemostasis is achieved, further exposure of the ICA may be needed based on the location of the injury to achieve distal and proximal control. In the event that the petrous or parapharyngeal ICA is injured, exposure of more proximal segments of the ICA is required in order to accomplish immediate hemostasis. Many techniques are available for managing arterial injury and can be classified into four categories: preservation of the artery, bypass, sacrifice, and endovascular management. Controlling bleeding, while also preserving the vessel, can be accomplished with suturing, bipolar coagulation, aneurysm clips, surgical packing, or a crushed muscle graft.[37,38] If the patient had demonstrated decreased collateral perfusion on a preoperative BTO, then a bypass may be performed preoperatively to reduce the risk of ischemic injury if the case has a high risk of an arterial injury. If the BTO demonstrated good circulation especially in cases with lesions that extend into the arterial wall, then sacrifice of the ICA is also an option to prevent bleeding.

Once bleeding is encountered, the first step should be to attempt to find the site of bleeding and evaluate for any immediate intervention. If the bleeding can be controlled using clips or bipolar cautery, this should be attempted first. The use of crushed autologous muscle graft to plug the site of arterial injury can be a very effective technique for stopping active arterial bleeding from ICA or another large vessel injury. It is important to avoid the use of injectable hemostatic matrix (i.e., Surgiflo) as this material may enter the artery and embolize distally, resulting in an ischemic stroke. If the bleeding is unable to be controlled and a BTO was performed preoperatively without any neurological sequelae, the ICA may be sacrificed. Although its use has not been widely investigated, the use of advanced imaging studies such as single photon emission computed tomography (SPECT) in conjunction with BTO may increase the sensitivity of detecting patients who may develop stroke after ICA sacrifice.[39] Adenosine, which has been previously demonstrated to successfully decompress complex aneurysms to facilitate clip application, can be used to induce transient hypotension to facilitate ICA injury repair.[40,41] Alternatively, cervical compression of the ipsilateral common carotid artery can aid in reducing the high-pressure vascular injury to facilitate nasal packing.[42] In cases where the nasal cavity can be packed, the procedure must be aborted, and the patient should immediately be taken to the angiography suite for diagnostic cerebral angiogram to evaluate the vessel anatomy and investigate for any vascular irregularities. If postoperative digital subtraction angiography (DSA) demonstrates active bleeding from the injury site or stenosis of the ICA, then after evaluating risks and benefits with the endovascular and surgical teams, endovascular interventions may be pursued. These include traditional stents, flow diverters, coils to control the active bleeding or repair the injured vessels, or ICA occlusion.

9.8.3 ACA Injury

As with ICA injury, the first step is to identify the site of bleeding and the artery at risk. Although much has been written about injury to the ICA, there is not much written regarding injury to the ACA. Once the site of bleeding is identified and confirmed to be from the ACA or one of its branches, techniques similar to repairing ICA injuries can be utilized. However, given the small caliber and difficulty in preserving the ACA after

injury, injury to this artery is more likely to result in vessel sacrifice. Initially, the artery may be partially or completely clipped or ligated with bipolar cautery. Again, it is important to avoid the use of injectable hemostatic matrix as it can embolize and cause stroke. Autologous crushed muscle graft can be effective at controlling the arterial bleeding. Once the bleeding is controlled, the patient may be taken to the angiography suite for potential intervention. These include vessel sacrifice, stenting, or coiling. In addition, any areas of decreased or absent filling can be identified for potential stroke.

9.9 Potential Complications

Postoperative monitoring of the patient for change in neurological examination is extremely important. All patients who encounter intraoperative vascular injury should receive a CT, CTA, and formal angiography of the head to check for postoperative complications such as hemorrhage, pseudoaneurysm formation, or a development of a hematoma indicating the need for further intervention to control the bleeding.[43] The formation of a pseudoaneurysm can occur after injury to an artery, and may form acutely or several weeks or months after surgery.[4] Therefore, both early (postoperatively) and late (4–6 weeks postoperative) imaging modalities (CTA, DSA) should be obtained. Although it is possible to repair a pseudoaneurysm through open microsurgical techniques by clip wrapping or bypass grafting, endovascular treatment can involve either vessel sacrifice/occlusion or possibly preservation/repair with a flow diverter.[4,44] Although uncommon, rupture of a pseudoaneurysm of the ICA or ACA is a potential postoperative complication that can present with profuse, life-threatening epistaxis.[45] In this case, the patient should be taken to the angiography suite for likely endovascular occlusion of the ICA, with or without a subsequent bypass depending on the presence of collateral circulation. In the context of hemorrhage secondary to arterial injury, cerebral vasospasm can also occur. This may be treated pharmacologically or with endovascular balloon angioplasty.[44]

9.10 Management Algorithm

9.10.1 *ICA*

- Identify site of bleeding with suction, saline irrigation, and hemostatic packing.
- Temporarily stop bleeding with suturing, bipolar coagulation, aneurysm clips, or surgical packing.
- Once bleeding is temporarily stopped, take patient to angiography suite to evaluate for endovascular intervention by diagnostic cerebral angiogram.
- Sacrifice vessel if it cannot be repaired.

9.10.2 *ACA*

- Identify site of bleeding.
- If artery cannot be preserved with sidewall bipolar cautery or clipping it may be ligated with similar techniques.
- Take patient to angiography suite to evaluate for endovascular intervention by diagnostic cerebral angiogram.
- Perform vessel sacrifice if bleeding cannot be stopped.

9.11 Root Cause Analysis (Post Hoc Analysis)

- The rate of injury to the ICA in endoscopic transsphenoidal surgery is inversely related to the surgeon's experience. A two-surgeon, four-handed approach is recommended. For EEAs, the use of smaller angled endoscopes should be attempted first, increasing the angulation only as necessary.
- For tumors that are in close proximity to the anterior cerebral vasculature, preoperative imaging must be studied to evaluate for the presence of a cortical cuff. This protective barrier of noneloquent brain matter separating the tumor from the vasculature makes EEAs more feasible.
- The type of tumor should be taken into careful consideration. In general, tumors with a firmer, more fibrous consistency present a challenge for endoscopic endonasal removal. Chondroid tumors that have eroded the bony carotid canal can make the ICA more vulnerable to injury during tumor removal.
- A thorough knowledge of the extracranial and intracranial vasculature is required prior to any surgical intervention.
- In the case of intraoperative arterial bleeding, it is important to identify the site of bleeding and to stop the bleeding with packing or clip ligation. It is important to avoid the use of injectable hemostatic matrix as this material may enter the artery and embolize distally, resulting in a stroke.

9.12 Conclusion

EEAs have the potential to result in a variety of complications, including major vascular injuries. To minimize the risk of vascular complications, one should perform a thorough review of preoperative imaging studies to understand the vascular anatomy in relation to the pathology. If the pathology involves or encases the ACAs and/or the ICAs, preoperative BTO can be considered to evaluate collateral flow in case the involved ICA is injured and subsequently requires sacrifice. In the case of tumors involving the ACAs, the presence of a cortical cuff must be investigated in the preoperative imaging when considering choosing an EEA versus an open approach. When a vascular complication does occur during an endoscopic procedure of the anterior skull base, the first step should be to attempt to find the site of bleeding and stop the bleeding with the aforementioned techniques. Immediate postoperative angiography should be performed to further assess status of the vessel injury and to employ any necessary interventional treatments. An experienced team with a two-surgeon, four-handed approach is recommended for complex pathologies in which vascular injuries may be encountered.

References

[1] Prevedello DM, Doglietto F, Jane JA, Jr, Jagannathan J, Han J, Laws ER, Jr. History of endoscopic skull base surgery: its evolution and current reality. J Neurosurg. 2007; 107(1):206–213

[2] Majmundar N, Kamal NH, Reddy RK, Eloy JA, Liu JK. Limitations of the endoscopic endonasal transcribriform approach. J Neurosurg Sci. 2018; 62(3):287–296

[3] Gardner PA, Tormenti MJ, Pant H, Fernandez-Miranda JC, Snyderman CH, Horowitz MB. Carotid artery injury during endoscopic endonasal skull base surgery: incidence and outcomes. Neurosurgery. 2013; 73(2) Suppl Operative: ons261–ons269, discussion ons269–ons270

[4] Romero ADCB, Lal Gangadharan J, Bander ED, Gobin YP, Anand VK, Schwartz TH. Managing arterial injury in endoscopic skull base surgery: case series and review of the literature. Oper Neurosurg (Hagerstown). 2017; 13(1):138–149

[5] Berker M, Aghayev K, Saatci I, Palaoğlu S, Onerci M. Overview of vascular complications of pituitary surgery with special emphasis on unexpected abnormality. Pituitary. 2010; 13(2):160–167

[6] Couldwell WT, Weiss MH, Rabb C, Liu JK, Apfelbaum RI, Fukushima T. Variations on the standard transsphenoidal approach to the sellar region, with emphasis on the extended approaches and parasellar approaches: surgical experience in 105 cases. Neurosurgery. 2004; 55(3):539–547, discussion 547–550

[7] Gardner PA, Kassam AB, Snyderman CH, et al. Outcomes following endoscopic, expanded endonasal resection of suprasellar craniopharyngiomas: a case series. J Neurosurg. 2008; 109(1):6–16

[8] Stippler M, Gardner PA, Snyderman CH, Carrau RL, Prevedello DM, Kassam AB. Endoscopic endonasal approach for clival chordomas. Neurosurgery. 2009; 64(2):268–277, discussion 277–278

[9] Frank G, Sciarretta V, Calbucci F, Farneti G, Mazzatenta D, Pasquini E. The endoscopic transnasal transsphenoidal approach for the treatment of cranial base chordomas and chondrosarcomas. Neurosurgery. 2006; 59(1) Suppl 1: ONS50–ONS57, discussion ONS50–ONS57

[10] Ciric I, Ragin A, Baumgartner C, Pierce D. Complications of transsphenoidal surgery: results of a national survey, review of the literature, and personal experience. Neurosurgery. 1997; 40(2):225–236, discussion 236–237

[11] Bouthillier A, van Loveren HR, Keller JT. Segments of the internal carotid artery: a new classification. Neurosurgery. 1996; 38(3):425–432, discussion 432–433

[12] DePowell JJ, Froelich SC, Zimmer LA, et al. Segments of the internal carotid artery during endoscopic transnasal and open cranial approaches: can a uniform nomenclature apply to both? World Neurosurg. 2014; 82(6) Suppl: S66–S71

[13] Osborn AG. Diagnostic Cerebral Angiography. (Lippincott Williams & Wilkins, Philadelphia, PA: 1999). AJNR Am J Neuroradiol. 1999; 20(9):1767–1769

[14] Renn WH, Rhoton AL, Jr. Microsurgical anatomy of the sellar region. J Neurosurg. 1975; 43(3):288–298

[15] Unal B, Bademci G, Bilgili YK, Batay F, Avci E. Risky anatomic variations of sphenoid sinus for surgery. Surg Radiol Anat. 2006; 28(2):195–201

[16] Hewaidi G, Omami G. Anatomic variation of sphenoid sinus and related structures in Libyan population: CT scan study. Libyan J Med. 2008; 3(3): 128–133

[17] Fujii K, Chambers SM, Rhoton AL, Jr. Neurovascular relationships of the sphenoid sinus. A microsurgical study. J Neurosurg. 1979; 50(1):31–39

[18] Hudgins PA, Browning DG, Gallups J, et al. Endoscopic paranasal sinus surgery: radiographic evaluation of severe complications. AJNR Am J Neuroradiol. 1992; 13(4):1161–1167

[19] Grigorian A, Rajaraman V, Hunt CD. Traumatic intracranial aneurysms complicating anterior skull base surgery. J Craniomaxillofac Trauma. 1998; 4(4):10–14

[20] Maniglia AJ. Fatal and major complications secondary to nasal and sinus surgery. Laryngoscope. 1989; 99(3):276–283

[21] Fliss DM, Gil Z. Atlas of Surgical Approaches to Paranasal Sinuses and the Skull Base. Springer; 2016

[22] Cavallo LM, Messina A, Cappabianca P, et al. Endoscopic endonasal surgery of the midline skull base: anatomical study and clinical considerations. Neurosurg Focus. 2005; 19(1):E2

[23] Han JK, Becker SS, Bomeli SR, Gross CW. Endoscopic localization of the anterior and posterior ethmoid arteries. Ann Otol Rhinol Laryngol. 2008; 117(12):931–935

[24] Abuzayed B, Tanriover N, Gazioglu N, et al. Endoscopic endonasal anatomy and approaches to the anterior skull base: a neurosurgeon's viewpoint. J Craniofac Surg. 2010; 21(2):529–537

[25] Kassam AB, Prevedello DM, Carrau RL, et al. Endoscopic endonasal skull base surgery: analysis of complications in the authors' initial 800 patients. J Neurosurg. 2011; 114(6):1544–1568

[26] Horowitz PM, DiNapoli V, Su SY, Raza SM. Complication avoidance in endoscopic skull base surgery. Otolaryngol Clin North Am. 2016; 49(1): 227–235

[27] Dusick JR, Esposito F, Malkasian D, Kelly DF. Avoidance of carotid artery injuries in transsphenoidal surgery with the Doppler probe and micro-hook blades. Neurosurgery. 2007; 60(4) Suppl 2:322–328, discussion 328–329

[28] Kassam AB, Gardner PA, Snyderman CH, Carrau RL, Mintz AH, Prevedello DM. Expanded endonasal approach, a fully endoscopic transnasal approach for the resection of midline suprasellar craniopharyngiomas: a new classification based on the infundibulum. J Neurosurg. 2008; 108(4):715–728

[29] Mason E, Gurrola J, II, Reyes C, Brown JJ, Figueroa R, Solares CA. Analysis of the petrous portion of the internal carotid artery: landmarks for an endoscopic endonasal approach. Laryngoscope. 2014; 124(9):1988–1994

[30] Ditzel Filho L, de Lara D, Prevedello DM, et al. Expanded endonasal approaches to the anterior skull base [J]. Otorhinolaryngol Clin 2011;3(3):176–183

[31] Koutourousiou M, Fernandez-Miranda JC, Wang EW, Snyderman CH, Gardner PA. Endoscopic endonasal surgery for olfactory groove meningiomas: outcomes and limitations in 50 patients. Neurosurg Focus. 2014; 37(4):E8

[32] Di Maio S, Cavallo LM, Esposito F, Stagno V, Corriero OV, Cappabianca P. Extended endoscopic endonasal approach for selected pituitary adenomas: early experience. J Neurosurg. 2011; 114(2):345–353

[33] Juraschka K, Khan OH, Godoy BL, et al. Endoscopic endonasal transsphenoidal approach to large and giant pituitary adenomas: institutional experience and predictors of extent of resection. J Neurosurg. 2014; 121(1):75–83

[34] Kulwin C, Schwartz TH, Cohen-Gadol AA. Endoscopic extended transsphenoidal resection of tuberculum sellae meningiomas: nuances of neurosurgical technique. Neurosurg Focus. 2013; 35(6):E6

[35] Oskouian RJ, Kelly DF, Laws ERJ, Jr. Vascular injury and transsphenoidal surgery. Front Horm Res. 2006; 34:256–278

[36] Ebner FH, Kuerschner V, Dietz K, Bueltmann E, Naegele T, Honegger J. Reduced intercarotid artery distance in acromegaly: pathophysiologic considerations and implications for transsphenoidal surgery. Surg Neurol. 2009; 72(5):456–460, discussion 460

[37] Valentine R, Wormald PJ. Controlling the surgical field during a large endoscopic vascular injury. Laryngoscope. 2011; 121(3):562–566

[38] Gardner PA, Snyderman CH, Fernandez-Miranda JC, Jankowitz BT. Management of major vascular injury during endoscopic endonasal skull base surgery. Otolaryngol Clin North Am. 2016; 49(3):819–828

[39] Tansavatdi K, Dublin AB, Donald PJ, Dahlin B. Combined balloon test occlusion and SPECT analysis for carotid sacrifice: angiographic predictors for success or failure? J Neurol Surg B Skull Base. 2015; 76(4):249–251

[40] Wang X, Feletti A, Tanaka R, et al. Adenosine-induced flow arrest to facilitate intracranial complex aneurysm clip ligation: review of the literature. Asian J Neurosurg. 2018; 13(3):539–545

[41] Fastenberg JH, Garzon-Muvdi T, Hsue V, et al. Adenosine-induced transient hypotension for carotid artery injury during endoscopic skull-base surgery: case report and review of the literature. Int Forum Allergy Rhinol. 2019; 9(9):1023–1029

[42] Valentine R, Wormald PJ. Carotid artery injury after endonasal surgery. Otolaryngol Clin North Am. 2011; 44(5):1059–1079

[43] Solares CA, Ong YK, Carrau RL, et al. Prevention and management of vascular injuries in endoscopic surgery of the sinonasal tract and skull base. Otolaryngol Clin North Am. 2010; 43(4):817–825

[44] Raymond J, Hardy J, Czepko R, Roy D. Arterial injuries in transsphenoidal surgery for pituitary adenoma; the role of angiography and endovascular treatment. AJNR Am J Neuroradiol. 1997; 18(4):655–665

[45] Biswas D, Daudia A, Jones NS, McConachie NS. Profuse epistaxis following sphenoid surgery: a ruptured carotid artery pseudoaneurysm and its management. J Laryngol Otol. 2009; 123(6):692–694

10 Dealing with Major Intraoperative Vascular Injury

Sean P. Polster, Paul A. Gardner, and Juan C. Fernandez-Miranda

Summary

Prevention and management of complications is a cornerstone of surgery. As endoscopic endonasal surgery gains popularity and is becoming the standard of care for sellar, parasellar, and medial middle fossa skull base access, its complications have been well studied with strategies that have improved over the last decade. Internal carotid artery (ICA) injury is a potentially devastating injury. Management algorithms and training paradigms have evolved for these injuries. Preoperative planning is paramount and may include a balloon test occlusion of the ICA. In this chapter we review the modern literature as well as the University of Pittsburgh series. It is clear that experienced teams with premeditated ICA injury protocols can provide effective management with potentially good outcomes. This chapter serves to review key elements in understanding vascular and endoscopic challenges, preoperative planning, landmarks, rescue steps as well as postoperative management and complication avoidance in the setting of middle fossa ICA injury. These principles are important to incorporate into training of all levels.

Keywords: ICA injury, internal carotid, middle fossa, endoscopic endonasal, multidisciplinary approach

10.1 Key Learning Points

- It is rare that internal carotid artery (ICA) injury is the result of a single error; multiple factors lead to poor outcomes.
- Preoperative checklist, imaging, realistic goals of surgery, and possibly balloon test occlusion are necessary to consider.
- Dual surgeons with dynamic endoscopy and bimanual dissection are key to avoiding and managing injury.
- Bipolar cautery, clip-based repair, and packing strategies should all be available options for repair of ICA injury.
- Muscle packing over an area of injury is often the most reliable technique and should be considered the first option for any sizeable or difficult to control injury.
- Cerebral perfusion is the end goal and should not be compromised. Indirect measurement with neurophysiologic monitoring can assist in decision-making.
- A multidisciplinary team is important for postoperative management.
- Digital subtraction angiography is necessary to diagnose and treat immediate and late complications.
- Although never the first option, if hemorrhage becomes truly life threatening, carotid sacrifice should be considered. A majority of patients will tolerate sacrifice of a single ICA.
- Older patients may tolerate sacrifice less well due to loss of collateral.

10.2 Introduction

Endoscopic endonasal surgery (EES) for treating paranasal and skull base pathology has grown in popularity over the last two decades, largely replacing microscopic approaches.[1] EES has led to decreased morbidity and improved patient outcomes secondary to the numerous advantages afforded by improved visualization, midline corridor with decreased neurovascular manipulation, avoidance of skin incision, and reduced postoperative pain with shorter hospital stays.[2,3,4] The evolution of EES has gone well beyond midline pituitary surgery to encompass an almost unrestricted access to the ventral skull base. Despite multiple advances in approach, technique, and equipment, much fear remains for the inexperienced operator when dealing with some of the potential complications, especially those of a vascular nature.

Encountering the ICA is extremely common during ESS. The lateral walls of the sella have a close relationship with the ICA. Protrusion of the ICA into the sphenoid sinus due to pneumatization has been reported to occur in about 70% of patients and frank dehiscence within the sphenoid sinus occurs in about 22% of patients.[5] Furthermore, advanced pathologies including sinonasal, middle, and posterior cranial fossa lesions may require exposure and/or mobilization of the ICA. This includes lesions of the petrous apex, cavernous sinus, clivus, infratemporal fossa, and parapharyngeal space all of which may have increased risk of injury.

ICA injury may result in varying degrees of morbidity and even death. Early complications include overwhelming hemorrhage/blood loss or carotid occlusion. Delayed manifestations include formation of pseudoaneurysm, vessel spasm, thrombosis, embolization, or formation of a caroticocavernous fistula which can all further complicate repair or treatment of the underlying pathology. In addition, repair or interventions aimed at treating large vessel injury have independent risk profiles that each carry additional risks and benefits. Therefore, the prevention and management of such injuries remain important considerations for EES operators in both the short- and long-term manifestations of ICA injury.

Injury to the ICA most often occurs within the middle fossa likely owing to the majority of pathologies suitable for EES occurring centrally (i.e., pituitary tumors). The incidence of accidental injury of the ICA during traditional skull base surgery has been reported to range as high as 3 to 8%.[6] Although the rate of ICA injury during EES pituitary surgery is low by comparison (less than 1%)[3] and has been documented largely in case reports, the incidence during expanded EES (those cases with exposure beyond the face of the sella) has a higher risk profile. These estimations are subject to publication bias, as systematic accounting of ICA injuries in the literature are lacking. A recent survey of experienced surgeons while attending the University of Pittsburgh Medical Center (UPMC) Skull Base Surgery Course reported that 20% of participants had encountered a carotid injury within the preceding 12 months.[7] Expanded approaches require wide exposure with the goal of further reach and more extensive resection with reports citing injury rates as high as 4 to 9%.[8,9] With the growing popularity of endoscopic endonasal cases ICA injury is in need of additional study.

Large vessel injury is a difficult to treat complication and has limited the novice from enjoying the maximal benefits of EES.

A learning curve exists to successfully deploying EES across a broad set of pathologies with advantages that outweigh this potential injury. Training paradigms have been proposed to avoid and address potential large vessel injury and allow for stepwise progression of comfort and skill for operators.[1,10] In this chapter, the literature reporting ICA injury is reviewed, and our team's own experience and a paradigm for complication avoidance and management of injury are presented.

10.3 Vascular Challenge

10.3.1 Anatomy of the Middle Fossa ICA

Within the middle fossa and skull base, the ICA has a three-dimensional course with consistent relationships to other anatomical landmarks. However, these may be distorted by pathology, prior surgery, irradiation, and anatomical variation. Understanding the impact of these factors and careful study of appropriate preoperative imaging studies to understand the relationship of each unique case is valuable.

Many classifications have been proposed, including the Fischer classification (1938) with a focus on describing the extracranial and intracranial segments, and the more modern and widely used classification schemes of Gibo et al and Rhoton as well as Bouthillier et al.[11,12,13,14,15] Yet, the key transcranial relationships do not fully address the cranial base from a ventral viewpoint. Alfieri and Jho reported a meaningful attempt to classify the segments of the ICA from an endoscopic endonasal perspective; however, their classification has multiple limitations.[16] Namely, it excludes segments of the ICA proximal to the foramen lacerum, and relies on sphenoid sinus pneumatization, a feature that is highly variable, for identifying landmarks of the ICA. Labib et al introduced a comprehensive classification scheme that is applicable to the expanded endonasal approaches.[17] These segments correspond to consistent anatomic landmarks that can be identified. These landmarks have been refined and ICA segments correlated to create a more modern nomenclature for endonasal operators (▶ Table 10.1). Wide variability in nomenclature is still found in the neurosurgical literature which can create uncertainty when converting between systems of transcranial, endovascular, or radiology-based naming schema. Preoperative imaging of vessels and knowledge of anatomical landmarks can be used in conjunction with Doppler ultrasound, indocyanine green fluoroscopy, optical/electromagnetic navigation, and contralateral anatomical symmetry to define patient-specific ICA anatomy along with pathology.

Table 10.1 Anatomical landmarks of the internal carotid artery

Segment	Endonasal anatomical landmark	Bouthillier classification[14]
Ascending/parapharyngeal	Eustachian tube	C1
Horizontal petrous	Vidian nerve	C2
Foramen lacerum	Medial pterygoid wedge	C3
Paraclival	Paraclival protuberance	C4
Paraclinoid	mOCR/lOCR	C5/6

Abbreviations: mOCR, medial optic carotid recess; lOCR, lateral optic carotid recess.

10.3.2 Endoscopic Aspects/Challenges

ICA injury management is technically challenging given the fact that it is a large, high-flow (estimated to be around 200–300 mL/min), high-pressure artery that if injured immediately compromises the surgical field.[18] This is amplified when using endoscopic visualization in a narrow corridor. Massive bleeding leads to a loss of orientation and obscures identification of the injury point. Restoration of visualization requires stepwise maneuvers to regain control of the field. Moreover, the lack of direct endonasal vascular suture repair excludes traditional treatment options. In addition, for novices, the optical characteristics of the endoscope, which are vastly different from those of the microscope, may make endoscopic anatomy particularly challenging. Specifically, the two-dimensional view of the endoscope interferes with traditional depth perception and has to be overcome with dynamic endoscopy relying on instrument relationships. These factors together can alter the perspective as well as depth perception of the ICA (▶ Fig. 10.1) and, combined with the nasal corridor, create a perceived lack of control.[17]

10.4 Injury Avoidance

10.4.1 Preoperative

"Intellectuals solve problems, geniuses prevent them"

(Albert Einstein)

Each clinical scenario, with unique anatomical variations and pathological distortions, needs to be thoroughly evaluated preoperatively. This starts with comprehensive neurological and rhinological assessments (in addition to anesthesia, endocrinology, ophthalmology, or others as deemed necessary). It is worthwhile to evaluate any high risk or complex case in a multidisciplinary clinic and tumor board setting (neuroradiology and even oncology as needed) where surgical planning is discussed between the primary surgeons to develop the operative plan including surgical challenges, overall surgical goal, reconstruction plan, and risk stratification. This plan is then further discussed with the operating room (OR) staff and anesthesia team for operative day readiness. Furthermore, these risks and potential complications are discussed with the patient on more than one occasion. Even the rare complication of large vessel injury is discussed in detailed with each patient as part of our informed consent process.

Computed tomography angiography (CTA) and magnetic resonance imaging (MRI) are part of the standard imaging protocol. Both modalities are important to highlight bony anatomy in relation to vascular anatomy as well as soft tissue and pathological involvement by MRI assessment. Devoted MR sequences are tailored to relevant anatomy with special skull base sequences (fast-spin echo, steady-state free procession, fine cut T2) or pituitary sequences (dynamic) depending on the clinical scenario. Unexpected pathology should always be considered when approaching sellar pathology (e.g., poorly pneumatized bone, dehiscence, ectatic/kissing carotids, carotid-clinoid ring, tumor invasion into adventitia, etc.). Typically, preoperative imaging can delineate vascular abnormalities such as an aneurysm, pseudoaneurysm,

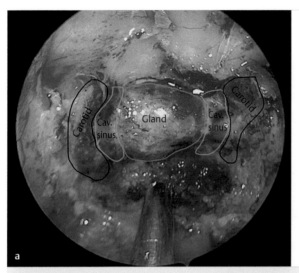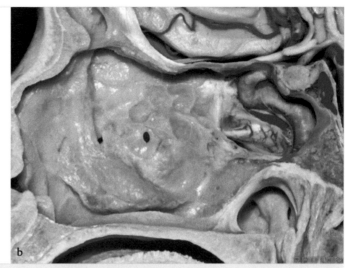

Fig. 10.1 **(a)** Endoscopic endonasal view in a transsphenoidal case delineating the position of the gland, cavernous sinus, and carotid arteries beneath the dura. **(b)** A Rhoton anatomical dissection showing the sagittal viewpoint of the same anatomy. The loss of the three-dimensional depth is significantly distorted by the endoscopic view; this may be more noticeable with the internal carotid artery (ICA). (Figure reproduced with permission from *The Rhoton Collection®.*)

or carotid-cavernous fistulae. If vascular abnormalities exist or cranial circulation is unclear, they can be further delineated with digital subtraction angiography.

Case selection depends on the experience of the surgical team. High-risk cases should be considered for a balloon test occlusion (BTO) of the ICA to assess collateral cerebral blood flow and evaluate for tolerance of sacrifice. BTO, however, can be associated with a 5 to 10% false-negative result. Imaging adjunct with perfusion CT, MR single-photon emission computed tomography (SPECT), transcranial Doppler, or other methods can be used to confirm/improve the result or be utilized if patient factors prohibit preoperative endovascular testing. BTO prior to high-risk ICA cases reduces the incidence of postoperative stroke compared with indiscriminate ICA sacrifice.[19,20] This topic is discussed in detail in Chapter 3.

In general, good surgical technique is also key in avoiding ICA injury; ensuring excellent visualization, orientation, keeping a clean surgical field, and proper working instruments are important factors. Experience and teamwork between the two surgical teams and an operative plan will allow seamless execution and avoid off-course surgery. Subcapsular tumor dissection and proper skeletonization of key anatomy also play a role so that normal anatomy can be maintained with delicate manipulation of sensitive structures. Gross ballistic movements or aggressive biting of bone should also be avoided as safer access can be achieved with diligent drilling or "egg shelling" of delicate anatomy, including the ICA. Exposure should be adequate to ensure proximal control in the event of an injury.

Neurophysiology is of critical importance as it serves as the only measure of cerebral perfusion while under anesthesia. Somatosensory evoked potentials (SSEPs) remain the mainstay of hemispheric perfusion which is important when employing interventions. In addition to guiding decisions on which interventions can be deployed, it is useful to guide management by the anesthesia team as further discussed in the following. The routine use of SSEPs should be considered on all endoscopic endonasal cases. Electroencephalography (EEG) can also be added in high-risk cases to aid in intraoperative decision-making if perfusion is compromised. Chapter 21 thoroughly discusses neurophysiological considerations associated with skull base vascular concerns.

10.4.2 Anatomical Risk

The relationship of the ICA to the sphenoid sinus has been morphometrically detailed in the neurosurgical and skull base literature.[21,22] Large vessel course and pneumatization patterns can be identified on preoperative imaging. Dehiscent ICA in the sphenoid sinus has been reported to occur in 4 to 22% of cases with 8 to 70% of patients having an ICA prominence into the sphenoid sinus.[23] The average intercarotid distance of the parasellar segment ICAs has been reported as 12 mm but can be less than 4 mm. These facts alone are not risk factors and if properly incorporated into a surgical plan can aid in early identification.[22] Bony septations within the sphenoid sinus can attach in a number of patterns, including midline, on the ICA, optic nerve, or multiple locations. However, it is important to realize that almost all septations (89%) extend or attach to bone over the ICA at some point.[24] These septations should be removed with caution, typically with the use of a high-speed drill, to avoid fracturing into the encased soft tissue at the distal aspect of the bone.

10.5 Impact of Pathologies

Ectasia or distortion of the anatomical course of the ICA by tumor compression or invasion may place the vessel at risk. This may or may not include adventitia invasion that can be seen with aggressive tumors (▶ Fig. 10.2). Invasion or flow-limiting stenosis of the ICA increases the risk and, depending on the pathology and goals of surgery, may necessitate a BTO in preparation for sacrifice or potential injury.

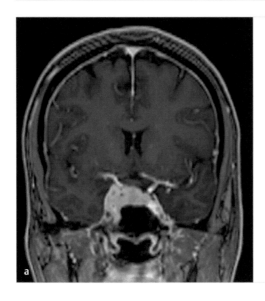
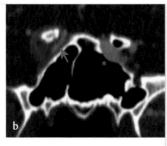
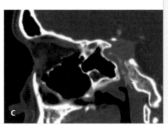

Fig. 10.2 **(a)** Preoperative magnetic resonance imaging (MRI) showing invasive spheno-cavernous meningioma. **(b, c)** Computed tomography (CT) angiogram (Top: coronal; Bottom: right parasagittal section) showing a right spheno-cavernous meningioma with internal carotid artery (ICA) invasion that has encased and restricted flow of the right ICA (*arrows*) as well as a dehiscent left ICA (*).

Specific pathologies have been suggested to pose additional risk for ICA injury. Tumors that have intimate contact with the ICA can disturb tissue planes which can increase risk of inadvertent injury. Additionally, lesions that extend beyond a single segment of the ICA (≥2), requiring exposure or mobilization of the carotids, is a cause to consider the case at an elevated risk as proposed by Al Qahtani et al.[25,26] Therefore, middle fossa and posterior fossa origin or growth extension pose a significant risk in comparison to anterior cranial fossa tumors. Encasement of the ICA by more than 120 degrees has been proposed as a risk factor for potential injury as it suggests loss of tissue planes, and early identification of surrounding anatomy proves more difficult. If the pathology is within the chondroid tumor family (chordomas and chondrosarcomas), there is an elevated risk profile for ICA injury;[3] this may also be related to the fact that these tumors are best treated with radical resection as they typically abut if not encase the ICA crossing periosteal planes. Hence, radical resection with curative intent is in itself a risk factor for ICA injury.

Finally, tumors may secrete factors that can affect the major vasculature. A common example is growth hormone (GH) secreting pituitary adenomas which are known to cause vascular ectasia with increased risk of ICA injury.[27]

10.5.1 Operator/Intraoperative

Utilizing the training paradigm proposed by Snyderman et al on the acquisition of surgical skills for endonasal skull base surgery, surgeons should be well prepared before tackling cases where ICA injury is at a more than moderate risk.[1] All endonasal surgery teams should be prepared and have forethought about a potential vascular injury; but, as case complexity increases and anatomical reach brings the likelihood of ICA injury to the forefront, management should be within a surgical team's skill set before embarking. This is also true for trainees who are supervised by senior surgeons; stepwise progression of skill and judicious supervision are required to achieve a balance of training the next generation of surgeon while ensuring a safe and effective outcome. Preparation can be furthered by mentorship with a more senior surgeon, training

courses, cadaveric dissection, and training models of ICA injury/repair.[28]

Surgical planning for cases that involve tumor invasion or distortion of the ICA requires planning a wide corridor that allows maximal working space for free bimanual dissection. Careful sharp dissection is used in areas of high risk with small careful movements, which can potentially allow for repair if a minor injury occurs. Dual surgeons with dynamic endoscopy (i.e., not using a static endoscope holding device) can play an immense but difficult to quantify role. Constant movement of the endoscope allows for an ideal view and ensures that endoscope placement does not impede dissection movement. In addition, constant cross-checking between two experienced surgeons working side by side prevents inevitable single operator error. Instrumentation choice or lack of proper instrumentation can also play a role in ICA injury. Typically, the drill is used to thin bone until it can be "flaked" away and is used with a "coarse" diamond bit (≤4 mm) and copious irrigation to prevent thermal injury and increase visualization. This bit is used initially on areas other than close to the ICA which serves to slightly dull it before it is used to *blue-line* over the ICA. We have also found great success with the occasional use of a "minimally invasive" drill attachment (MIS curved 13 or 16 cm) that has a curved shaft and protected drill bit shaft that can improve reach and visualization. Other powered instruments such as ultrasonic aspirators can be of value for focal bone removal in close proximity to the ICA but should be used with a great deal of caution in combination with frequent assessment with Doppler ultrasound, image guidance, and even indocyanine green (ICG) fluoroendoscopy. Microdebriders and monopolar electrocautery should only be used outside of the sphenoid sinus. Use of Kerrison or pituitary rongeurs can also be high-risk maneuvers as they allow for pulling or biting of poorly visualized tissue. In addition, all necessary instrumentation should be present in case of injury, for example, hemostatic agents or bipolar cautery devices. It is essential to have knowledgeable scrub nurses that understand the surgical methods and the proper set-up and handling of instrumentation.

Additional factors that add risk but are hard to predict include the degree of adherence of the lesion to the ICA which can be influenced by previous surgery, irradiation, or bromocriptine therapy.[29] These have all been reported to be risk factors in ICA injury.[25,30] Given that these factors will likely require real-time operative assessment, the goals of surgery should be considered if manipulation of nearby adherent structures proves to add significant risk without clear clinical benefit to the patient. Even though one proximate cause of injury can be identified, multiple factors are at play. A disastrous complication is seldom the result of an isolated circumstance and is likely multifactorial.

10.6 Case Example

A recent review of the running case series at the University of Pittsburgh has identified a total of 18 ICA injuries, representing an event rate of 0.46% ($n = 18/3889$). 17/18 cases involved tumors that had grown beyond the sella and all were considered Level III, IV, or V in complexity (as described by Snyderman et al) meaning that all cases were of an advanced degree of difficulty on the learning curve for endoscopic endonasal skull base surgery. The most frequent location was in the cavernous segment ($n = 7$, 39%) followed by the paraclival segment ($n = 5$, 28%). Injury most commonly occurred during tumor dissection ($n = 10$, 56%). Pathologies included adenoma ($n = 5$, 28%), chordoma ($n = 5$, 28%), meningioma ($n = 5$, 28%), and three others (17%). Five patients (28%) had prior surgery with three (17%) having undergone prior irradiation. Bipolar electrocautery was attempted in all cases of ICA injury but most required other treatments. Aneurysm clips were used in nine cases (50%) and packing (muscle and/or cotton) in the remainder. Clipping or packing was combined with a muscle patch in six (33%) cases. All cases underwent immediate postoperative digital subtraction angiography (DSA) which in 14 cases (78%) required no subsequent intervention. Of the four remaining cases, two (11%) were treated with coil embolization, one (6%) with stent placement, and one (6%) with thrombectomy. At 1-month follow-up, pseudoaneurysm formation was detected in three (17%) cases, one treated with observation and two with stent placement. Two (11%) of the ICA injuries resulted in death with the remainder having no neurological deficits at 1-month postoperative.

We further highlight a video case that reviewed elements that contributed to injury (**Video 10.1**).

10.7 Management Strategy/ Management Algorithm

The first step of ICA injury management is realization that an arterial injury has occurred. To the novice, minor arterial bleeding may be mistaken as venous bleeding and managed inappropriately with injection of hemostatic material. The cavernous sinus can bleed profusely and in a pulsatile fashion; typically, this is significantly less than that of the ICA or a perforator and the blood of the ICA has a distinctive arterial color. Whenever bleeding is encountered from the medial cavernous sinus, the question of origin should be addressed and never assumed. Further, when an ICA injury occurs, the lens of the endoscope is often splashed with blood and loss of visualization

occurs either from direct contamination or when the surgical field fills with blood.

Once it has been identified that a large caliber vessel has been injured, the surgeon should notify the OR team. In an ideal situation, this should activate a readily available protocol of actions (▶ Fig. 10.3). The core of this includes the surgeons, the anesthesia team, and the OR staff (scrub and circulating nurse, neurophysiologist). The subsequent steps need to occur in an effective manner and often simultaneously.

10.7.1 The Surgeons

The surgeons should regain control of the surgical field with suction to clear the blood and identify the bleeding point for further assessment. This is best done with two surgeons working to dynamically clear the blood and maintain view. Four hands allow for the endoscope, two suctions, and a working instrument to be deployed in concert, which may be necessary as single suction may be insufficient. The dual suctions should be on separate lines so that there is always one functioning suction.

Direct pressure on the injury site should be the next action to reduce blood loss and deploy the plan. The area of pressure should be as focused as possible, narrowing down to using a single cottonoid, or focal packing material to cover the injury point with suction so that subsequent salvage techniques can be attempted. Indiscriminate packing should be avoided to avoid injury to adjacent structures and minimize risk of blood tracking intracranially through a dural defect. If all else fails, packing should be judiciously employed to stop exsanguination for ensuing emergent neuroendovascular intervention. Packing is the bail-out option if the clinical scenario deteriorates (▶ Fig. 10.4). Packing options can include muscle (preferred first layer on the artery), resorbable (gelfoam, Nasopore, Posisep) or nonresorbable (cotton based) materials, Merocels, and balloons (Foley) depending on the clinical situation.

10.7.2 Cautery

If the bleeding point can be controlled and visualized, primary attempts at sealing the vessel injury should be undertaken. Bipolar cautery can be attempted first depending on the size of the injury. Small side wall injuries or perforator avulsions can be sealed, as previously described by Kassam et al[31] who illustrated longitudinal violation of the side wall being repaired with cautery. This is done by placing a suction directly onto a segment of the artery which allows for bipolar cautery to create a seal. The suction and cautery are then moved together along the injury. Given the size of the ICA, this ideally preserves flow and distal perfusion with minimal stenosis. Cautery should be an early line attempt with the goal of salvage while maintaining patency but can also be used if needed as a method of ligation to seal off the artery in case of an irreparable injury.

10.7.3 Suture/Clip Repair/Ligation

If bleeding cannot be easily controlled or to provide more distinct control, additional access to more proximal and distal points on the artery should be exposed in order to attempt more advanced salvage techniques. This can provide sites of

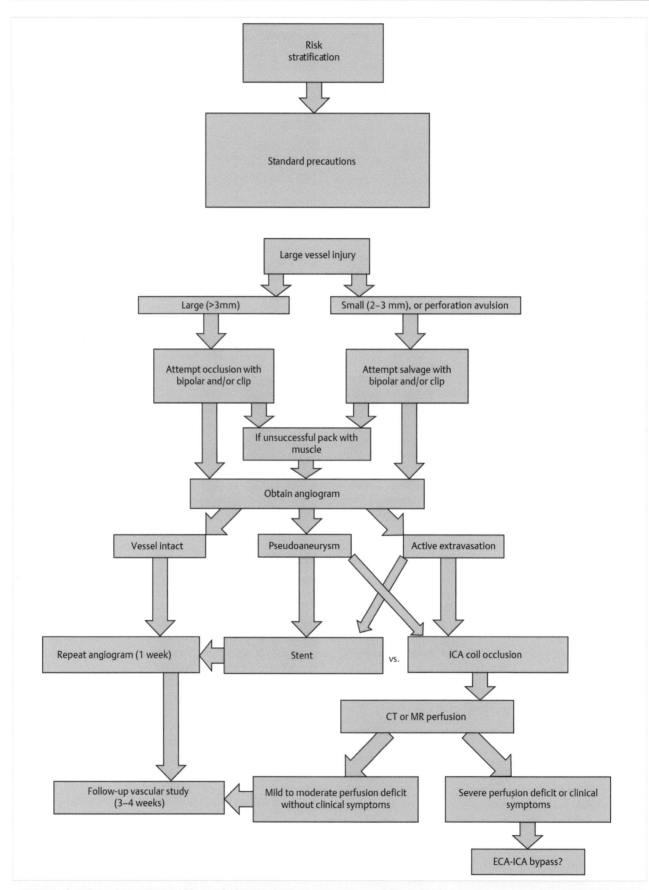

Fig. 10.3 Algorithm summarizing internal carotid artery (ICA) injury management considerations.

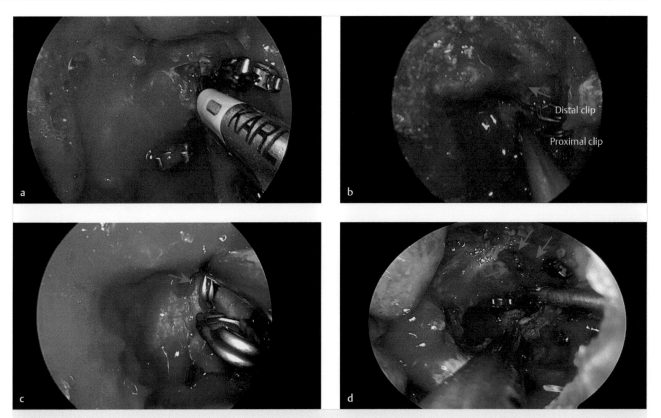

Fig. 10.4 Repair techniques: **(a)** Bipolar cautery with clip application. **(b)** Internal carotid artery (ICA) occlusion with application of clips at the proximal and distal segments of paraclival carotid artery (*arrow* denotes cavernous segment). **(c)** Angled clip application pinching off injury point (seen within clip) with preservation of ICA (*arrows*). **(d)** Muscle patch applied over injury point (*arrows*), harvested from the nasopharynx, with trapping clips in place (cavernous distal and paraclival proximal).

temporary or permanent ligation. If properly planned, proximal and distal control may allow for trapping of the artery. If not, consideration of gaining such control will depend on the site of injury and/or tumor involvement of proximal or distal segments. For example, injury of the lacerum segment of the ICA has little hope for endonasal proximal control and wide cavernous encasement may prevent direct identification of proximal or distal control points. For proximal control in such cases, pre-planning with a small cervical cutdown to the ICA can provide for rapid and definitive proximal control (external carotid artery [ECA]-ICA distal collaterals notwithstanding) (▶ Fig. 10.5). Compression of the ipsilateral ICA in the neck should always be performed to decrease flow and occasionally provide some degree of proximal control. This must be performed by a physician who is confidant in the location of the cervical ICA and familiar with the degree of compression required. Proximal endovascular control may be an option but is time consuming and most endovascular interventions are difficult or impossible using only C-arm fluoroscopy available in an OR. A hybrid suite may overcome this limitation but has its own challenges even if available.

Primary clip repair presents an attractive salvage technique. Straight or angled clips can be applied directly to the side wall to "pinch off" the area of injury and leave a reduced lumen with patency. If repair of the vessel wall defect cannot be achieved, then clip ligation is a reasonable option. However, this can present multiple dilemmas as it may affect cerebral perfusion

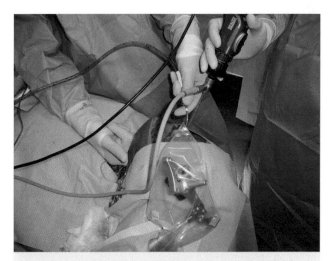

Fig. 10.5 Preparation technique for internal carotid artery (ICA) cutdown/compression point for proximal control. A small, transverse incision is used and can provide immediate proximal control with clip placement.

and definitively closes off any further endovascular access to the site of injury. Furthermore, proximal occlusion will not control retrograde bleeding. SSEPs and mean arterial pressure (MAP) should be judiciously assessed. If test occlusion is per-

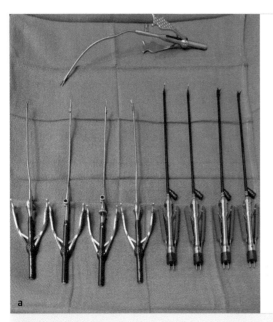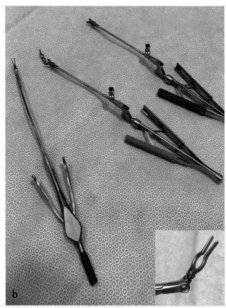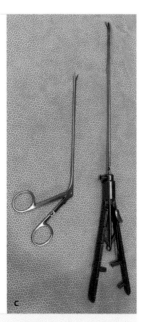

Fig. 10.6 (a) Endoscopic instrument set with malleable dissection forceps (top), rigid instruments (left), and angled bipolar instruments (right). (b) Endoscopic clip appliers; insert showing ability to rotate a straight clip in the applier. (c) Endonasal needle driver and grasper for use with barbed endoscopic suture.

formed, relative hypotension should be included to see if SSEPs show any pressure dependence.

Multiple commercial endoscopic (single shaft) clip appliers (Mizuho, Lazic) are available that allow for placement of a variety of clips at different working angles for precise application of clips with the intent of repair or ligation (▶ Fig. 10.6). Sundt-Keyes clips can also be applied in an attempt to secure the injury but are often large and may not line up well with the tortuous course of the carotid siphon. Familiarization with your institution's resources should be routinely undertaken with the team.

Direct suturing is another extraordinarily advanced technique that can be attempted; however, it has the drawback of being technically demanding and time consuming. Special commercially available needle holders and tying instruments are available but technically demanding to use (▶ Fig. 10.6). This is not recommended unless the surgical team has dedicated significant time in a cadaver lab or other model to ensure that they can reliably apply this technique. In addition, it requires definitive proximal and distal control as ongoing bleeding would make this technique virtually impossible.

10.7.4 Packing

Packing Materials

Packing can be done with hemostatic agents and direct pressure. Cotton can additionally be used to add bulk and create a plug that stops the egress of blood. Muscle is an excellent hemostatic agent; with gentle crushing, muscle endogenously releases Ca^{++} which is a potent activator of the clotting cascade. Muscle is uniquely effective at stopping bleeding and may be the preferred option.[32] Harvest points should be identified preoperatively. Endonasal harvest can be achieved from

the nasopharynx near midline via the longus capitis and rectus capitis anterior muscles which provide an easy and endoscopically accessible point for muscle harvest. The temporalis, rectus abdominus, or lateral thigh can all also provide muscle and may be easily prepped into the sterile field at the beginning of any surgery. Hemostatic agents such as Surgicel® or Avitene® will be ineffective agent in the setting of large arterial bleeding and are only used as a superficial dressing after control is obtained. Morselized, flowable gelfoam (Surgifoam®, Floseal®, Surgiflo®, etc.) should be strictly avoided in any arterial injury given its potential to embolize. It is extremely effective against low-flow, local venous bleeding but presents a clear embolic risk when used on arterial injury. This can result in an irreversible devastating embolization of the cerebral arterial circulation. Other agents have been described including Teflon and methyl methacrylate patch, Syvek marine polymer, and fibrin glue.[4,9,33]

Any compressive packing needs to be evaluated for potential contraindications, most notably if the dura has already been opened. Channeling of blood to the subdural space can occur with catastrophic results as well as compression of sensitive neural structures.

10.7.5 Anesthesia Team

The anesthesia team should aim to assist in maintaining cerebral perfusion. This is done in part by replacing blood as necessary as well as blood components. Significant hemorrhage and local consumption will deplete clotting factors. MAP goals should not be compromised as this is contrary to the vital goal of maintaining cerebral perfusion. A balance of adequate perfusion while allowing for vessel repair or tamponade can be guided by SSEPs. Anesthesia can modify blood pressure to maintain symmetric SSEPs; reactionary significant lowering of

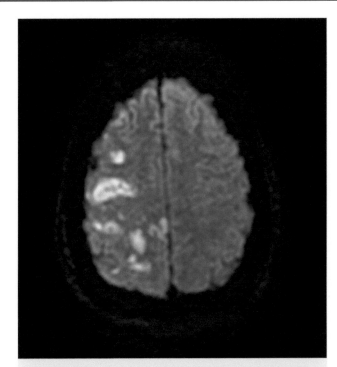

Fig. 10.7 Diffusion weighted magnetic resonance image of a case demonstrating embolic phenomenon originating from hypoperfusion during injury and repair of an internal carotid artery (ICA). To prevent this, once ICA injury has been identified we avoid the use of potential embolic material (i.e., flowable gelfoam), anticoagulate when performing repeated manipulation, and avoid prolonged ICA occlusion if associated with neurophysiology changes (as in this case).

the systolic blood pressure should be avoided unless guided by neurophysiology. Temporary reduction in flow can be achieved with proximal compression in the neck (digital compression of the ipsilateral carotid artery) or administration of adenosine.[34] Adenosine has the advantage of reducing flow with a short half-life and avoiding rebound hypertension, tachycardia, or tachyphylaxis.[35] Adenosine is dosed at 0.3 to 0.4 mg/kg of ideal body weight to achieve approximately 30 to 60 seconds of arrest or hypotension in patients under anesthesia with re-mifentanil/low-dose volatile anesthetic and propofol-induced burst suppression.[34] MAP may be transiently and intentionally dropped to allow for control in settings where it is not easily maintained or to test perfusion in the setting of temporary occlusion.

Additionally, the seemingly paradoxical use of heparin should be considered in any situation requiring frequent or repetitive arterial manipulation, as this can lead to local thrombus which can then embolize (▶ Fig. 10.7).

10.7.6 OR Staff (Technicians, Nurses, Neurophysiology, Blood Bank, and Additional Resources)

Once an ICA injury has occurred, the OR team should notify the OR control station that additional resources may be needed. The blood bank should also be notified that additional resources may be required beyond what is immediately available, especially if mass transfusion protocols are not already in place at your institution. Neurointerventional services should also be

made aware as soon as possible that an ICA injury has occurred. The biplane suite should be reserved with proper staffing as if this were a stroke code.

The OR staff should be trained in emergency situations that call for additional resources beyond normal operating conditions. They should be made aware of equipment location and ideally in-service drills should be performed to identify potential hazards. Mobilization of specialty resources, such as endoscopic clip appliers or adenosine, needs to occur promptly and should not distract the surgeon. Calling in an additional circulator or scrub nurse can be very valuable given the need for equipment, blood checks, and rapid action. If additional surgeons are available to assist with critical maneuvers such as carotid compression in the neck or muscle harvest, they should be rapidly notified.

Electrophysiology is only helpful if already in place. We routinely employ electrophysiology with SSEPs at a minimum. Electrophysiology leads should be maintained if the patient is transported to a different location for endovascular intervention and continual monitoring should be employed as a measure of adequate cerebral perfusion throughout all steps of ICA control and repair.

Endovascular intervention generally requires leaving the OR for the biplane suite. The OR and associated staff should prepare for return to the OR after endovascular treatment as additional procedures may be necessary. Femoral or radial access points should be prepared for access with anesthesia assessment for suitability given other lines of access. Ideally this communication should occur in advance of transporting the patient to the biplane suite. Heparinization or other anticoagulation may be required for endovascular treatment. In general, tumor removal should not proceed in favor of evaluation of the extent and impact of injury. Rare situations with a minor injury and easy control could be considered for a short period of further dissection.

10.7.7 Neurointerventional/ Endovascular Assessment and Treatment

Nearly all patients who suffer an ICA injury require DSA. CTA may miss small but important changes and offers no potential for rapid intervention. It may be considered if an injury is minor and easily controlled or if DSA is not available. If DSA shows a normal vessel then repeat DSA or CTA should be performed before and after packing is removed and in a more delayed fashion, as discussed below.

Endovascular assessment provides two advantages:
- Diagnosis/assessment of the injury and distal flow assessment.
- Interventions with either repair (i.e., maintaining flow) or sacrifice.

Diagnostic DSA can aid in delineating the site of injury, the degree of stenosis, and the relative distal or collateral flow. If no flow is present and depending on the intraoperative action taken the vessel can be further secured with coil embolization. If the vessel remains patent and can be safely navigated, then additional interventions can be undertaken. Decision on endovascular intervention should include input from the operating surgeon to help guide decision-making in the endovascular suite (see Chapter 17, "Endovascular Options to Treat Iatrogenic Vascular Injury and Tumor Involvement of the Skull Base").

Balloon occlusion, either at the level of injury or with proximal and distal balloons, can be used for temporary control.

Stenting or flow diversion is ideally used to maintain patency but may be difficult given the anatomy of the ICA siphon. Complications following stent placement within the ICA show about a 4% risk of stroke within the first 30 days[36] from in-stent thrombosis or occlusion. Patients treated with stenting or flow diversion will require dual antiplatelet administration which could pose short-term complications as well as implications for future treatments or return to the OR. If packing is employed, its impact needs to be considered depending on its current or future impact on the area of injury.

If endovascular options fail to restore patency of the ICA and occlusion cannot be tolerated, a remaining viable option would be to bypass the injured segment via a transcranial approach. Success of this has not be widely reported and has multiple hurdles, not the least of which is the prolonged ischemic time required prior to revascularization, even in the best of hands. In these dire situations, realistic expectations should be discussed (▶ Fig. 10.3).

10.8 Delayed Complications

The original goals of surgery may have not been achieved and now require reassessment for potential intervention. The risk profile of reoperation needs to be taken into account. Even if the carotid artery is sacrificed it still may present surgical challenges including packing, clips, and back bleeding that can be a significant concern. Furthermore, this also dramatically changes the risk profile to the contralateral ICA. If stenting was utilized, then anticoagulation/antiplatelet treatment needs to be paramount if additional operative interventions are considered.

10.8.1 Vasospasm

In ICA injury and manipulation of the vessel in addition to endovascular intervention, the potential for vasospasm is real and can lead to additional complications. Vasospasm can occur immediately upon ICA injury or in a delayed fashion.[37] Acute awareness of this and its delayed manifestations need to be noted as it should be considered on the differential if clinical decline occurs. In addition, any intracranial subarachnoid hemorrhage (SAH) that results in a major vascular injury should be treated in a similar fashion to aneurysmal SAH.

10.8.2 Pseudoaneurysm Formation/ Carotid-Cavernous Fistula

The most frequent complication following parasellar ICA injury/rupture is formation of a pseudoaneurysm, which is a tear through all the layers of the artery with contained flow into the surrounding tissue. In the context of iatrogenic injury and repair, the aneurysm is formed and maintained by the packing or external repair. It has been reported by Laws et al that this can be minimized by utilizing muscle as a direct covering that can allow for healing of the vessel.[37] Pseudoaneurysm can occur in a delayed fashion and may not be identified on acute imaging. Imaging intervals need to be set up to identify this potential complication and prompt treatment is warranted if identified. A typical timeline for repeat DSA would include ultra-early

(within 48 hours), early (within a week), and late (after 6 weeks). Rupture of a pseudoaneurysm can have disastrous outcomes and also require immediate control of the airway and bleeding control. This is subsequently treated with endovascular intervention or sacrifice. Carotid artery thrombosis can also occur in a delayed fashion with risk depending on the injury and interventions taken.

Any postoperative epistaxis mandates endoscopic examination of the nasal cavity. Similarly, an immediate angiogram is recommended if the patient is at potential risk of carotid blow out.

If bleeding of the ICA is contained within the cavernous sinus it can result in the formation of a carotid cavernous fistula (CCF). This is a rare occurrence and with close vascular follow up as well as aggressive treatment of pseudoaneurysms this late sequela is often prevented. The more relevant presentation is when an unnoticed carotid injury occurs during prior transsphenoidal surgery. Patients with a history of any transsphenoidal surgery or near exposure of the cavernous ICA should have CCF in the differential diagnosis. Typically, the presentation includes chemosis and proptosis and is treated with endovascular intervention.[38] Patients who undergo EES with skull base defects or exposure of the carotid arteries should be labeled as special patients who have oral or nasal instrumenting (i.e., nasogastric tubes, intubation, deep mucosal swabbing, etc.) only done by skull base/ENT teams.

10.9 Root Cause Analysis and Lessons Learned

10.9.1 Review of the Modern Literature (Search Strategy)

A systematic search of the PubMed/MEDLINE database was completed by utilizing PRISMA based criteria to assess the modern literature over the last 5 years to understand the recently published experience for ICA injury. Search terms were "carotid injury" and "endoscopic surgery"; only English-language articles were used. This resulted in 140 unique entries which were all reviewed for content by analyzing available abstracts. Those deemed not relevant were excluded based on criteria previously proposed.[39] A total of 22 published manuscripts were included for review that had available patient/intervention information (▶ Table 10.2).

AlQahtani et al report a case series with 28 cases collected across 11 centers. They identify anatomical considerations that are deemed to increase risk. These include dehiscent and prominent ICAs, invasive tumors, use of unfamiliar instruments, and lack of a multidisciplinary team. Overall, they conclude that ICA injury is associated with more than one risk factor and human error is a key element in a cascade leading to ICA injury.[26] Zhang et al reviewed a case series of 20 patients with mostly pituitary adenomas and chordomas. They developed a treatment algorithm related to endovascular management that showed a high preservation rate of 83.3% with the use of the Willis covered stent. This was compared to the previously reported rate of 20% with the Jostent graft in a single center experience. They also attribute the success of this series to the use of a hybrid OR that allows early endovascular diagnosis and treatment after local bleeding is controlled.[40]

Table 10.2 Systematic review of the modern literature for carotid injury and endoscopic surgery

Author Year	Type of study	Location of injury	Operative interventions	Endovascular management	Morbidity outcome	Case reported risk factors
AlQahtani 2020	Case series (11 centers) (n = 28/7160)	Parasellar ICA: 17 (61%) Paraclival ICA: 7 (25%) Parapharyngeal ICA: 2 (4%) Paraclinoid ICA: 2 (4%)	Packing: 10 (36%) Muscle patch: 15 (54%) Transcervical carotid ligation: 3 (11%)	Coil embolization: 14 (50%) Endovascular stenting: 6 (21%) No endovascular intervention: 8 (29%)	Survival without neurological deficits: 22 (78%), survival with neurological deficits: 3 (11%), postoperative MI:1 (4%), death in OR: 2 (7%)	Dehiscent ICA canal, bulging of the vessel, ICA displaced by the lesion, sphenoid septa with attachment to the ICA canal, distance between ICAs, vessel wall abnormality, tumor encasement, 6/28 (21%) cases were with a single surgeon
Safaee 2019	Case report (n = 1)	Cavernous ICA	Cottonoid	Coil embolization	No postoperative symptoms	Chondrosarcoma, cavernous sinus invasion
Wang 2019	Case series (n = 2)	Cavernous ICA	Bipolar electrocautery and muscle patch (longus capitis)	None	No postoperative deficits: 2/2	Complete tumor encasement, cavernous sinus invasion
Nariai 2019	Case report (n = 1)	Cavernous ICA	N/A	Pipeline stent placement	No postoperative deficits	Rathke's cleft cyst
Fastenberg 2019	Case report (n = 1)	Cavernous ICA	Packing, dural sealant and muscle	BTO followed by sacrifice with particle embolization	Basal ganglia ischemia without obvious long-term consequence, transient CN VI palsy	Cavernous sinus and sella invasion, superior and lateral displacement of the ICA Tumor encasement
Tang 2019	Case series on EES for nasopharyngeal carcinoma (n = 1/55)	N/A	N/A	Stenting	No postoperative deficits	Cavernous sinus invasion, tumor encasement
Nasi 2019	Case report (n = 1)	Cavernous ICA	N/A	Detachable balloon (removed 4 days later) + coils	No postoperative deficits	N/A
Lum 2019	Case report (n = 1)	Paraclival ICA	Sphenoid sinus packing	Stenting attempted—failed due to thrombosis, BTO, coil embolization	Multifocal watershed infarcts, right hemiparesis + expressive dysphagia (resolved at 12-week follow-up)	N/A
Zhang 2020	Single institution retrospective analysis of all EES cases (n = 20/3658)	N/A	Nasal packing: 20/20 (100%)	No: 9/20 Covered stent placement: 6/11 5/11: Parent artery occlusion	19/20: Outcome with mrs 3 or better 1/20: Death in OR	N/A
Giorgianni 2019	Case report (n = 1)	Cavernous ICA	Sphenoid sinus packing + Surgicel	BOT and flow diverter stent placement	No postoperative deficits	Cavernous sinus invasion, history of bromocriptine therapy
Wedemeyer 2019	Retrospective analysis of Rathke's cleft cyst operations (n = 1/112)	N/A	N/A	Coil embolization	No postoperative deficits	N/A

(Continued)

Table 10.2 (Continued) Systematic review of the modern literature for carotid injury and endoscopic surgery

Author Year	Type of study	Location of injury	Operative interventions	Endovascular management	Morbidity outcome	Case reported risk factors
Ryu 2018	Single center retrospective series of nasopharyngeal cancers (n = 1/9)	N/A	N/A	Coil embolization	No postoperative deficits	N/A
Duek 2017	Case report (n = 1)	Cavernous ICA	Cottonoid, Surgicel, muscle (temporalis muscle)	No	No postoperative deficits	N/A
Karadag 2017	Case report (n = 1)	Cavernous ICA	Nasal packing	Flow diverting stent	No postoperative deficits	Acromegaly with distortion of local anatomy and decreased distance between ICAs, cavernous sinus invasion and tumor encasement
Romero 2017	Single center retrospective analysis of all EES (n = 1/800)	Cavernous ICA	Nasal packing	BTO, coil embolization	No postoperative deficits	Carotid injury is a rarely encountered injury
Zoli 2018	Single center retrospective analysis of EES treated chordomas (n = 2/65)	N/A	N/A	Coil embolization: 2/2	No postoperative deficits	Chordomas in given location present additional risk
Zhang 2016	Retrospective case series performed by a single rhinologist (2/12797)	Parasellar ICA	Surgicel + Fascia lata muscle patch: 2/2 (100%)	No: 2/2	No postoperative deficits: 2/2	Additional risk when invasion of ICA wall by tumor
Chin 2016	Systematic literature review (190 articles) (n = 50)	Cavernous: 34/50 (68%) Ophthalmic: 3/50 (6%) Petrous: 2/50 (4%) Lacerum: 2/50 (4%) Clinoidal: 2/50 (4%) Unknown: 7/50 (14%)	Nasal packing (+/− crushed muscle or other hemostatic material): 36/56 (64%) Bipolar cautery: 4/56 (7%) Clip sacrifice: 4/56 (7%) (3 endoscopic) Unknown: 6/56 (11%)	Yes: 27/50, coil embolization or detachable balloon: 17/50	No postoperative deficits: 38/50 Transient neurologic deficits (gone at 3-month follow-up): 4 Permanent neurologic deficits: 1 Death: 2 Unknown: 5	The majority of patients were managed with a good outcome
Cobb 2015	Case report (n = 1)	Cavernous ICA	Gelfoam, Surgiseal, bipolar cautery, packing, muscle patch (hemostasis not achieved)	Temporary balloon occlusion to allow for suture	No postoperative deficits	Cavernous sinus invasion adds risk
Smith 2015	Single center retrospective analysis of ACTH secreting pituitary adenomas and silent corticotrophs (n = 1/82)	N/A	N/A	Coil embolization	No postoperative deficits	Acromegaly may add additional risk

(Continued)

Table 10.2 (Continued) Systematic review of the modern literature for carotid injury and endoscopic surgery

Author Year	Type of study	Location of injury	Operative interventions	Endovascular management	Morbidity outcome	Case reported risk factors
Padhye 2015	Retrospective multicenter analysis of patients who required endoscopic management of intranasal major arterial hemorrhage (n = 8/9)	Cavernous: 6/8 (75%) Paraclinoidal: 1/8 (13%) Paraclival: 1/8 (13%)	Tensor fascia lata muscle: 6/8 Temporalis muscle: 1/8 (13%) Rectus abdominis: 1/8(13%)	Endovascular stent: 2/8	No postoperative deficits: 6/8 Pseudoaneurysm requiring stenting: 1/8 Carotid dissection managed by observation: 1/8	Factors that add risk: Midlying carotid or carotid aneurysm: 3/8 Tumor encasement: 1/8 Dehiscent canal: 1/8
Mortimer 2015	Case series on management of pseudoaneurysm (n = 1)	Cavernous	Bipolar cautery, surgical packs	No	Pseudoaneurysm found on MRI 3 days postoperative treated with coil occlusion	Delayed injury manifestation still poses injury potential
UPMC case series 1998–2020	Injuries to the ICA from institutional case series (n = 18/3889)	Cavernous: 7/18 (39%) Paraclival: 5/18 (28%)	Bipolar cautery: 18/18 (100%) Aneurysm clips: 9/18 (50%) Packing: 9/18 (50%) Clipping or packing were combined with muscle patch: 6/18 (34%)	Angiogram without Intervention: 14/18 (78%) Coil embolization: 2/18 (11%) Stent placement: 1/18 (6%) Thrombectomy: 1/18 (6%)	At 1-month follow-up: Pseudoaneurysm formation: 3/18 (17%) No postoperative neurological deficit related to ICA injury: 12/18 (67%) Minor deficits: 4/18 (22%) Death: 2/18 (11%)	More difficult cases with invasive tumors and aggressive surgical plan have the highest risk. Bipolar cautery is the best salvage option with subsequent clip application. Successful ICA repair in the majority of cases with good outcomes

Abbreviations: ACTH, adrenocorticotropic hormone; BTO, balloon test occlusion; EES, endoscopic endonasal surgery; ICA, internal carotid artery; MRI, magnetic resonance imaging; N/A, information not available; OR, operating room; UPMC, University of Pittsburgh Medical Center; mrs, modified Rankin Scale.
Note: *Additional factors assayed but not consistently reported in the listed manuscripts include pharmacological management, prior surgery and prior radiation.

They identified radical resection of an adherent lesion with involvement of the ICA and lesions that require wide exposure to be high-risk cases for ICA injury. Chin et al reviewed 50 cases of ICA injury, with the cavernous segment representing the most common site of injury (68%) and pituitary adenoma and chondroid tumors representing the most common pathologies. The authors detail the various methods of bleeding control including packing, clip sacrifice, and bipolar coagulation.[39] Padhye et al reviewed nine cases with a surgical team trained in large vessel injury with a protocol in place. They report that an experienced team was able to control bleeding and have superior outcomes. This article describes the cavernous segment as the most frequently injured segment as well.[41]

The UPMC experience as outlined above shows a similar experience to that reported in the modern literature over the past 5 years. The cavernous segment was the most commonly injured, which likely reflects the sheer volume of transsphenoidal exposures compared to other segments of the ICA that are encountered with less frequency. Bipolar cautery was also reported to be a reasonable first attempt at repair with reports of success, followed by clipping and packing and ultimately endovascular intervention.

Overall, neurological outcomes were reported to be variable with the majority being good and death a rare event in the modern era. In the literature review of 76 patients, 5 mortalities were reported and 2 in the UPMC series. Mortality is likely underreported however, as this may be a deterrent to publication.

The additional single patient case reports in ▶ Table 10.2 further reinforce similar lessons with the cavernous segment being the most commonly injured site and intraoperative techniques proving successful at stopping bleeding with subsequent endovascular assessment/intervention. These case reports and series are subjected to publication bias as more injuries are likely to have occurred than what have been reported.

The overall theme, from reviewing the modern literature and our institution's case series, confirms that although ICA injury can occur in any endoscopic endonasal procedure, more aggressive tumors or more aggressive resection goals pose an elevated risk. A predefined strategy appears to be an important aspect for successful carotid injury repair and, if executed properly, can result in good outcomes in most cases. Devastating outcomes remain a distinct possibility and ICA injuries should be considered and discussed during preoperative planning and consent. Surprisingly, previously identified risk factors are absent in the modern literature, namely, prior radiation or the use of bromocriptine, while acromegaly was considered a risk factor in two case reports in the modern literature. With so few case reports and lack of standardization of reporting it is difficult to draw concrete conclusions. The underreporting of carotid injury during EES was recently highlighted in a study estimating that at least 20% of surgeons encountered such injury within a 12-month period of time. This was obtained via survey of experienced operators who had participated in the UPMC skull base course or as members of the Skull Base Congress.[7] It is clear that this topic requires extensive study and operators should be educated on its occurrence and management.

This chapter has attempted to distil the lessons learned from our own case series and those in the literature into a preoperative check list as well as an intraoperative management algorithm, which is the only consistently reported improvement in management (▶ Table 10.3). Any operator who encounters an ICA injury is encouraged to complete a root cause analysis exercise to leverage the event into a systematic learning experience (▶ Fig. 10.8).

Table 10.3 Preoperative check list and risk stratification considerations

- Surgical planning with vessel imaging (typically CTA and MRI) to identify risk factors for injury
- If considered high risk, digital subtraction angiography and balloon test occlusion (BTO) can be considered
- Preoperative risk stratification should include:
    - Results of BTO (if deemed necessary)
    - Age of patient
    - Comorbidities
    - Pathology
    - Tumor invasion and/or adherence
    - Surgical goal (resection for cure versus palliative debulking/decompression)
    - Adjuvant treatments available (radiation)

Preoperative planning

- Neuroendovascular team available on day of surgery
- Anesthesia:
    - Senior anesthesia team with EEA and complex case experience
    - Reliable IV access
    - Arterial access
    - Catheter angiogram access (femoral or radial access points)
    - Neck access for compression
    - Abdomen and thigh prep for fat, muscle, and/or facia
    - Blood products (4 units immediately available)
    - Pharmacological intervention (IC-Green, adenosine 0.3 mg/kg, vasoactive agents for blood pressure control)
- Technical adjuncts:
    - Image guidance system
    - Endonasal Doppler ultrasound probe
    - Neuro-electrophysiology (somatosensory evoked potentials)
- Preferred instruments:
    - Cautery device(s) (bipolar)
    - Two suction devices with an additional "back up" suction with independent source
    - Hemostatic agents (Surgicel, gelfoam, liquid/injectable gelfoam, novel agents)
    - Endoscopic vessel repair kit (clips and angled appliers) (▶ Fig. 10.6)
- Injury action plan:
    - See intraoperative algorithm (▶ Fig. 10.3)

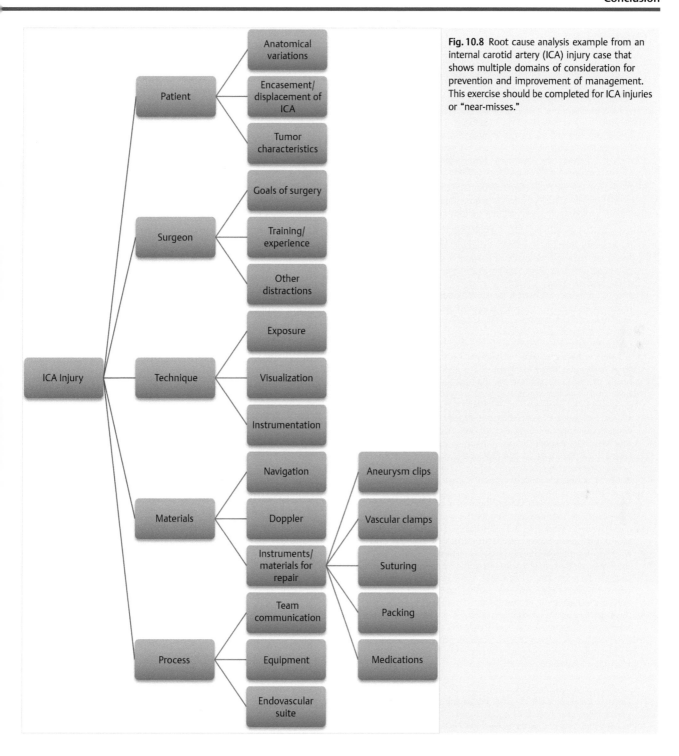

Fig. 10.8 Root cause analysis example from an internal carotid artery (ICA) injury case that shows multiple domains of consideration for prevention and improvement of management. This exercise should be completed for ICA injuries or "near-misses."

10.10 Conclusion

As the popularity of endoscopic endonasal techniques grows, surgeons should be well versed in management of ICA injuries. Careful preoperative planning, defined roles, team surgery, adequate instrumentation, and careful progression through the endonasal learning curve can all help to prevent or successfully manage such injuries. Check lists and algorithms should be reviewed and practiced in advance. Close clinical and radiologic monitoring of the patient is important to prevent early and late complications. These themes have been consistently reported in the literature and have improved outcomes.

References

[1] Snyderman C, Kassam A, Carrau R, Mintz A, Gardner P, Prevedello DM. Acquisition of surgical skills for endonasal skull base surgery: a training program. Laryngoscope. 2007; 117(4):699–705

[2] Padhye V, Murphy J, Bassiouni A, Valentine R, Wormald PJ. Endoscopic direct vessel closure in carotid artery injury. Int Forum Allergy Rhinol. 2015; 5(3):253–257

[3] Gardner PA, Tormenti MJ, Pant H, Fernandez-Miranda JC, Snyderman CH, Horowitz MB. Carotid artery injury during endoscopic endonasal skull base surgery: incidence and outcomes. Neurosurgery. 2013; 73(2) Suppl Operative:ons261–ons269, discussion ons269–ons270

[4] Valentine R, Wormald PJ. Carotid artery injury after endonasal surgery. Otolaryngol Clin North Am. 2011; 44(5):1059–1079

[5] Renn WH, Rhoton AL, Jr. Microsurgical anatomy of the sellar region. J Neurosurg. 1975; 43(3):288–298

[6] Inamasu J, Guiot BH. Iatrogenic carotid artery injury in neurosurgery. Neurosurg Rev. 2005; 28(4):239–247, discussion 248

[7] Rowan NR, Turner MT, Valappil B, et al. Injury of the carotid artery during endoscopic endonasal surgery: surveys of skull base surgeons. J Neurol Surg B Skull Base. 2018; 79(3):302–308

[8] Frank G, Sciarretta V, Calbucci F, Farneti G, Mazzatenta D, Pasquini E. The endoscopic transnasal transsphenoidal approach for the treatment of cranial base chordomas and chondrosarcomas. Neurosurgery. 2006; 59(1) Suppl 1:ONS50–ONS57, discussion ONS50–ONS57

[9] Gardner PA, Kassam AB, Snyderman CH, et al. Outcomes following endoscopic, expanded endonasal resection of suprasellar craniopharyngiomas: a case series. J Neurosurg. 2008; 109(1):6–16

[10] Lavigne P, Faden D, Gardner PA, Fernandez-Miranda JC, Wang EW, Snyderman CH. Validation of training levels in endoscopic endonasal surgery of the skull base. Laryngoscope. 2019; 129(10):2253–2257

[11] Alikhani P, Sivakanthan S, van Loveren H, Agazzi S. Paraclival or cavernous internal carotid artery: one segment but two names. J Neurol Surg B Skull Base. 2016; 77(4):304–307

[12] Rhoton AL, Jr. The cavernous sinus, the cavernous venous plexus, and the carotid collar. Neurosurgery. 2002; 51(4) Suppl:S375–S410

[13] Rhoton AL, Jr. The supratentorial arteries. Neurosurgery. 2002; 51(4) Suppl:S53–S120

[14] Bouthillier A, van Loveren HR, Keller JT. Segments of the internal carotid artery: a new classification. Neurosurgery. 1996; 38(3):425–432, discussion 432–433

[15] Gibo H, Lenkey C, Rhoton AL, Jr. Microsurgical anatomy of the supraclinoid portion of the internal carotid artery. J Neurosurg. 1981; 55(4):560–574

[16] Alfieri A, Jho HD. Endoscopic endonasal cavernous sinus surgery: an anatomic study. Neurosurgery. 2001; 48(4):827–836, discussion 836–837

[17] Labib MA, Prevedello DM, Carrau R, et al. A road map to the internal carotid artery in expanded endoscopic endonasal approaches to the ventral cranial base. Neurosurgery. 2014; 10 Suppl 3:448–471, discussion 471

[18] Cebral JR, Castro MA, Putman CM, Alperin N. Flow-area relationship in internal carotid and vertebral arteries. Physiol Meas. 2008; 29(5):585–594

[19] Mathis JM, Barr JD, Jungreis CA, et al. Temporary balloon test occlusion of the internal carotid artery: experience in 500 cases. AJNR Am J Neuroradiol. 1995; 16(4):749–754

[20] Gonzalez CF, Moret J. Balloon occlusion of the carotid artery prior to surgery for neck tumors. AJNR Am J Neuroradiol. 1990; 11(4):649–652

[21] Gibelli D, Cellina M, Gibelli S, et al. Relationship between sphenoid sinus volume and accessory septations: a 3D assessment of risky anatomical variants for endoscopic surgery. Anat Rec (Hoboken). 2020; 303(5):1300–1304

[22] Rhoton AL, Jr. The sellar region. Neurosurgery. 2002; 51(4) Suppl:S335–S374

[23] Fujii K, Chambers SM, Rhoton AL, Jr. Neurovascular relationships of the sphenoid sinus. A microsurgical study. J Neurosurg. 1979; 50(1):31–39

[24] Fernandez-Miranda JC, Prevedello DM, Madhok R, et al. Sphenoid septations and their relationship with internal carotid arteries: anatomical and radiological study. Laryngoscope. 2009; 119(10):1893–1896

[25] Hatam A, Greitz T. Ectasia of cerebral arteries in acromegaly. Acta Radiol Diagn (Stockh). 1972; 12(4):410–418

[26] AlQahtani A, London NR, Jr, Castelnuovo P, et al. Assessment of factors associated with internal carotid injury in expanded endoscopic endonasal skull base surgery. JAMA Otolaryngol Head Neck Surg. 2020; 146(4):364–372.

[27] Sivakumar W, Chamoun RB, Riva-Cambrin J, Salzman KL, Couldwell WT. Fusiform dilatation of the cavernous carotid artery in acromegalic patients. Acta Neurochir (Wien). 2013; 155(6):1077–1083, discussion 1083

[28] Pacca P, Jhawar SS, Seclen DV, et al. "Live cadaver" model for internal carotid artery injury simulation in endoscopic endonasal skull base surgery. Oper Neurosurg (Hagerstown). 2017; 13(6):732–738

[29] Raymond J, Hardy J, Czepko R, Roy D. Arterial injuries in transsphenoidal surgery for pituitary adenoma; the role of angiography and endovascular treatment. AJNR Am J Neuroradiol. 1997; 18(4):655–665

[30] AlQahtani A, Castelnuovo P, Nicolai P, Prevedello DM, Locatelli D, Carrau RL. Injury of the internal carotid artery during endoscopic skull base surgery: prevention and management protocol. Otolaryngol Clin North Am. 2016; 49(1):237–252

[31] Kassam A, Snyderman CH, Carrau RL, Gardner P, Mintz A. Endoneurosurgical hemostasis techniques: lessons learned from 400 cases. Neurosurg Focus. 2005; 19(1): E7.

[32] Padhye V, Valentine R, Paramasivan S, et al. Early and late complications of endoscopic hemostatic techniques following different carotid artery injury characteristics. Int Forum Allergy Rhinol. 2014; 4(8):651–657

[33] Fukushima T, Maroon JC. Repair of carotid artery perforations during transsphenoidal surgery. Surg Neurol. 1998; 50(2):174–177

[34] Fastenberg JH, Garzon-Muvdi T, Hsue V, et al. Adenosine-induced transient hypotension for carotid artery injury during endoscopic skull-base surgery: case report and review of the literature. Int Forum Allergy Rhinol. 2019; 9(9):1023–1029

[35] Bendok BR, Gupta DK, Rahme RJ, et al. Adenosine for temporary flow arrest during intracranial aneurysm surgery: a single-center retrospective review. Neurosurgery. 2011; 69(4):815–820, discussion 820–821

[36] Henry M, Amor M, Klonaris C, et al. Angioplasty and stenting of the extracranial carotid arteries. Tex Heart Inst J. 2000; 27(2):150–158

[37] Laws ER, Jr. Vascular complications of transsphenoidal surgery. Pituitary. 1999; 2(2):163–170

[38] Cossu G, Al-Taha K, Hajdu SD, Daniel RT, Messerer M. Carotid-cavernous fistula after transsphenoidal surgery: a rare but challenging complication. World Neurosurg. 2020; 134:221–227

[39] Chin OY, Ghosh R, Fang CH, Baredes S, Liu JK, Eloy JA. Internal carotid artery injury in endoscopic endonasal surgery: a systematic review. Laryngoscope. 2016; 126(3):582–590

[40] Zhang Y, Tian Z, Li C, et al. A modified endovascular treatment protocol for iatrogenic internal carotid artery injuries following endoscopic endonasal surgery. J Neurosurg. 2019; 132(2):343–350

[41] Padhye V, Valentine R, Sacks R, et al. Coping with catastrophe: the value of endoscopic vascular injury training. Int Forum Allergy Rhinol. 2015; 5(3):247–252

11 Dealing with Major Vascular Injuries During Endonasal Posterior Fossa Surgery

Pierre-Olivier Champagne, Thibault Passeri, Eduard Voormolen, Anne-Laure Bernat, Rosaria Abbritti, and Sébastien Froelich

Summary

Dealing with major vascular injury during endoscopic endonasal posterior fossa surgery can be fearsome and complex. This chapter gives an overview of the readiness, prevention, and surgical management of such instances.

Keywords: Posterior fossa, endoscopic endonasal surgery, vascular injury

11.1 Key Learning Points

- Dealing with major vessel injury during endonasal posterior fossa surgery can prove more complex than with a parasellar internal carotid artery (ICA) injury.
- Careful identification of high-risk cases helps prepare for a major vascular injury.
- Adequate exposure helps to prevent and control major vessel injury during endoscopic endonasal surgery.
- Applying pressure with a cottonoid on the site of bleeding is a good first step to gain initial control of the field and prepare for definitive control.
- Options for obtaining definitive control over an injury depend on many factors including intradural or extradural localization.

11.2 Introduction

Major vascular injury remains one of the most feared and dangerous complications in endoscopic endonasal surgery. Refinement of endoscopic endonasal surgery allowed expansion of these surgical approaches outside the sella. With new corridors and accessible anatomy came new risks, such as injury to major vascular structures other than the parasellar internal carotid arteries (ICAs). Major vascular injury to the posterior fossa can be particularly hazardous to manage endoscopically, due to the presence of perforators, highly eloquent neuronal tissue and nerves, and deep location. This chapter aims at providing an overview of the management of major vascular injury during endonasal posterior fossa surgery, with special attention to injury of paraclival ICAs, vertebrobasilar arteries, and their branches.

11.3 Preoperative Considerations

Being prepared to face a major vascular injury can make a significant difference in the outcome of said injury. The most important preoperative aspect resides in being able to recognize high-risk cases.[1,2,3] Proximity of the operated lesion to major vascular structures, ranging from simple contact to encasement and invasion, can significantly increase the risk of vascular injury and special attention should be paid to preoperative imaging (such as computed tomography [CT] angiogram) to assess the vascular relationships between the lesion and major vessels and anatomical variations. Previous surgery in the area can also increase vascular risk via scarring between the vessels and surrounding structures and also by giving the operator fewer anatomical landmarks to rely on during surgical approach. History of irradiation in the area can also heighten the risk of vascular injury via scarring and weakening of the vessel wall. Existing vascular conditions such as an aneurysm (or pseudoaneurysm) or visible vascular wall anomalies should also be considered significantly increased risk. All of those factors can be easily identified with careful examination of preoperative imaging and complete patient's past medical history.

Related pathologies presenting a risk for major vessel injury during endoscopic endonasal surgery to the posterior fossa include craniopharyngiomas (which usually puts at risk the posterior communicating arteries and perforators), chordomas and chondrosarcomas (which put at risk the vertebrobasilar complex and the cavernous ICA—in case of infiltration of the cavernous sinus), petrous apex lesions such as cholesterol granulomas (which put at risk mainly the paraclival ICAs), clival meningiomas, and petroclival (controversial for endoscopic endonasal approach [EEA]) meningiomas (which put at risk the vertebral basilar complex).

If a procedure is deemed high risk, for example, a multioperated lesion with previous irradiation, the vascular risk should be weighted in the risk-benefit assessment and depending on circumstances the decision could be either to not operate, choose another treatment strategy (radiation instead of surgery), choose another surgical approach, or transfer the case to a highly experienced team. In cases of high risk of paraclival ICA injury, a useful preoperative adjunct is to perform a balloon test occlusion (BTO). This test can predict to a certain degree if sacrifice of the ICA will lead to a stroke. However, BTO should be done by an experienced endovascular team with rigorous criteria. BTO of the vertebral arteries can also be performed, although it is by far less often used.[4] It can be performed in those cases with very highly asymmetric vertebral arteries, when the dominant one is involved or in case of absence of communication between the contralateral vertebral artery and the vertebrobasilar junction.[5,6]

Right before surgery for high-risk cases, the proper equipment (such as an adequate bipolar, endoscopic clips and single shaft clip appliers) should be available in the room and both the nursing team and anesthesiology team should be aware of the risk and should prepare accordingly by having blood products and extra suctions ready. In case of high risk of vascular injury, the neurointerventional team should also be aware and prepared. In the best scenario, the surgical team discuss in advance the possibility of a major vascular injury and a plan of action is already defined together with the neurointerventional team in the event of said injury.

11.4 Surgical Avoidance of Injury

The best way to manage major vascular injury in endoscopic endonasal surgery (EES) is to avoid them. A major aspect resides in localizing the high-risk vessel and working zone. Depending on various factors such as patient's anatomy (e.g., sphenoid sinus pneumatization), tumor extent, and scarring, major vessels might be hard to visualize from the start. In these instances, relying on adjuncts such as image guidance (CT angiography, magnetic resonance imaging [MRI], and merged images) and Doppler ultrasound is paramount to help localize the vessels. These adjuncts, combined with in-depth study of preoperative imaging and careful, stepwise dissection technique, help minimize the risk of intraoperative injury.

Another important aspect is the degree of aggressiveness of lesion dissection from vessels. Depending on intrinsic factors such as tumor texture and vessel frailty, some small piece of tumor should be left on the vessel if its dissection is deemed too dangerous. Dissection of tumor from any vessel should be done as much as possible in a bimanual fashion using the same microsurgical principles as in open surgery in a clear field with maximal visualization of the vessel. One of the worst-case scenarios is a major vascular injury in the context of minimal access to it. To prevent this, potentially dangerous maneuvers on vessels should be performed once maximal safe exposure has been obtained, either through tumor resection and/or bony removal. The extent of exposure obtained should ideally allow for proximal and distal control of the involved vessel with aneurysm clips. When dealing with anterior circulation vessels, having paraclival carotids exposed for proximal control can prove useful. Ease of paraclival ICA exposure also greatly depends on the patient's sinus pneumatization and has to be taken into consideration. Unfortunately, for posterior circulation vessels, early access to the vertebrobasilar might prove more arduous due to their inferior intradural localization. It is also important to remember that around a fragile vessel, almost any instrument has the potential to cause an injury and dissection should always be carried out with the utmost care. A pure diamond drill burr with continuous irrigation is recommended when removing bone over the cavernous ICA, and when using a Kerrison rongeur to remove the remaining thin shell of bone, care must be taken to be subperiosteal with the foot of the instrument and to constantly keep a close view of the side of the instruments while closing. Sharper instruments such as scissors and retractable blade pose a higher risk of injury, especially if not inserted under direct visualization. For dissection of the tumor away from the tumor or vessel away from the tumor, gentle repetitive strokes with a blunt suction will often be more than enough to safely resect tumor in contact with a vessel. For more adherent tumor, sharp dissection using a suction for counter-traction and scissors will also be useful, although bearing more risk for injury. Very gentle manipulation of calcified tumor lying next or around a major vessel without traction is mandatory in order to avoid direct vessel injury or avulsion of small collaterals embedded into the bloc (especially for highly calcified chondrosarcomas). ▶ Fig. 11.1 illustrates a case of an endoscopic endonasal removal of a clival chordoma adherent to the basilar artery and its branches, exemplifying the aforementioned principles.

11.5 Surgical Management

In the event of a major vascular injury, one of the first steps is letting everyone know it happened as fast and as clearly as possible. The anesthesiology team should expect intense and prolonged blood loss and act accordingly, scrub personnel directly assisting the surgeon should devote all of their attention to the procedure and instruments request, and circulating personnel should bring aneurysm clips if not already in the room. It is important to remember that an operator's hasty and disorganized reaction to a major bleeding can sometimes cause more harm than the bleeding itself. In that regard, it is of upmost importance to remain as calm as possible. Adequate preparation and good communication with operating room personnel help to diminish the stress associated with such events. Help from another experienced surgeon, if available, should also be sought immediately. Having another operator can help to delegate the tasks, share the burden, and elaborate solutions. The additional surgeon can also drive the endoscope and bring cottonoid or hemostatic agent into the field while the operator is controlling the bleeding with tamponade and using his or her two hands. This can prove invaluable especially for less experienced surgeons.

11.5.1 Bleeding Localization and Control

Like in any bleed, the first step is to localize it. Bringing a cottonoid into the field and applying it with a suction at the site of the injury with enough pressure to stop the bleeding is a good way to do so. However, in case of intradural injury, pressure on the vessel should also be carefully applied in order not to damage the brainstem or cranial nerves behind it.

In case of a major bleeding, a significant volume of Surgicel, cottonoids, or other packing may have been applied for tamponade to control it. In this case it is more difficult to get perception of the amount of pressure on the surrounding structures which are hidden by the packing. These should be progressively taken out in order to locate the bleeding source and reapply the smallest possible Surgicel and/or cottonoid over it. Depending on the amount of bleeding, another surgeon holding/driving the endoscope and a second suction can be helpful to help take control of the field.

The "chopstick technique" used by the senior author can also be used and allows for bimanual manipulation with a single operator holding both the endoscope and the instruments.[7] One of the main advantages of the chopstick is to have no sword conflict with the endoscope and to allow for a very short distance between the tip of the endoscope and the tip of the instruments. The very close view of the tip of the instruments allows a precise control of the movements of the instruments and reduces the two-dimensional effect of the endoscope. The close view of the tip of the instruments also helps to reduce the risk of injury.

Once control is taken, this allows time to reassess the situation and surroundings. At that moment the following questions should be answered: Is the injury intradural or extradural? Can this vessel be safely sacrificed? What are the proximal and distal control options for the injured vessel?

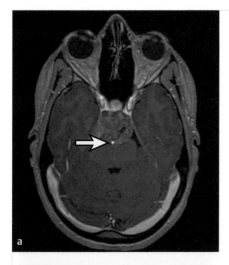

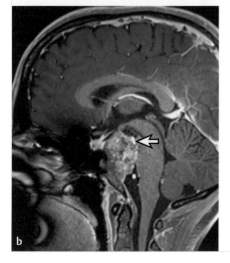

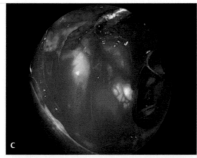

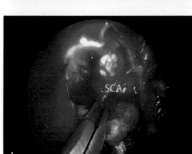

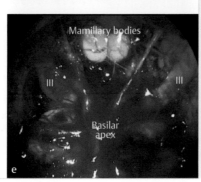

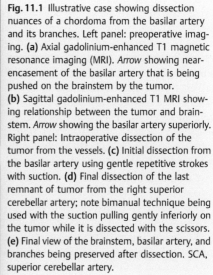

Fig. 11.1 Illustrative case showing dissection nuances of a chordoma from the basilar artery and its branches. Left panel: preoperative imaging. **(a)** Axial gadolinium-enhanced T1 magnetic resonance imaging (MRI). *Arrow* showing near-encasement of the basilar artery that is being pushed on the brainstem by the tumor. **(b)** Sagittal gadolinium-enhanced T1 MRI showing relationship between the tumor and brainstem. *Arrow* showing the basilar artery superiorly. Right panel: Intraoperative dissection of the tumor from the vessels. **(c)** Initial dissection from the basilar artery using gentle repetitive strokes with suction. **(d)** Final dissection of the last remnant of tumor from the right superior cerebellar artery; note bimanual technique being used with the suction pulling gently inferiorly on the tumor while it is dissected with the scissors. **(e)** Final view of the brainstem, basilar artery, and branches being preserved after dissection. SCA, superior cerebellar artery.

Regardless of whether bleeding is of intradural or extradural origin, adequate visualization of the injured vessel is essential to help gain more definitive hemostasis. Although this can be challenging since the operator has to keep control over the bleeding while exposing the proximal and distal parts of the vessel, it should be attempted by either removing additional bone (e.g., exposing more proximal paraclival ICA), removing tumor, or dissecting arachnoid membranes. The goal is to visualize properly the site of injury and to have enough access proximally and distally to be able to occlude the vessel if needed. If potentially dangerous vessel dissection was kept for the end, this step is usually already done and proper visualization of the vessel and the injury is already obtained.

11.5.2 Extradural Bleeding

Major vascular injury management is different if it is present intradurally or extradurally. During EEA to the posterior fossa, the extradural vessels most at risk are the paraclival ICAs. The management of paraclival ICA injury follows the usual principles of ICA injury, which is the most commonly injured major vessel during EES and the injury on which the most literature has been written.[8] After gaining control of the field and proper exposure, a nonocclusive hemostatic method should be

attempted. In cases of smaller injury, bipolar electrocautery on low setting can be attempted to close the vessel wall defect without occluding the vessel itself. The other preferred method is the application of a tangential clip to close the opening. During these attempts, significant blood loss should be expected and keeping contact with the anesthesiology team to ensure that resuscitation keeps up with the blood loss is paramount. To help visualize the defect, intravenous adenosine can be used to temporally arrest circulation.[9] Perfect coordination with the anesthesiology team is essential in order to arrest the flow only when the operator is ready to place the clip, maximizing the time during which the field will be free of blood.

If these maneuvers prove unsuccessful, local tamponade of the defect to stop the bleeding should be the next option. Sacrifice of the vessel should be considered only if a previous BTO was performed, confirming that sacrifice of the vessel is safe, or if no other option is available to control an ongoing bleeding putting the patient's life at risk. Various materials have been reported for local tamponade, with cottonoid (gauze) being the most widely used, mainly because of its availability.[2] Other reported materials include Teflon,[10] crushed muscle,[11,12,13] Gelfoam, and oxidized cellulose.[13,14,15] One disadvantage of cottonoids is that they do not resorb and could promote infection if left in place. In that regard biocompatible and resorbable agents or autologous materials are better. Muscle has the advantages of good biocompatibility and crushing it could promote local blood clot formation via the release of calcium.[16,17] The main disadvantage of muscle resides in the fact that it must be harvested while keeping control over the injury. A possible tactic is to have one operator harvest the muscle as soon as the injury occurs while the others either compress the injury with a cottonoid or try other hemostatic methods. Muscle access should be anticipated during the preparation of the surgical field and draping. Common sites for muscle harvesting include the thigh and the temporalis muscle (which is closer to the nose). Regardless of the agent, the goal of local tamponade should be to stop the bleeding without occluding the vessel.[18] However, vessel occlusion is not uncommon and even sometimes unavoidable.[11,18,19]

Other methods of vessel control have also been reported, such as the direct closure of the vessel using a Sundt-type clip.[18] A combination of the aforementioned techniques can also be used. For example, if a clip managed to significantly reduce the blood flow from the injury, adding some gentle local packing on the remaining bleeding might help to gain complete hemostasis.

If despite all of these maneuvers the bleeding is still ongoing, packing to control the bleeding as much as possible should be performed and emergent measures to bring the patient to the angiography suite to occlude the vessel should be taken.[14,20]

11.5.3 Intradural Bleeding

Management of intradural injury to major arteries in the posterior fossa such as the vertebrobasilar arteries and their branches differs in some aspect from extradural injury. First, blood extravasation can result in significant subarachnoid hemorrhage. Keeping this in mind, suctioning the outgoing blood is even more important in the event of an intradural injury. Another particularity is that most of these vessels, the basilar artery in particular, cannot be sacrificed without risking a significant posterior circulation stroke.[21] In the context of basilar artery injury, every effort must be made to preserve the vessel. The presence of surrounding nervous structures such as the brainstem and cranial nerves can also make surgical control of the bleeding much more arduous. Packing over the vessel can also be much more difficult, since pressure from packing can damage surrounding nervous structures and there is no bony buttress against which the vessel can be tucked. A large amount of packing can not only harm surrounding structures but also prevent adequate skull base defect reconstruction, leading almost inevitably to cerebrospinal fluid (CSF) leak.

Once control is achieved, in most instances the procedure has to be stopped. If a prompt and nonocclusive control has been achieved, for example, with a tangential clip over a paraclival ICA in a patient who suffered acceptable blood loss, continuation of the surgery can be considered. This decision requires a deep understanding of the risks and benefits of pursuing the surgery (▶ Fig. 11.2).

11.6 Closure and Reconstruction

Closure and reconstruction options will vary according to the type of vascular control achieved, material used, and degree of dural opening. Depending on which material has been used to control bleeding (clip or resorbable material), the planned reconstruction technique for the case may vary. Having tissue covering over exposed ICAs should also be kept in mind. Protruding clips can also erode through tissues used for reconstruction. In these cases, using fat to increase the distance between the clip tip and the layers of covering material can help to prevent this. Filling the sphenoid sinus and covering it with a nasoseptal flap (NSF) after having removed the mucosa is also an option to prevent erosion from a clip protruding into the sphenoid sinus. If nonresorbable material such as a cottonoid has been left in place in a definitive fashion, it should be covered by a vascularized flap to separate it from the nasal cavity. If a cottonoid is left in place with the plan to remove it, reconstruction can be delayed after definitive control (endovascular occlusion) is gained. In these cases, depending on the urgency to go to the angio suite, the coverage can span from oxidized cellulose and cottonoid or fat to a septal flap if it is readily available. In cases of major bleeding requiring emergent endovascular treatment, an early second look surgery (either immediately after or the day after) is usually required.

11.7 Postoperative Management

Postoperative management essentially revolves around avoiding complications related to the injury, such as pseudoaneurysm formation, stroke, rebleeding, and the consequences of subarachnoid hemorrhage such as hydrocephalus and vasospasm.

A systematic immediate postoperative angiogram (digital subtraction angiography [DSA]) should be performed after any endoscopic endonasal major vessel injury, preferably with the patient still under general anesthesia. The goals are multiple: assessment of blood flow distal to the injury, assessment of injured vessel patency (occlusion or stenosis), and eliminating any ongoing blood extravasation or the formation of early pseudoaneurysm. With the patient still under general anesthesia, necessary interventional techniques can be performed. Active extravasation can be treated with occlusion of the vessel (preferably with a BTO showing good collateral circulation and no repercussion on neuromonitoring if available), flow diversion, covered stent, or glue/coil embolization (with or without stent) if a pseudoaneurysm is present. Significant stenosis, if thought to impact on distal blood flow, can be treated with stenting or balloon angioplasty.

A follow-up angiogram (or CT angiogram) should be performed within a week after the injury and at 1 month and 6 months, to rule out the formation of a pseudoaneurysm.

If intradural bleeding occurred, leading to subarachnoid bleeding, an immediate CT scan should also be obtained to evaluate the extent of subarachnoid hemorrhage and potential ventricular dilatation. The potential for vasospasm should also be kept in mind in those patients. In case of massive subarachnoid hemorrhage, the use of stents requiring antiplatelet therapy should be avoided if possible as it may complicate the management of any subsequent hydrocephalus with external ventricular drain (EVD) placement.

If nonabsorbable material such as cottonoid has been used for packing, the question of when and if at all it should be removed remains controversial and understudied. Although the retained material poses a risk of infection, it should be weighed

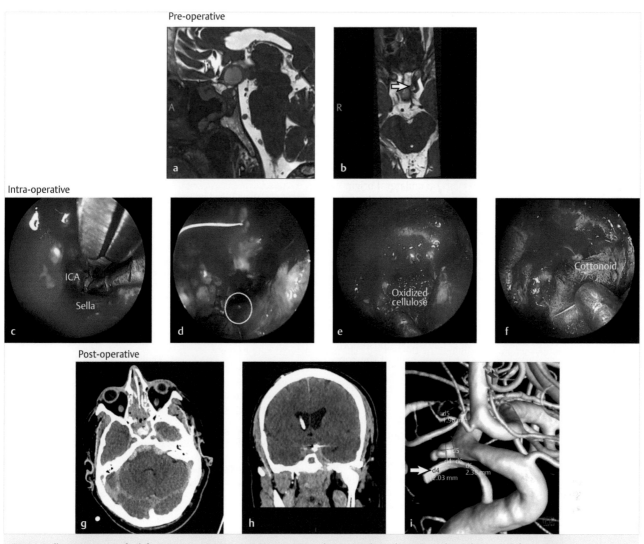

Fig. 11.2 Illustrative case of a left posterior communicating artery injury during a redo endoscopic endonasal approach for a recurrent craniopharyngioma. **(a, b)** Preoperative imaging showing the recurrent cystic component as well as the left posterior communicating artery passing in front of the cyst (*arrow*), making it at high risk of injury during cyst opening. **(c–f)** Intraoperative management of the injury. **(c)** Scissors inadvertently injured the posterior communicating artery while attempting to fenestrate the cyst. **(d)** Initial control of the field with the suction. Circle represents the site of ongoing blood flow. **(e)** First layer of local packing with oxidized cellulose. **(f)** Second layer of packing with cottonoid, achieving final hemostasis. **(g)** Postoperative computed tomography (CT) scan showing local blood clot as well as diffuse subarachnoid hemorrhage. **(h)** Ventricular dilatation with external ventricular drainage in place. **(i)** Immediate postoperative angiogram showing a pseudoaneurysm at the end of the injured vessel, which was embolized. *Arrow* showing cottonoid left in place.

against the risk of rebleeding when removing it. If endovascular treatment (such as occlusion of the vessel) has been added, the risk of bleeding is lower and should favor reintervention for removal of the foreign body. However, in the presence of a fragile vessel with poor proximal and distal control, it might be wiser to leave the foreign body in place. If a decision to re-explore and remove is made it is best to go back in the first couple of days to avoid scarring and adherences as much as possible.

11.8 Illustrative Case (▶ Fig. 11.2)

A 57-year-old man presented with a suprasellar cystic recurrence of a craniopharyngioma following a first endoscopic endonasal removal 5 months prior. Neurological examination revealed new significant bitemporal vision loss secondary to chiasmatic compression. The decision was made to reintervene via the same corridor with the goal of surgery being to decompress the cyst to relieve symptoms and allow radiation therapy. Injury to the left posterior communicating artery occurred when attempting to fenestrate the cyst with scissors. Risk factors pertaining to this case include fibrosis and adherence due to previous surgery as well as medial displacement of the posterior communicating artery by the tumor. One of the main reasons the injury happened is because the vessel was displaced medially and splayed on the cyst's surface; it was mistaken for a part of the cyst wall when trying to fenestrate it with the scissors. Control was achieved using local compression with oxidized cellulose and a single cottonoid which was left in place.

The previous NSF was used for closure in a single layer, covering completely the defect and cottonoid. Immediate postoperative catheter-based angiogram revealed no filling of the vessel with adequate retrograde filling of the perforators coming from the distal posterior communicating artery. A pseudoaneurysm at the proximal end of the occluded vessel was treated using coils. Significant subarachnoid hemorrhage leading to ventricular dilatation mandated the placement of a temporary EVD. The patient recovered with no new neurological deficit and the cyst was drained a month later via a supraorbital approach.

11.8.1 Management Analysis and Root Cause Analysis of the Presented Case

Management of the bleeding in the above case was done according to the aforementioned principles. After localizing the bleeding with a single cotton and a suction, some dissection was attempted to improve visualization, confirming the bleeding to be from the posterior communicating artery instead of the ICA. After attempts at clipping, final control was achieved with local compression. This was immediately followed by a postoperative angiogram and placement of an EVD.

A combination of factors contributed to the injury. These included: patient's factors (recurrent tumor, aberrant anatomy), surgical strategy (limited exposure), and operator factors (a trainee performed the surgery). Careful analysis of these factors can lead to recognition in the future.

11.9 Conclusion

Major vascular injuries during endonasal posterior fossa surgery represent highly challenging situations. Often, especially when dealing with an intradural injury, vessel sacrifice is not possible without causing significant neurological damage. Due to the presence of perforator arteries to the brainstem, the deep location, and the presence of surrounding critical neurological structures, dealing with intradural posterior fossa vascular injury can be treacherous. The risk and consequences of vascular injury must be considered in surgical decision-making when considering EEA to the posterior fossa and must be weighted in regard to the surgical team's degree of comfort in managing them.

References

[1] Snyderman CH, Fernandez-Miranda J, Gardner PA. Training in neurorhinology: the impact of case volume on the learning curve. Otolaryngol Clin North Am. 2011; 44(5):1223–1228

[2] Valentine R, Wormald PJ. Carotid artery injury after endonasal surgery. Otolaryngol Clin North Am. 2011; 44(5):1059–1079

[3] AlQahtani A, Castelnuovo P, Nicolai P, Prevedello DM, Locatelli D, Carrau RL. Injury of the internal carotid artery during endoscopic skull base surgery: prevention and management protocol. Otolaryngol Clin North Am. 2016; 49(1):237–252

[4] Guimaraens L, Cuellar H, Sola T, Vivas E. Temporary balloon occlusion test of the left vertebral artery using parenchymography as tolerance predictor. A case report. Neuroradiol J. 2008; 21(1):115–119

[5] Sorteberg A, Bakke SJ, Boysen M, Sorteberg W. Angiographic balloon test occlusion and therapeutic sacrifice of major arteries to the brain. Neurosurgery. 2008; 63(4):651–660, 660–661

[6] Zoarski GH, Seth R. Safety of unilateral endovascular occlusion of the cervical segment of the vertebral artery without antecedent balloon test occlusion. AJNR Am J Neuroradiol. 2014; 35(5):856–861

[7] Labidi M, Watanabe K, Hanakita S, et al. The chopsticks technique for endoscopic endonasal surgery—improving surgical efficiency and reducing the surgical footprint. World Neurosurg. 2018; 117:208–220

[8] Rowan NR, Turner MT, Valappil B, et al. Injury of the carotid artery during endoscopic endonasal surgery: surveys of skull base surgeons. J Neurol Surg B Skull Base. 2018; 79(3):302–308

[9] Fastenberg JH, Garzon-Muvdi T, Hsue V, et al. Adenosine-induced transient hypotension for carotid artery injury during endoscopic skull-base surgery: case report and review of the literature. Int Forum Allergy Rhinol. 2019; 9(9):1023–1029

[10] Fukushima T, Maroon JC. Repair of carotid artery perforations during transsphenoidal surgery. Surg Neurol. 1998; 50(2):174–177

[11] Raymond J, Hardy J, Czepko R, Roy D. Arterial injuries in transsphenoidal surgery for pituitary adenoma; the role of angiography and endovascular treatment. AJNR Am J Neuroradiol. 1997; 18(4):655–665

[12] Weidenbecher M, Huk WJ, Iro H. Internal carotid artery injury during functional endoscopic sinus surgery and its management. Eur Arch Otorhinolaryngol. 2005; 262(8):640–645

[13] Ahuja A, Guterman LR, Hopkins LN. Carotid cavernous fistula and false aneurysm of the cavernous carotid artery: complications of transsphenoidal surgery. Neurosurgery. 1992; 31(4):774–778, discussion 778–779

[14] Biswas D, Daudia A, Jones NS, McConachie NS. Profuse epistaxis following sphenoid surgery: a ruptured carotid artery pseudoaneurysm and its management. J Laryngol Otol. 2009; 123(6):692–694

[15] Dolenc VV, Lipovsek M, Slokan S. Traumatic aneurysm and carotid-cavernous fistula following transsphenoidal approach to a pituitary adenoma: treatment by transcranial operation. Br J Neurosurg. 1999; 13(2):185–188

[16] Gardner PA, Snyderman CH, Fernandez-Miranda JC, Jankowitz BT. Management of major vascular injury during endoscopic endonasal skull base surgery. Otolaryngol Clin North Am. 2016; 49(3):819–828

[17] Padhye V, Valentine R, Paramasivan S, et al. Early and late complications of endoscopic hemostatic techniques following different carotid artery injury characteristics. Int Forum Allergy Rhinol. 2014; 4(8):651–657

[18] Laws ER, Jr. Vascular complications of transsphenoidal surgery. Pituitary. 1999; 2(2):163–170

[19] Oskouian RJ, Kelly DF, Laws ERJ, Jr. Vascular injury and transsphenoidal surgery. Front Horm Res. 2006; 34:256–278

[20] Kocer N, Kizilkilic O, Albayram S, Adaletli I, Kantarci F, Islak C. Treatment of iatrogenic internal carotid artery laceration and carotid cavernous fistula with endovascular stent-graft placement. AJNR Am J Neuroradiol. 2002; 23(3):442–446

[21] Mattle HP, Arnold M, Lindsberg PJ, Schonewille WJ, Schroth G. Basilar artery occlusion. Lancet Neurol. 2011; 10(11):1002–1014

12 Vascular Challenges in Anterior Skull Base Open Surgery

Vinayak Narayan and Anil Nanda

Summary

A variety of standard microsurgical approaches and techniques have been developed over decades to deal with anterior skull base pathologies. The most feared complication of anterior cranial base surgery is vascular injury and its consequences. This chapter provides an overview of relevant surgical anatomy of the anterior skull base, common anterior, and anterolateral skull base approaches, pathologies involving anterior cranial base vasculature, relevant vascular challenges, common vascular complications, and microsurgical techniques to avoid such complications.

Keywords: Vascular, skull base, anterior, complications, tumor

I profess to learn and to teach anatomy not from books but from dissections, not from the tenets of philosophers but from the fabric of nature.

William Harvey (De Motu Cordis, 1628)

12.1 Key Learning Points

- Among the various microsurgical approaches, the common approaches which help in the surgical management of anterior cranial base lesions are transbasal, frontotemporal, and transsphenoidal approaches.
- Vascular complications are the most feared complications in anterior skull base surgery and include both arterial and venous (channels/sinus) complications.
- Vascular complications may manifest via hemorrhage, vasospasm, embolism or thrombosis, pseudoaneurysm, or vessel stenosis.
- The selection of the ideal approach is the most crucial step in anterior skull base surgery.
- The anterior cerebral artery (ACA), its branches, and the anterior communicating artery (AComA) complex are often involved in anterior skull base and suprasellar tumors.
- The incidence of internal carotid artery (ICA) injury during transsphenoidal surgery varies from 0.2 to 2%.
- Anatomic proximity, tumor infiltration, surgical error, prior radiotherapy, inadequate preoperative imaging or interventions like cerebral angiogram or embolization, and suboptimal use of neurosurgical adjuncts such as neuronavigation or micro-Doppler are common reasons for vascular injury.
- The indications for surgery should be clear, surgical strategies must be tailored according to the pathology, and goals of surgery well-defined.
- Avoiding direct injury to the brain and vessels involves the use of surgical adjuncts, adequate exposure via skull base approach, minimal brain retraction, and optimum brain relaxation.
- Internal debulking of tumor and bimanual, extracapsular dissection are among the most important microneurosurgical techniques to avoid devastating vascular complications.
- Careful patient selection, meticulous preoperative planning, proper understanding of the regional anatomy, firsthand radiological knowledge of anatomical variations, safe handling of critical neurovascular structures, intraoperative anticipation of vascular injury, and strict postoperative surveillance are the keys to avoid such complications and achieve the best overall outcome.

12.2 Introduction

Skull base approaches are designed to expose and treat complex skull base pathologies optimally while reducing the extent of retraction and manipulation of normal neurovascular structures. A complete understanding of the complex vascular anatomy of the anterior skull base is crucial prior to attempting surgical treatment of any vascular or skull base pathologies in this region. The anterior approaches to the skull base include transsphenoidal, transbasal or extended transbasal, transmaxillary or extended transmaxillary, and transoral approaches. The anterolateral approaches include frontotemporal orbitozygomatic, subtemporal transzygomatic and preauricular subtemporal-infratemporal approaches. The major complications arising out of skull base surgeries are vascular injury, cranial nerve injury, brainstem damage, cerebrospinal fluid (CSF) leak, and varying extent of cosmetic deformity among which vascular complications might be the most dreadful nightmare for a neurosurgeon. In this chapter we focus on the vascular challenges which can be encountered while performing an anterior skull base open surgery and the techniques to prevent it.

12.3 Surgical Vascular Anatomy of Anterior Cranial Base

The anterior cranial base is formed by ethmoid, sphenoid, and frontal bones. It has endocranial and exocranial surfaces which are connected by canals and foramina, through which numerous vascular structures pass. The anterior cranial fossa faces the frontal lobes with gyri recti medially and the orbital gyri laterally, along with the branches of the anterior cerebral arteries (ACAs) medially and middle cerebral arteries laterally.[1] Another set of vessels traversing the anterior cranial base are anterior and posterior ethmoidal arteries, supraorbital arteries, and supratrochlear arteries through the anterior and posterior ethmoidal foramina, supraorbital foramen, and supratrochlear foramen, respectively. The optic canal transmits the ophthalmic artery along with the optic nerve. The main arterial supply to the orbit is the ophthalmic artery. The wide collateralization network of ophthalmic artery makes its sacrifice well tolerated in most situations as long as the collateral vessels are intact. These collateral vessels include leptomeningeal collaterals, duro-arteriolar collaterals, and periventricular collaterals commonly arising from anterior ethmoidal, posterior ethmoidal, and lacrimal arteries.[2] The collateralization is also enhanced by the orbital plexus linking the ophthalmic artery with facial, middle meningeal, and maxillary arteries and the rete mirabile caroticum connecting internal and external carotid arteries.[3]

The main venous drainage of the orbit is through the superior and inferior ophthalmic veins. The intracranial view of the anatomical bony landmarks of the anterior cranial base is demonstrated in ▶ Fig. 12.1. The sellar region is very much related to the main trunk and early branches of internal carotid artery (ICA). The distance separating the medial margin of the carotid artery and the lateral surface of the pituitary gland is an important consideration in anterior cranial base approaches (transsphenoidal surgery).[4] The distance between the gland and artery varies from 1 to 7 mm (average, 2.3 mm). The intercarotid distance between cavernous carotid arteries is 15 to 17 mm in normal individuals and increases from 20 to 22 mm in patients with pituitary adenoma.[3,4,5]

The perforating branches of the ACA include the recurrent artery of Heubner (RAH) and subcallosal-hypothalamic perforating branches, while the cortical branches include fronto-orbital artery (FOA) and frontopolar artery (FPA). Its anatomical course and variations are particularly relevant when performing microsurgical resection of meningiomas located at tuberculum sellae, planum sphenoidale, and olfactory groove. The FOA is the first cortical branch of the ACA, typically arising within the first 5 to 10 mm of the A2 segment, and runs along the orbital surface of the frontal lobe to supply the olfactory bulb and tract, gyrus rectus, and orbital gyri, while the FPA is the second cortical branch, larger in diameter, and courses in the interhemispheric fissure to supply the medial and ventral surfaces of the frontal pole.[5] The FOA is related to the olfactory tract and sulcus while the FPA relates to the interhemispheric fissure. A normal anterior communicating artery (AComA) could be defined as an anastomosis between the left and right ACA through a single lumen. Najera et al report the location of AComA above the anterior half of the optic chiasm in 20% of cases, an anatomic variation that could increase the risk of vascular injury.[5] The authors also mention the origin of RAH within 5 mm of the AComA in most cases. RAH could be encountered anterior to the A1 segment in almost half of the cases, while in the remaining the RAH may be positioned above or behind the A1 segment.[5]

In the endocranial surface of the anterior cranial base, the foramen caecum in the midline provides the passage of the emissary vein.[1] The inferior frontal veins drain the orbital surface of the frontal lobe. They are mainly divided into two groups—anterior group and posterior group. The anterior group veins take their course toward the frontal pole and empty into the superior sagittal sinus. The anterior veins comprise both anterior orbitofrontal and frontopolar veins. The posterior group drains to join the veins at the medial part of the sylvian fissure which later converge on the anterior perforated substance to form the basal vein. The posterior group comprises the olfactory and posterior orbitofrontal veins. The inferior frontal veins and the areas they drain are as follows: the anterior orbitofrontal vein drains the anterior part of the gyrus rectus and the anteromedial part of the orbital gyri, the posterior orbitofrontal veins drain the posterior portion of the orbital surface of the frontal lobe, and the olfactory vein drains the olfactory sulcus

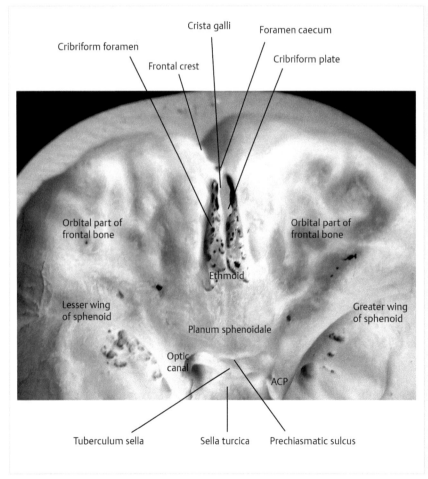

Fig. 12.1 Image demonstrating the overview of bony landmarks of anterior cranial base (intracranial view). ACP, anterior clinoid process.

and the adjacent part of the gyrus rectus and medial orbital gyri.[6] The cavernous sinuses are located on either side of the sphenoid sinus, sella, and pituitary gland.[4] Venous sinuses that interconnect the paired cavernous sinuses may be found in the margins of the diaphragma and around the gland and termed anterior/posterior intercavernous sinus based on location. If both anterior and posterior intercavernous sinuses coexist, they together constitute the circular sinus.[4]

12.4 Pathologies Involving Anterior Cranial Base, Surgical Approaches, and Associated Vascular Challenges

A large spectrum of neurosurgical disorders affects the anterior cranial base. The common pathologies affecting the base include benign and malignant tumors, arteriovenous fistula/malformations, CSF fistula, congenital malformations, traumatic brain injury, bony lesions, and infectious pathologies. The benign tumors such as planum sphenoidale meningioma (PSM), olfactory groove meningioma (OGM), tuberculum sella meningioma (TSM), and malignant tumors like esthesioneuroblastoma, chondrosarcoma, and other sinonasal malignancies can also involve the skull base. Osseous pathologies such as fibrous dysplasia, congenital malformations such as encephalocele, infectious pathologies like tuberculous osteomyelitis or meningitis, or paranasal fungal infections extending to the anterior cranial base are other possibilities. Many of these lesions can reach enormous size and result in encasement of major vessels and other neural structures. The management strategy of each pathology varies and may not always be primarily surgical.

Various intracranial approaches to the anterior skull base have been described before. Among these, the common approaches we use for the microsurgical management of the aforementioned lesions include transbasal, pterional, or frontotemporal, and transsphenoidal approaches. In transbasal or subfrontal approaches, the anatomical variations of the anterior ethmoidal artery (AEA) create a big challenge. Abdullah et al reported that AEA is closely related to the skull base in 62.7% of cases (grades I and II) and courses freely in the ethmoid sinus below the skull base in the remaining 37.3% (grade III). In the former group, 42.5% of the artery is completely within the skull base (grade I) while another 20.2% course at the level of skull base with some degree of bony protrusion (grade II). Sometimes, the AEA is located below the skull base with a mesentery connecting it to skull base. If the AEA is not recognized as being in a mesentery, the artery might be accidentally injured while clearing sinonasal septations at the skull base, especially in sinonasal infiltrative malignant or infective pathologies.[7]

The ACA, its branches, and the AComA complex are often involved in anterior skull base and suprasellar tumors.[5] The ACAs become separated as far as the AComA complex allows as the tumor enlarges. As a result, the ACAs could be found posterosuperior and lateral to OGMs.[8] The medial orbitofrontal and frontopolar branches may become incorporated into the tumor capsule. The FOA is the most frequently involved vessel in anterior skull base meningiomas, particularly in OGMs, since this artery runs along the olfactory sulcus. We have observed that OGMs may initially displace the FOAs laterally and then later encase them, while the FPAs are typically attached to the upper pole of the tumor within the interhemispheric fissure.[5] Apart from the common sources of blood supply such as anterior/posterior ethmoidal arteries and sphenoidal branch of middle meningeal artery, the pial branches of ACA and AComA also constitute potential additional vascular challenges in giant anterior cranial base tumors. The anterior and posterior ethmoidal arteries provide the major blood supply in olfactory groove meningioma. Early dissection of the tumor from the frontal lobe and visualization of the ACAs are the key steps to avoid catastrophic vascular complications in such scenarios. However, the absence of an arachnoid plane between the tumor and the surrounding vessels may predict more difficult resection and higher risk of vascular injury.

Tumors that originate from the tuberculum sellae or planum sphenoidale displace the optic nerves superiorly and laterally, the optic chiasm superiorly and posteriorly, the ICAs laterally, the anterior cerebral and communicating arteries superiorly, and the pituitary gland inferiorly.[9] The blood supply for TSM is typically from the posterior ethmoidal arteries; with increasing size, arterial supply is parasitized from the AComA, ACA, McConnell capsular arteries, and dural hypophyseal vessels.[10] The approach selection (microsurgical/endoscopic) in TSM is largely guided by the involvement of internal carotid, anterior cerebral, or AComA.[11] Bifrontal or pterional/orbitozygomatic approaches are better in vessel encasement cases. While resecting esthesioneuroblastoma or other sinonasal malignancies with intracranial extension, it is critical to understand both the neurovascular structures involved (especially the ACAs and their branches) and the presence of subpial invasion to avoid inadvertent injuries.[9] When operating in the suprachiasmatic region, injury to the AComA branch, subcallosal artery (ScA), can lead to severe cognitive and memory dysfunction due to basal forebrain involvement. ScA can be considered as one of the most important perforators of the AComA complex, apart from hypothalamic and chiasmatic arteries.[12]

In a frontotemporal approach, after opening the sylvian fissure, the stem of the ICA and its branches, the ACA complex, middle cerebral artery complex and optic nerve need to be identified and meticulously preserved while operating the lesion. Circumferential encasement of the major arterial complex or perforator vessels stands as a major challenge in any skull base surgery, especially in large or giant meningioma resection.[13] Also, the identification of perforator vessels versus tumor feeders is crucial in avoiding complications. A preoperative angiogram may give a fair clue of the vascularity and anatomy of tumor feeders and also help to differentiate them from the perforators which should be preserved intraoperatively. Tracing the vessel to the parent artery and dissection along the subarachnoid plane also help to preserve the perforator vessels. The transsphenoidal approach to midline sellar and suprasellar lesions is limited laterally by bilateral ICAs, and the common vascular structures which may sustain inadvertent injury are the sphenopalatine artery and branches, ICA, basilar artery, and intercavernous sinus. Ectasia of the cavernous ICA and kissing carotids are significant challenges to the transsphenoidal approach, making the surgical corridor narrow and the dural opening difficult.[14] The use of micro-Doppler and careful dural opening help to overcome such challenges. This dolichoectasia may be seen in the pituitary fossa, sphenoid bone, or sinus and is commonly seen in acromegaly patients. Protrusion of the ICA into the sphenoid sinus is also relatively common (25–30%). Dehiscence of the bony sphenoidal wall of the ICA is seen in 10% cases.[15] Another rare challenge that needs to be anticipated is the association of aneurysm (ICA or its branches) and pituitary adenoma. The variations in the anatomy of the intercavernous sinus also pose significant surgical challenge in microsurgical transsphenoidal approaches. This can often be managed with injection of flowable Gelfoam or tissue glue.

In the subfrontal approaches, the anterior superior sagittal sinus (SSS) is commonly ligated to release the anterior falx. The anterior SSS includes veins that drain the medial, lateral, and basal surfaces of the frontal lobe.[16] The frontopolar veins have a single trunk, but variations such as multiple tributaries near the SSS also exist.[17] Many approaches require ligation of the anterior one-third of SSS for resection of midline anterior cranial fossa meningiomas. However, it is not safe in all cases. The length, caliber, and tributaries probably determine the area of frontal lobe drained by a vein into the anterior one-third of SSS. Longer, larger veins and veins with more tributaries drain a larger area. Acutely angulated veins also carry more blood from the posterior and eloquent areas of frontal lobe.[18] So the quantification of venous drainage based on preoperative contrast-enhanced magnetic resonance (MR) venogram could provide information on choosing midline basal versus lateral approaches.

12.5 Vascular Complications in Anterior Cranial Base Surgery

Vascular complications are the most feared complications in anterior cranial base surgery and includes both arterial and venous (channels/sinus) complications. Ischemic complications are caused by hemodynamic insufficiency, embolization, vasospasm, radiation vasculopathy, and venous anomaly.[19] Arterial injuries are frequently evident in the immediate postoperative period, whereas venous injuries typically present days later, resulting in congestive edema, hemorrhage, and seizures. Close anatomic proximity of the lesion with vessels is the main reason for inadvertent injury. Other causes are infiltration of tumor into adjacent vasculature, error in surgical technique, prior radiotherapy, inadequate preoperative imaging or interventions like cerebral angiogram or embolization, and suboptimal use of neuronavigation or micro-Doppler.[20] Intraoperative arterial injury may lead to catastrophic sequelae, which may range from hemorrhage, vasospasm, embolism or thrombosis, and sometimes delayed complications like pseudoaneurysm or arterial (ICA) stenosis. Carotid pseudoaneurysmal formation and eventual rupture may occur as a result of excessive adventitial dissection. This complication is usually sudden and fatal and may occur intraoperatively or postoperatively. Tuchman et al report the interval to diagnosis following surgery varied between 0 days and 10 years.[21] Performing computed tomography (CT) angiography 2 to 3 days after surgery in suspected cases may detect the pseudoaneurysm as immediate postoperative imaging may be negative in many cases except for active extravasation. Stroke arising due to thrombotic occlusion of the ICA or

embolism into distal vessels can also be a major concern. Sometimes the blunt injury of perforator vessels during dissection may lead to its vasospasm of varying severity in the postoperative period. Meticulous sharp dissection, maintaining arachnoid plane, avoiding vessel traction, and placement of papaverine-soaked Gelfoam over the perforator vessels are some of the techniques which can be used to avoid the postoperative vasospasm. The stagnation of arterial flow is common after surgical resection of basal arteriovenous malformation (AVM) and may result in retrograde thrombosis of feeding arteries leading to hypoperfusion. This happens especially if the AVM is large, patient is old, or the feeding arteries long. Similar stagnation can affect the venous system as well, though the neurologic deficit from venous thrombosis may be reversible, unlike arterial occlusion.

The incidence of ICA injury during transsphenoidal surgery varies from 0.2 to 2% in large series.[22,23] Arterial bleeding can also come from ICA branches such as the inferior hypophyseal artery or small capsular artery.[24,25] Injury to the sphenopalatine or posterior nasal artery is not rare in this approach (3.4%) though it is usually manageable with careful localization and coagulation of these arteries if transected.[26] Sometimes torrential bleed may happen while opening the sellar dura due to the venous channels over the entire face of the sellar dura in cases of pituitary microadenoma. As the bleeding may be in the form of diffuse ooze and difficult to localize to any specific vessel, flowable Gelfoam or glue may be the most beneficial tools in such situations. The anatomic relationship between the AComA complex/proximal ACA branches and tumors is a fundamental issue when dealing with large suprasellar lesions.[5] The main source of permanent neurological deficit after suprasellar meningioma surgery, other than visual loss, is intraoperative injury to the ACA or its branches.[5] Kassam et al reported a case of avulsion of FOA during the resection of an OGM in which the patient developed a delayed A2 pseudoaneurysm which ruptured and resulted in permanent right hemiparesis and cognitive deficits.[27]

The RAH supplies key territories including the anterior part of caudate nucleus, putamen, outer segment of the globus pallidus, and even the anterior limb of internal capsule. Inadvertent injury or occlusion may cause faciobrachial monoparesis, if the branch supplying the anterior limb of the internal capsule is compromised, and aphasia, if the artery is on the dominant side.[5] The neurological deficits associated with the injury of posterior perforating arteries from the AComA include incapacitating memory deficits and personality changes. Fortunately, there is a very low risk of injuring these vessels whenever the pathology is ventral to the AComA; lesions such as complex adenomas with subarachnoid invasion or meningiomas may occupy the space behind the AComA putting the subcallosal perforating arteries at risk.[5]

Obliteration of a patent SSS may impair venous return and induce edema in the part of the brain where venous drainage is obstructed, especially in tumors with significant peritumoral frontal lobe edema. Even in the anterior third of the sinus, long considered to be less critical, sinus ligation could result in sacrifice of the draining veins, leading to significant frontal lobe venous congestion, edema, or infarction. Furthermore, in these patients with large anterior cranial base tumors, there is increased intracranial pressure due to the presence of a large mass and secondary decreased venous return. Preoperative contrast-enhanced MR venogram provides necessary information on the status of the location/caliber of draining veins and their tributaries which helps in choosing the ideal approach and further surgical planning.

12.6 How to Avoid Arterial and Venous Complications?

Surgeons must be proficient with various surgical approaches to the anterior skull base and knowledgeable of their specific potential risks and benefits. The selection of the ideal approach is one of the most crucial steps in skull base surgery. Surgical strategies must be tailored according to each case based on location, nature and size of the lesion, relationship with surrounding neurovascular structures, extent of dural attachment (meningioma), and surgeon's expertise. The approach should also achieve the goals of minimal brain retraction, proper exposure of the lesion/neurovascular structures, especially toward the tumor base at the skull base surface, and also the ability to cut off or reduce tumor blood supply. Preoperative angiogram provides the opportunity to perform embolization prior to the lesion resection, especially in highly vascular lesions. If major vessel injury or sacrifice is anticipated, the patient should be well prepared for possible arterial clip reconstruction or bypass surgery or sinus reconstruction surgeries. In hypercoagulable high-risk conditions such as Cushing's disease, perioperative anticoagulant prophylaxis may help in reducing the incidence of thrombotic or embolic complications.[28] Minimal handling of vessels and avoiding prolonged brain retraction can avoid these complications to a great extent. The regional cerebral blood flow can decrease to the point of ischemia when brain retraction pressures exceed 20 mm Hg.[29,30] Clinical studies demonstrated CSF drainage as an effective method in decreasing the retraction pressure required. Also, the use of multiple retractors reduces the pressure applied by each retractor. The vigilant monitoring of retraction pressures using strain-gauge retractors may also be helpful, especially while applying over arteries and cranial nerves. Strict airway and oxygenation maintenance as well as adequate fluid and electrolyte balance are yet other preventive measures to avoid complications in skull base surgery and may play a role in venous infarct management.

Internal debulking of tumor and bimanual, extracapsular dissection are the most important microneurosurgical techniques to avoid devastating vascular complications in anterior cranial base lesions. Meningiomas of the anterior cranial fossa represent 12 to 20% of all intracranial meningiomas.[31] While performing a frontotemporal approach for OGM, the initial debulking and exposure of the basal dura mater provide the opportunity to coagulate and divide the feeding arteries. This, as well as splitting of the sylvian fissure, provides better visualization of the ICA bifurcation at the posterolateral aspect of tumor, with subsequent identification of the ACA complex, optic chiasm, and optic nerves. Changes in head rotation intraoperatively provide varying angles of visualization of ACA complex and thereby its preservation. In the subfrontal transbasal microsurgical approach, the dura mater of the anterior cranial base is dissected free from the underlying bone and the dural basal vessels can be then coagulated and divided. This is a very crucial step for early devascularization of an anterior

skull base tumor. Comparing the lateral approach to anterior bifrontal approach, the senior author reported the experience from the personal series of 57 patients and suggested that lateral (pterional/frontotemporal) approaches resulted in less frontal lobe damage, less encephalomalacia (as measured by ratio of porencephalic cave volume to tumor volume) in the hemisphere contralateral to the tumor, and better olfactory preservation in comparison to anterior approaches.[32] Preoperative ethmoidal artery ligation can play a major role in the surgical excision of large-to-giant anterior skull base meningiomas.[33]

The advantages of sharp arachnoid dissection over blunt dissection have already been reported. Zygourakis et al in their study report that following the arachnoid plane and dissection along the arachnoid planes in the suprasellar cistern to protect the AComA complex, often separated from the tumor capsule by an arachnoid sheath, may help prevent complications. Also, when portions of the tumor are wrapped around the A1 and AComA, a small portion of tumor can be left unresected if it cannot be easily separated from the associated perforating arteries. ACA encasement and sagittal sinus invasion may be the predictive factors favoring open microsurgical resection over endonasal approach and should be weighed more heavily than tumor size, distance to optic chiasm, sellar invasion, or surgical approach when predicting the morbidity of a surgery for PSMs or OGMs.[34]

Based on diameter alone, the RAH could be mistaken for the FOA. The RAH, FOA, and FPA can be differentiated according to their origin, course, and destination. The key landmarks for these three arteries are the A1 segment, the olfactory tract, and the interhemispheric fissure, respectively. While the FOA distally drifts away from the A1 segment, the RAH remains parallel to A1.[5] In cases of giant olfactory groove meningiomas with complete encasement of the FOA, its intraoperative sacrifice may have little clinical consequences as the vascular territory may have already been compromised by the tumor growth.[5] Suprasellar meningiomas with potential vascular encasement are a relative contraindication for endoscopic endonasal surgery. The FOA is the most commonly encountered vessel when resecting sinonasal tumors with anterior skull base invasion, and selective coagulation of its feeders to the olfactory tracts is required for complete oncological resection. As 20% of FOAs supply the frontal pole, care should be taken to preserve the FOA when possible; this is not always simple or possible given the tendency (85%) of the FOA to cross the olfactory tract.[5]

Preservation of normal vasculature, while maintaining the ability of the surgeon to attain the greatest visibility, is an important factor when choosing an approach. The transbasal approach allows access to the origin of the anterior SSS, allowing for maximum draining vein preservation, thereby avoiding venous infarction. Maximal preservation of the draining veins should be considered while resecting large anterior skull base lesions. Borghei-Razavi et al reported the advantage of removing the orbital bar while performing the transbasal approach as it offers a trajectory allowing ligating the most anterior aspect of the SSS without risking injury to any of the veins draining into the sinus.[16] The other techniques for avoiding basal venous injury are providing adequate extension of the patient's head, release of CSF, and using epidural dissection so that the dura can be opened in a low subfrontal fashion rather than over the frontal pole, thereby preserving the majority of venous integrity. The complication rate of venous infarctions can also be decreased by performing extended bifrontal craniotomies with bilateral orbital osteotomies rather than traditional bicoronal craniotomies.[16] The technique of extradural posterior mobilization of the sphenoparietal sinus has been described to achieve adequate retraction of the frontal lobe intradurally without sacrificing the frontobasal bridging veins.[35] Goldschmidt et al reported the use of near-infrared vein finder technique to define cortical veins, pathological dural veins, and venous sinus anatomy prior to dural opening, and it offers a real-time image independent of brain shift.[36] Consideration of venous drainage is important when selecting the approach for patients with midline anterior cranial fossa meningiomas, since removal of such tumors would require a low trajectory to gain access to the base of the tumor. The variation in the origin of the first and second veins draining into SSS should also be an important factor when deciding the approach.[16] Although the transbasal approach can be performed with the preservation of the SSS, a unilateral approach such as the pterional approach can bypass the risk to injure SSS or basal draining veins entirely. Consequently, these results are important to consider when choosing an optimal approach for resection of such tumors as these patients are at increased risk of venous infarction.

There may not be a single best approach for the resection of anterior cranial base lesions. Multiple different approaches may be used for anterior cranial base tumor or AVM resection including pterional, subfrontal, and orbitofrontal approaches. Each approach has its own benefits and disadvantages. Avoiding direct injury to the brain and vessels involves the use of surgical adjuncts, adequate exposure, and optimum brain relaxation. Minimizing the use of retractors to preserve veins is essential. Intraoperative imaging modalities such as digital subtraction angiography (DSA), indocyanine green video angiography, or micro-Doppler are efficient adjuncts to check for the patency of vessels after tackling the pathology. There exists no precise vascular assessment today which can predict the occurrence of vascular complications accurately. Postoperative adjuncts include DSA, transcranial Doppler, CT/MR angiography, and physiologic modalities such as positron emission tomography (PET), hexamethylpropyleneamine oxime (HMPAO SPECT), 133Xe clearance, xenon-enhanced CT (Xe/CT), perfusion CT (PCT), and diffusion-weighted/MR perfusion imaging.[37] Significant limitations remain in the management of cerebrovascular anatomy and physiology in anterior cranial base microsurgery. Patient-related factors (age, comorbidities, medications), pathology-related factors (symptoms, size, location, configuration), anticipation of potential cerebrovascular complications, and, most importantly, the experience of the surgeon are paramount to successful outcome. Most importantly, as in the case of any skull base surgery, the natural history of disease and the effectiveness of alternate mode of treatments must be weighed against the morbidity of surgical procedure.

12.7 Illustrative Case Example

12.7.1 Case History and Examination

A 36-year-old woman presents with mild to moderate dull headache and progressive bilateral blurring of vision for 3 months. On examination, visual acuity was 6/60 in both eyes with bitemporal field defects. She was evaluated with MRI of the brain and was diagnosed with a sellar-suprasellar lesion, possibly pituitary adenoma (► Fig. 12.2). Her endocrinology profile revealed the tumor was a nonfunctioning tumor. In view of large size of tumor and progressive worsening of symptoms, she was planned for surgical resection of the lesion.

12.7.2 Management Strategy and Complications

The patient was scheduled for transnasal transsphenoidal microsurgical resection of the tumor. The tumor was firm in consistency. During tumor decompression, sudden torrential bleeding started from the superior aspect of the operative field (**Video 12.1**). The volume of bleed was significant and ICA tear was suspected. The patient's blood pressure increased to 230/180 mm Hg. Head elevation was done, depth of anesthesia was increased, hyperventilation was provided, and mannitol infusion was started. Ipsilateral carotid compression was attempted. To achieve hemostasis, the bleeding source was first attempted to be localized, but could be not be clearly defined. The surgical cavity was then packed with Gelfoam, oxidized cellulose, and fat. Hemostasis was achieved with great difficulty. Fibrin sealant glue was also applied in the packed operative region. Postoperative CT brain imaging revealed diffuse subarachnoid hemorrhage, blood in the basal cisterns, cerebral edema, and residual tumor (► Fig. 12.2). Following CT, patient was taken to neurointerventional suite for a four-vessel digital subtraction angiogram. It showed intact ICA and nonfilling of the distal basilar artery with active extravasation of contrast (► Fig. 12.2). Due to the poor prognosis, no further intervention was attempted. She did not regain consciousness after surgery and died on the second postoperative day. The final histopathology of the tumor was reported as fibrosarcoma.

12.7.3 Other Options to Control Intraoperative Severe Bleeding in This Case

Several maneuvers have been discussed in the literature to aid in the control of bleeding. Head elevation and controlled hypotension are two options which can be considered immediately following torrential bleed. The technique of ipsilateral carotid compression has been described and it provides a little more time for adequate nasal packing.[38] Bilateral carotid artery compression in the neck with concurrent surgical widening of the sphenoid sinus ostium to facilitate nasal pack placement has also been reported.[39] The major packing agents available in literature are muscle patch, teflon, Gelfoam, fibrin glue, oxidized cellulose, oxygel, muslin gauze, and methyl methacrylate patches.[38,40] Some surgeons prefer to use fascia lata, sternocleidomastoid, or quadriceps muscle patches along with fibrin glue and oxidized cellulose for hemostasis though gauze is still most commonly used. However, the data from sheep model by Valentine et al reports muscle patch as the best primary hemostatic agent.[41] The surgeon should always keep in mind the possibility of vascular occlusion/stenosis and its disastrous consequences which can happen due to overpacking.[42]

Vessel occlusion appears to be the safest and most reliable method to stop bleeding though it carries the risk of stroke.

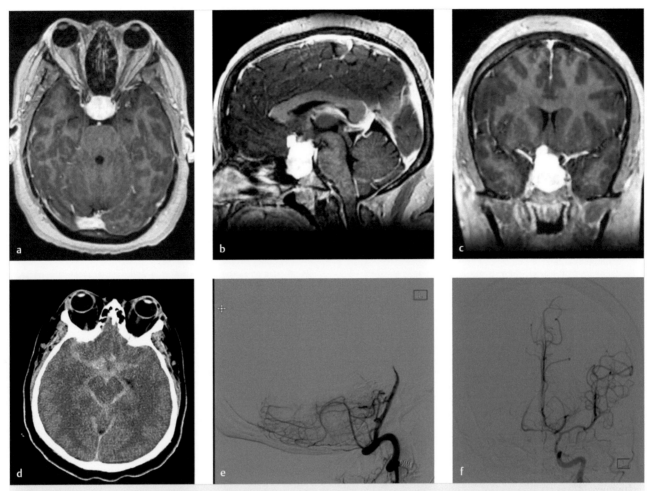

Fig. 12.2 **(a)** Gadolinium (Gd)-enhanced axial magnetic resonance imaging (MRI) brain image showing sellar-suprasellar lesion (pre-op). **(b)** Gd-enhanced sagittal MRI brain image showing sellar-suprasellar lesion (pre-op). **(c)** Gd-enhanced coronal MRI brain image showing sellar-suprasellar lesion (pre-op). **(d)** Noncontrast axial computed tomography (CT) brain image showing diffuse subarachnoid hemorrhage (SAH) and cerebral edema (post-op). **(e)** Left vertebral injection angiogram image showing nonfilling of distal basilar artery and extravasation of contrast (post-op). **(f)** Left carotid injection angiogram image showing normal filling of internal carotid artery (ICA), anterior cerebral artery (ACA), and middle cerebral artery (MCA) branches (post-op).

If direct clipping of the vessel is not possible, tamponade with packing agents can be considered as a temporary measure until the definite endovascular treatment is achieved.[43] In such cases, serial angiographic evaluation may be needed to follow the dynamic nature of these arterial lesions.

12.7.4 Root Cause Analysis of the Vascular Injury

The injury in this particular case could be due to the aggressive manipulation of the tumor in the sellar region. The aberrant anatomy of the vessels and the error in surgical technique contributed to the inadvertent vascular injury. The use of intraoperative Doppler probe or indocyanine green angiography while attempting decompression can give clues regarding the position of major vessels. The use of ultrasonic aspirator should be avoided near the cavernous sinus or close to vessels as it may be difficult to visualize its tip sometimes. The tumor capsule should not be removed until it is well dissected off the surrounding structures. The basic principles of internal decompression and extracapsular

dissection need to be strictly followed to avoid intraoperative vascular complications. Also, overpacking could have been the possible cause for the inadvertent vascular occlusion. The intraoperative diagnosis of fibrosarcoma could have changed our surgical goals due to the technical difficulties arising from the firm consistency of tumor, potential invasiveness, and poor surgical outcome despite multimodality treatment.

12.8 Conclusion

Surgical resection remains the mainstay of effective treatment for both benign and malignant lesions of the anterior cranial fossa and a variety of microsurgical approaches have been designed to treat these pathologies. Choosing the best surgical trajectory along with utilization of microsurgical technical advances and vascular adjuncts helps in safe maximal resection and provide better long-term outcomes. Vascular injury represents a potentially fatal complication of cranial base surgery. Internal debulking of tumor and bimanual, extracapsular dissection are among the most important microneurosurgical techniques to avoid such devastating complications. Proper patient selection, team approach, understanding the regional anatomy, selecting the best surgical corridor, meticulous handling of neurovascular structures, adequate release of CSF, sharp arachnoid dissection, minimal use of fixed retraction, optimum use of operative adjuncts including neuronavigation, intraoperative anticipation of vascular injury, proper clip reconstruction techniques, and postoperative surveillance for catastrophic hemorrhage or infarcts are the strategies to avoid cerebrovascular complications in anterior skull base microsurgeries.

References

[1] Rhoton AL, Jr. The anterior and middle cranial base. Neurosurgery. 2002; 51(4) Suppl:S273–S302

[2] Robert T, Cicciò G, Sylvestre P, et al. Anatomic and angiographic analyses of ophthalmic artery collaterals in moyamoya disease. AJNR Am J Neuroradiol. 2018; 39(6):1121–1126

[3] Liebeskind DS. Collateral circulation. Stroke. 2003; 34(9):2279–2284

[4] Rhoton AL, Jr. The sellar region. Neurosurgery. 2002; 51(4) Suppl:S335–S374

[5] Najera E, Truong HQ, Belo JTA, Borghei-Razavi H, Gardner PA, Fernandez-Miranda J. Proximal branches of the anterior cerebral artery: anatomic study and applications to endoscopic endonasal surgery. Oper Neurosurg (Hagerstown). 2019; 16(6):734–742

[6] Rhoton AL, Jr. The cerebral veins. Neurosurgery. 2002; 51(4) Suppl:S159–S205

[7] Abdullah B, Lim EH, Mohamad H, et al. Anatomical variations of anterior ethmoidal artery at the ethmoidal roof and anterior skull base in Asians. Surg Radiol Anat. 2019; 41(5):543–550

[8] Aguiar PH, Tahara A, Almeida AN, et al. Olfactory groove meningiomas: approaches and complications. J Clin Neurosci. 2009; 16(9):1168–1173

[9] Gardner PA, Kassam AB, Rothfus WE, Snyderman CH, Carrau RL. Preoperative and intraoperative imaging for endoscopic endonasal approaches to the skull base. Otolaryngol Clin North Am. 2008; 41(1):215–230, vii

[10] Raza SM, Effendi ST, DeMonte F. Tuberculum sellae meningiomas: evolving surgical strategies. Curr Surg Rep. 2014; 2:73

[11] Nanda A, Ambekar S, Javalkar V, Sharma M. Technical nuances in the management of tuberculum sellae and diaphragma sellae meningiomas. Neurosurg Focus. 2013; 35(6):E7

[12] Najera E, Alves Belo JT, Truong HQ, Gardner PA, Fernandez-Miranda JC. Surgical anatomy of the subcallosal artery: implications for transcranial and endoscopic endonasal surgery in the suprachiasmatic region. Oper Neurosurg (Hagerstown). 2019; 17(1):79–87

[13] Narayan V, Bir SC, Mohammed N, Savardekar AR, Patra DP, Nanda A. Surgical management of giant intracranial meningioma: operative nuances, challenges, and outcome. World Neurosurg. 2018; 110:e32–e41

[14] Pereira Filho A de A, Gobbato PL, Pereira Filho G de A, Silva SB da, Kraemer JL. Intracranial intrasellar kissing carotid arteries: case report. Arq Neuropsiquiatr. 2007; 65 2A:355–357

[15] Hewaidi G, Omami G. Anatomic variation of sphenoid sinus and related structures in Libyan population: CT scan study. Libyan J Med. 2008; 3(3):128–133

[16] Borghei-Razavi H, Raghavan A, Eguiluz-Melendez A, et al. Anatomical variations in the location of veins draining into the anterior superior sagittal sinus: implications for the transbasal approach. Oper Neurosurg (Hagerstown). 2020; 18(6):668–675

[17] Sampei T, Yasui N, Okudera T, Fukasawa H. Anatomic study of anterior frontal cortical bridging veins with special reference to the frontopolar vein. Neurosurgery. 1996; 38(5):971–975

[18] Sahoo SK, Ghuman MS, Salunke P, Vyas S, Bhar R, Khandelwal NK. Evaluation of anterior third of superior sagittal sinus in normal population: identifying the subgroup with dominant drainage. J Neurosci Rural Pract. 2016; 7(2):257–261

[19] Origitano TC, al-Mefty O, Leonetti JP, DeMonte F, Reichman OH. Vascular considerations and complications in cranial base surgery. Neurosurgery. 1994; 35(3):351–362, discussion 362–363

[20] Gardner PA, Snyderman CH, Fernandez-Miranda JC, Jankowitz BT. Management of major vascular injury during endoscopic endonasal skull base surgery. Otolaryngol Clin North Am. 2016; 49(3):819–828

[21] Tuchman A, Khalessi AA, Attenello FJ, Amar AP, Zada G. Delayed cavernous carotid artery pseudoaneurysm caused by absorbable plate following transsphenoidal surgery: case report and review of the literature. J Neurol Surg Rep. 2013; 74(1):10–16

[22] Berker M, Aghayev K, Saatci I, Palaoğlu S, Önerci M. Overview of vascular complications of pituitary surgery with special emphasis on unexpected abnormality. Pituitary. 2010; 13(2):160–167

[23] Sylvester PT, Moran CJ, Derdeyn CP, et al. Endovascular management of internal carotid artery injuries secondary to endonasal surgery: case series and review of the literature. J Neurosurg. 2016; 125(5):1256–1276

[24] Isolan GR, de Aguiar PHP, Laws ER, Strapasson ACP, Piltcher O. The implications of microsurgical anatomy for surgical approaches to the sellar region. Pituitary. 2009; 12(4):360–367

[25] Laws ER, Jr, Kern EB. Complications of trans-sphenoidal surgery. Clin Neurosurg. 1976; 23:401–416

[26] Ciric I, Ragin A, Baumgartner C, Pierce D. Complications of transsphenoidal surgery: results of a national survey, review of the literature, and personal experience. Neurosurgery. 1997; 40(2):225–236, discussion 236–237

[27] Kassam AB, Prevedello DM, Carrau RL, et al. Endoscopic endonasal skull base surgery: analysis of complications in the authors' initial 800 patients. J Neurosurg. 2011; 114(6):1544–1568

[28] Boscaro M, Sonino N, Scarda A, et al. Anticoagulant prophylaxis markedly reduces thromboembolic complications in Cushing's syndrome. J Clin Endocrinol Metab. 2002; 87(8):3662–3666

[29] Andrews RJ, Bringas JR. A review of brain retraction and recommendations for minimizing intraoperative brain injury. Neurosurgery. 1993; 33(6):1052–1063, discussion 1063–1064

[30] Rosenørn J, Diemer NH. Reduction of regional cerebral blood flow during brain retraction pressure in the rat. J Neurosurg. 1982; 56(6):826–829

[31] Morales-Valero SF, Van Gompel JJ, Loumiotis I, Lanzino G. Craniotomy for anterior cranial fossa meningiomas: historical overview. Neurosurg Focus. 2014; 36(4):E14

[32] Nanda A, Maiti TK, Bir SC, Konar SK, Guthikonda B. Olfactory groove meningiomas: comparison of extent of frontal lobe changes after lateral and bifrontal approaches. World Neurosurg. 2016; 94:211–221

[33] Aref M, Kunigelis KE, Yang A, Subramanian PS, Ramakrishnan VR, Youssef AS. The effect of preoperative direct ligation of ethmoidal arteries on the perioperative outcomes of large anterior skull base meningiomas surgery: a clinical study. World Neurosurg. 2018; 120:e776–e782

[34] Zygourakis CC, Sughrue ME, Benet A, Parsa AT, Berger MS, McDermott MW. Management of planum/olfactory meningiomas: predicting symptoms and postoperative complications. World Neurosurg. 2014; 82(6):1216–1223

[35] Hasegawa H, Inoue T, Sato K, Tamura A, Saito I. Mobilization of the sphenoparietal sinus: a simple technique to preserve prominent frontobasal bridging veins during surgical clipping of anterior communicating artery aneurysms: technical case report. Neurosurgery. 2013; 73(1) Suppl Operative:E124–E127, discussion ons128–ons129

[36] Goldschmidt E, Faraji AH, Jankowitz BT, Gardner P, Friedlander RM. Use of a near-infrared vein finder to define cortical veins and dural sinuses prior to dural opening. J Neurosurg. 2019(August):1–8

[37] Mills JN, Mehta V, Russin J, Amar AP, Rajamohan A, Mack WJ. Advanced imaging modalities in the detection of cerebral vasospasm. Neurol Res Int. 2013; 2013:415960

[38] Valentine R, Wormald P-J. Carotid artery injury after endonasal surgery. Otolaryngol Clin North Am. 2011; 44(5):1059–1079

[39] Weidenbecher M, Huk WJ, Iro H. Internal carotid artery injury during functional endoscopic sinus surgery and its management. Eur Arch Otorhinolaryngol. 2005; 262(8):640–645

[40] Inamasu J, Guiot BH. Iatrogenic carotid artery injury in neurosurgery. Neurosurg Rev. 2005; 28(4):239–247, discussion 248

[41] Valentine R, Boase S, Jervis-Bardy J, Dones Cabral JD, Robinson S, Wormald PJ. The efficacy of hemostatic techniques in the sheep model of carotid artery injury. Int Forum Allergy Rhinol. 2011; 1(2):118–122

[42] Raymond J, Hardy J, Czepko R, Roy D. Arterial injuries in transsphenoidal surgery for pituitary adenoma; the role of angiography and endovascular treatment. AJNR Am J Neuroradiol. 1997; 18(4):655–665

[43] Romero ADCB, Lal Gangadharan J, Bander ED, Gobin YP, Anand VK, Schwartz TH. Managing arterial injury in endoscopic skull base surgery: case series and review of the literature. Oper Neurosurg (Hagerstown). 2017; 13(1):138–149

13 Dealing with Vascular Injury During Middle Fossa Surgery

Rami O. Almefty, Michael Mooney, and Ossama Al-Mefty

Summary

Vascular injury is one of the most feared complications of skull base surgery with potentially devastating ischemic or hemorrhagic consequences. The best management strategy is avoidance with thorough preparation and eliminating undue risk. A plan should be in place to deal with vascular injury and, in the event it occurs, the surgeon must remain calm and efficiently execute the plan. When possible, primary suture repair is the best solution. For injuries of the petrous or cavernous carotid artery, which may be encountered during middle fossa surgery, access to proximal and distal control is highly advantageous for dealing with the injury and minimizes its consequences. In this regard, carotid injury through the middle fossa approach is more manageable and amenable to reconstruction than injury through other approaches. The ability to immediately revascularize with bypass can be performed in the open surgical field, allowing reperfusion as soon as possible. In cases where bypass is not pursued, endovascular treatment with a covered stent can provide an immediate and durable treatment with vessel preservation, although this requires the administration of dual antiplatelet agents, which come with their own risks for postoperative bleeding. Endovascular intervention is also beneficial in obtaining proximal carotid control, if the neck or the horizontal petrous carotid is not available in the field.

Keywords: Skull base, internal carotid artery, temporal bone, endovascular, pseudoaneurysm, cerebral bypass, covered stent

13.1 Key Learning Points

- Vascular injury in skull base surgery is best managed by avoidance.
- Excellent understanding of the relevant anatomy and a thorough study of the pathologic anatomy is critical for avoiding vascular injuries.
- The petrous and cavernous portions of the internal carotid artery are of primary concern in middle fossa approaches.
- The critical step in safely operating along the middle fossa and cavernous sinus is proximal and distal control of the carotid artery.
- Branches from the petrous or cavernous segment of the internal carotid artery are noncritical, except for a persistent trigeminal artery or an early origin of the ophthalmic artery from the cavernous segment with a poor retinal collateral supply.
- A previously irradiated internal carotid artery develops radiation-induced angiopathy, characterized by diminution of the muscular layer and fragility of the vessel wall, which makes the vessel more susceptible to rupture during dissection.
- Carotid artery sacrifice may lead to morbidity and mortality despite reassuring temporary occlusion testing.
- If arterial injury is suspected intraoperatively, catheter angiography should be performed.

- If the initial angiogram is negative, repeat, delayed angiography is needed to ensure there is no delayed pseudoaneurysm development.
- Revascularization should always be considered and applied over a permanent occlusion of the carotid, particularly for cases in which no detailed temporary occlusion study with cerebral blood flow was performed.
- Endovascular reconstruction of an iatrogenically injured petrous and cavernous carotid arteries with vessel preservation can be accomplished with the use of covered stents. Flow-diverting devices are being increasingly used, but they do not provide immediate protection of the lesion and therefore in locations where there are no critical branches, a covered stent is a more optimal solution.
- If permanent carotid occlusion is deemed necessary, microsurgical clipping immediately proximal to the ophthalmic artery origin is the preferred method of vascular sacrifice. This strategy prevents thrombus formation and subsequent embolization from the occluded vessel and is possible through the exposure from the middle fossa approach.

13.2 Introduction

Vascular injuries are one of the most feared complications of skull base surgery with potentially devastating hemorrhagic or ischemic complications. Skull base surgeons should enter every skull base operation with a plan to avoid vascular injury and a separate plan to manage it, should it occur. Indeed, the best management of vascular injuries is avoidance, which is best accomplished with a thorough understanding of the normal and pathologic anatomy. Skull base anatomy requires an in-depth three-dimensional understanding of critical neurovascular structures, which is best mastered through considerable time spent in the dissection lab. If one idea could be imparted from this chapter, it should be a call to those seeking the trust and responsibility of caring for patients with skull base pathology, to spend the time in the dissection lab to learn skull base anatomy and its many variations. Regardless of the approach or technology used, this is the skull base surgeon's best tool in avoiding vascular injuries. When dealing with pathology, however, it is insufficient, as the "normal" anatomy is frequently distorted. It must be combined with a detailed preoperative study of the pathologic anatomy. In the case of skull base tumors, this should include magnetic resonance imaging (MRI), computed tomography (CT), and vascular imaging. We have found dynamic computed tomography angiography (CTA) particularly useful in studying vascular anatomy (▶ Fig. 13.1).[1]

13.3 Vascular Control and Injury Avoidance

Skull base approaches based on or including a middle fossa dissection are valuable for a variety of skull base pathologies. The key to

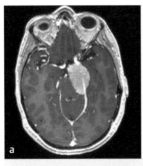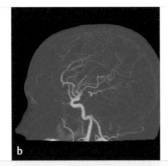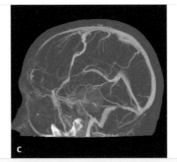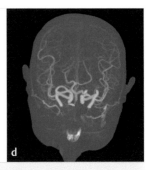

Fig. 13.1 Petroclival meningioma evaluated with preoperative dynamic computed tomography (CT) angiogram. (a) Axial T1-weighted magnetic resonance imaging (MRI) demonstrating a left-sided petroclival meningioma with extension into the middle fossa. (b) Dynamic CT angiogram, lateral view, demonstrating the arterial (b) and venous (c) phases. (d) Dynamic CT angiogram, submental view, demonstrating an intact circle of Willis.

safely working along the middle fossa is control of the internal carotid artery. The internal carotid artery enters the intracranial compartment from the neck via the carotid canal in the temporal bone (▶ Fig. 13.2). It then travels along the petrous portion of the temporal bone in the middle cranial fossa before ascending into the cavernous sinus between the foramen lacerum and petrolingual ligament. Within the carotid canal of the petrous bone, the carotid artery travels in a lateral to medial direction as it proceeds from posterior to anterior. The middle meningeal artery arising from the foramen spinosum is a reliable landmark in the middle fossa dissection. Once it is identified, the greater superficial petrosal nerve, which overlies the carotid artery, can be found just medially. The textbook representation is for the carotid artery to be entirely within a bony canal; however, bony dehiscence is not uncommon and extreme care must be taken to avoid injury of an exposed carotid artery.

Once the location of the carotid artery is established, control is sought. Although it should be included in the prepared field, the cervical carotid artery is not needed for obtaining control. Instead, we have adopted the Wascher and Spetzler technique of placing a small Fogarty balloon within the carotid canal.[2] If there is not already a complete uncovering of the bony canal, the bone is often paper thin at its most anterior aspect just prior to entering the cavernous sinus, and enough room to insert the Fogarty balloon is easily exposed with a diamond drill bit under copious irrigation or with a sharp dissector with its blunt end facing toward the canal. For dissection within the cavernous sinus, distal control is established at the clinoidal segment of the carotid artery after removal of the anterior clinoid process.

Another important anatomical consideration for managing vascular complications of the petrous and cavernous carotid is the lack of critical branches. The petrous carotid artery is inconsistent in the number and type of branches, and not infrequently there are no branches at all. Branches that do occur from the petrous carotid are the caroticotympanic branch, vidian artery, and periosteal arteries. The cavernous portion of the carotid artery supplies branches to the surrounding dura, tentorium, and redundant supply to the hypophysis.[3,4,5,6] Although these small branches may not provide a critical function, they may be implicated in the injury as they may avulse from the carotid artery leading to brisk arterial bleeding and if unrecognized, eventual pseudoaneurysm development.[7] In the

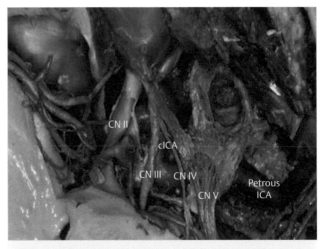

Fig. 13.2 Cadaveric dissection (right side) demonstrating the course of the petrous and cavernous internal carotid artery in relation to its surrounding cranial nerve and bony anatomy. cICA, cavernous segment of the internal carotid artery; CN, cranial nerve; ICA, internal carotid artery.

rare cases involving a persistent trigeminal artery, the surgeon must be wary of this critical arteries origin anywhere between the petrous and cavernous carotid artery segments.

13.4 Related Pathologies

- Neoplastic:
  - Meningioma:
    - Cavernous sinus.
    - Petroclival.
    - Middle fossa.
  - Schwannoma:
    - Trigeminal.
    - Vestibular.
  - Pituitary adenoma.
  - Chordoma.
  - Chondrosarcoma.
- Vascular:
  - Posterior circulation aneurysm.
  - Brainstem cavernous malformations.

- Nonneoplastic:
  - Petrous apex cholesterol granuloma.
  - Tegmen defect.
- Infectious:
  - Mucormycosis.
  - Aspergillosis.

13.5 Case Example

A 69-year-old female previously underwent surgery and radiation of a petrous meningioma at an outside institution (▶ Fig. 13.3). She presented with tumor progression and worsening facial function and underwent a transtemporal approach for re-resection. The petrous ridge was severely hyperostotic and drilled extensively. During drilling brisk arterial bleeding was encountered, which was controlled with gentle packing with Gelfoam. Surgery was completed and a complete resection accomplished. Following surgery, she was taken for catheter angiography, which showed a subtle irregularity without definitive pseudoaneurysm formation or contrast extravasation (▶ Fig. 13.3b). The patient remained at her neurologic baseline with stable facial nerve function. Given the concern for arterial injury, despite the apparent reassuring initial angiogram, follow-up CTA and then catheter angiography was performed at postoperative days 3 and 7, respectively. On the follow-up angiogram there was a clear pseudoaneurysm formation (▶ Fig. 13.3c). The pseudoaneurysm was successfully treated endovascularly with a covered coronary stent, the Graftmaster Jostent (Abbott Vascular, Santa Clara, California, USA) which remained widely patent on 8-month follow-up (▶ Fig. 13.3d).

13.6 Management Strategy

As emphasized earlier, the key to successfully dealing with an intraoperative vascular injury is careful planning. At each step of the operation, vascular control should be established and a plan for dealing with injury mentally rehearsed. Encountering copious arterial bleeding intraoperatively can be an alarming experience; however, it is critical to remain calm and execute the plan. In the case example, the bleeding was at the petrous carotid, an extradural location, and from a small caliber defect believed to be from an avulsion of a small branch artery, so it

could be controlled with packing. It should be noted that if major arterial bleeding occurs in the subarachnoid space, packing should be avoided as it can lead to subarachnoid hemorrhage and malignant cerebral edema. In these instances, the injured segment is best trapped and repaired with fine suture. This repair is similar to other microvascular anastomotic work, including the use of 8-0 to 10-0 Prolene suture, depending on vessel wall thickness and surgeon's preference, and running or interrupted suturing technique, depending on the extent and configuration of the injury.

Bleeding that occurs from the petrous or cavernous carotid that may occur during middle fossa surgery may not be so readily identified and exposed. In these cases where primary repair is not possible, packing with hemostatic material may be able to achieve hemostasis while the next steps for repair are planned. A variety of hemostatic materials can be utilized based on the exact nature of the injury and the surgeon's preference, including, Surgicel, Surgicel Fibrillar, Surgicel Nu-Knit, Gelfoam, or other similar materials. In some cases, Gelfoam coupled with Tisseel fibrin sealant can achieve hemostasis when other options have failed. Once the bleeding is controlled and the operation either completed or terminated based on the individual circumstances, a formal angiogram should be obtained. In cases that are particularly high risk for carotid artery injury, a hybrid neurosurgical operating suite equipped with biplane angiography and/or intraoperative imaging capabilities can be utilized and femoral sheath placement at the initiation of the procedure can be considered (▶ Fig. 13.4). At our institution, select cases are performed in our Advanced Multimodality Image Guided Operating (AMIGO) suite, which is equipped with both intraoperative CT and MR capabilities.

In the event that the initial angiogram is negative, follow-up, delayed angiography is needed to confirm that a pseudoaneurysm does not develop. In the event of pseudoaneurysm development, the classical management has been carotid artery sacrifice. Although that is a definitive solution to the pseudoaneurysm, clearly the ideal management would allow for vessel preservation, as carotid artery sacrifice has significant morbidity and mortality.[8,9,10,11,12,13] High-flow cerebrovascular bypass or intracranial stenting options allow for treatment of the lesion while maintaining (or recreating) the carotid circulation, although each strategy carries its own unique challenges (see Chapters 5 and 6). Lesion embolization and flow diversion are alternatives that

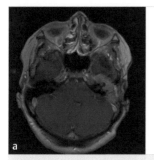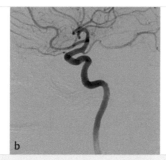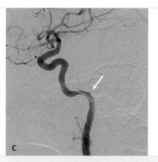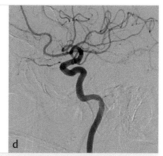

Fig. 13.3 Petrous meningioma with intraoperative carotid injury. **(a)** Axial T1-weighted magnetic resonance imaging (MRI) demonstrating a recurrent left-sided petrous meningioma. **(b)** Immediate postoperative angiogram, lateral view, with no evidence of pseudoaneurysm. **(c)** Repeat postoperative angiogram 7 days after surgery demonstrating clear pseudoaneurysm formation at the posterior aspect of the petrous carotid (*arrow*). **(d)** Postoperative angiogram 8 months after stent placement, demonstrating patency of the carotid artery with no evidence of aneurysm recurrence.

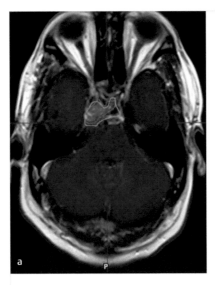
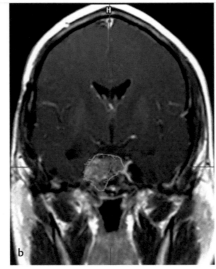
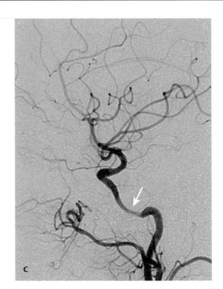
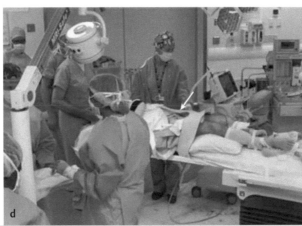

Fig. 13.4 Case example: Recurrent chordoma of the petrous temporal bone. (a, b) Axial and coronal magnetic resonance (MR) images demonstrating the recurrent tumor; outlines indicate segmentation from MR (blue) and computed tomography (CT) images (purple). (c) Preoperative digital subtraction angiography demonstrating stenosis and flow limitation in the petrous internal carotid artery (arrow) secondary to recurrent chordoma. (d) Intraoperative photograph of the preoperative preparation for this case, which included femoral sheath placement (*arrow*) for intraoperative angiography or endovascular intervention, if needed.

are relatively well established for other uses, but their immediacy and durability in the treatment of pseudoaneurysms is questionable[8] as they depend on an intact endothelial wall and allow for continued flow into the site of injury until delayed thrombosis occurs. Treatment with a covered stent avoids these shortcomings and allows for immediate lesion elimination and vessel preservation, and this is our preferred management. Unfortunately, the existing widely available covered stents are not specifically designed for intracranial use and can be technically difficult to deploy along the curves of the carotid artery. However, promising results have been reported[7,8,14,15,16] and should improve with further device development.

13.7 Potential Complications

Although treatment of pseudoaneurysms with a covered stent allows for immediate lesion exclusion and vessel preservation, it is not without risk. In addition to the standard risks of

endovascular procedures such as contrast adverse events, radiation exposure, and access complications, a unique challenge is faced in the setting of the immediate postoperative period. A covered stent is highly thrombogenic and at high risk for distal emboli and stent occlusion, which may lead to stroke. In order to mitigate this risk, dual antiplatelet therapy is necessary, but increases the risk of hemorrhagic complications. This risk is justified to preserve the carotid artery.

13.8 Management Algorithm

- Commit to cadaveric dissection to best understand skull base anatomy.
- Extensively study the preoperative images including vascular studies to understand and predict the pathologic anatomy.
- Plan surgery with vascular control in mind.
- Constantly assess and rehearse a plan for vascular complication management as the case proceeds.

- In the event of vascular injury, obtain control.
- If possible, primarily suture repair the injury.
- If primary repair is not possible, hemostasis must be achieved through the use of packing material and hemostatic adjuncts.
- If the site of injury cannot be adequately delineated or exposed, obtain an angiogram.
- If carotid patency cannot be maintained by primary repair or stenting and carotid sacrifice is necessary, one should proceed to immediate revascularization with bypass, particularly in the absence of documented adequate cerebral collateral circulation.
- In the event of negative angiogram, follow-up angiography should be performed to continue to assess for pseudoaneurysm formation.
- If a pseudoaneurysm develops in the petrous or cavernous carotid artery where there are no critical branches, endovascular treatment with placement of a covered stent can be pursued.

13.9 Root Cause Analysis—Common Factors Leading to Carotid Artery Injury

- Prior radiation weakening the artery wall and scarring the surgical planes.
- Prior operation further obscuring the anatomy and scarring the surgical planes.
- Extensively hyperostotic bone requiring extensive drilling.
- Bony dehiscence of the carotid canal.
- Over reliance on intraoperative navigation for carotid identification.
- Surgeon's experience or surgical technique in proximity to the carotid artery.

13.10 Conclusion

Although middle fossa surgery can pose a significant challenge to the skull base surgeon, vascular injuries can largely be avoided through both thorough knowledge of the vascular anatomy of the skull base and careful surgical planning. In cases when an injury is encountered, further resection should not be sought at the expense of undue risk to critical vascular structures. A predetermined plan and anticipation are needed to deal with a vascular injury safely and effectively and, when possible, primary repair is the best solution. In the event of a known or suspected intraoperative arterial injury, immediate postoperative catheter angiography is needed to evaluate for the presence of a pseudoaneurysm. If negative, repeat angiography should be performed to exclude the possibility of delayed pseudoaneurysm. Iatrogenic pseudoaneurysms can be treated safely and effectively with the endovascular placement of covered stents, with high-flow bypass, or carotid sacrifice reserved for cases where endovascular treatment is not feasible.

References

[1] Bi WL, Brown PA, Abolfotoh M, Al-Mefty O, Mukundan S, Jr, Dunn IF. Utility of dynamic computed tomography angiography in the preoperative evaluation of skull base tumors. J Neurosurg. 2015; 123(1):1–8

[2] Wascher TM, Spetzler RF, Zabramski JM. Improved transdural exposure and temporary occlusion of the petrous internal carotid artery for cavernous sinus surgery. Technical note. J Neurosurg. 1993; 78(5):834–837

[3] Martins C, Yasuda A, Campero A, Ulm AJ, Tanriover N, Rhoton A, Jr. Microsurgical anatomy of the dural arteries. Neurosurgery. 2005; 56(2) Suppl:211–251, discussion 211–251

[4] Osawa S, Rhoton AL, Jr, Tanriover N, Shimizu S, Fujii K. Microsurgical anatomy and surgical exposure of the petrous segment of the internal carotid artery. Neurosurgery. 2008; 63(4) Suppl 2:210–238, discussion 239

[5] Quisling RG, Rhoton AL, Jr. Intrapetrous carotid artery branches: radioanatomic analysis. Radiology. 1979; 131(1):133–136

[6] Yasuda A, Campero A, Martins C, Rhoton AL, Jr, de Oliveira E, Ribas GC. Microsurgical anatomy and approaches to the cavernous sinus. Neurosurgery. 2008; 62(6) Suppl 3:1240–1263

[7] Almefty R, Dunn IF, Aziz-Sultan MA, Al-Mefty O. Delayed carotid pseudoaneurysms from iatrogenic clival meningeal branches avulsion: recognition and proposed management. World Neurosurg. 2017; 104:736–744

[8] Sylvester PT, Moran CJ, Derdeyn CP, et al. Endovascular management of internal carotid artery injuries secondary to endonasal surgery: case series and review of the literature. J Neurosurg. 2016; 125(5):1256–1276

[9] Fox AJ, Viñuela F, Pelz DM, et al. Use of detachable balloons for proximal artery occlusion in the treatment of unclippable cerebral aneurysms. J Neurosurg. 1987; 66(1):40–46

[10] Swearingen B, Heros RC. Common carotid occlusion for unclippable carotid aneurysms: an old but still effective operation. Neurosurgery. 1987; 21(3): 288–295

[11] Larson JJ, Tew JM, Jr, Tomsick TA, van Loveren HR. Treatment of aneurysms of the internal carotid artery by intravascular balloon occlusion: long-term follow-up of 58 patients. Neurosurgery. 1995; 36(1):26–30, discussion 30

[12] Roski RA, Spetzler RF, Nulsen FE. Late complications of carotid ligation in the treatment of intracranial aneurysms. J Neurosurg. 1981; 54(5): 583–587

[13] Origitano TC, al-Mefty O, Leonetti JP, DeMonte F, Reichman OH. Vascular considerations and complications in cranial base surgery. Neurosurgery. 1994; 35(3):351–362, discussion 362–363

[14] Kim BM, Jeon P, Kim DJ, Kim DI, Suh SH, Park KY. Jostent covered stent placement for emergency reconstruction of a ruptured internal carotid artery during or after transsphenoidal surgery. J Neurosurg. 2015; 122(5): 1223–1228

[15] Leung GK, Auyeung KM, Lui WM, Fan YW. Emergency placement of a self-expandable covered stent for carotid artery injury during trans-sphenoidal surgery. Br J Neurosurg. 2006; 20(1):55–57

[16] Li MH, Li YD, Gao BL, et al. A new covered stent designed for intracranial vasculature: application in the management of pseudoaneurysms of the cranial internal carotid artery. AJNR Am J Neuroradiol. 2007; 28(8): 1579–1585

14 Posterior Fossa During Open Skull Base Surgery

David L. Penn, Marte Van Keulen, and Nicholas C. Bambakidis

Summary

In any skull base operation where the operative corridor can be small, deep, and poorly lit, any major vascular injury is a challenge to manage and successfully control. This is particularly true for procedures in the posterior fossa where all the aforementioned conditions can exist and the surgeon is surrounded by highly delicate and sensitive structures, such as the brainstem and cranial nerves. Injury to arterial or venous structures presents its own set of challenges. Arterial injuries can require much more complex techniques, such as microsuturing or bypass to repair while venous bleeding can often be stopped using tamponade with thrombogenic materials. The postoperative complications of arterial injury are often immediate and can cause devastating neurologic sequelae while, in contrast, the consequences of venous injury can be more delayed and unpredictable. The present chapter will review the relevant normal and variant anatomy of the posterior fossa to help surgeons avoid major intraoperative injuries and discuss techniques for controlling bleeding as well as manage some of the downstream consequences.

Keywords: Posterior fossa surgery, vascular injury, dural venous sinus thrombosis, vascular anatomy, anatomical variants

14.1 Key Learning Points

- Understanding the key vascular anatomy and common anatomical variants relevant to open skull base surgery in the posterior fossa is key to avoiding and dealing with vascular injury.
- Identification and direct visualization of the source of bleeding are paramount to appropriately controlling and repairing injuries when they occur. Brain relaxation and wide bony exposure can be key to achieving this in the posterior fossa.
- Preparation can be key to controlling arterial bleeding. Having the necessary equipment and hemostatic agents in the room and being ready before catastrophic injuries occur can help control these events and give surgeons the time and tools to appropriately repair them.
- Posterior communicating artery and vertebral artery dominance are important collateral relationships to understand in each patient undergoing posterior fossa surgery.
- Basilar artery injury may be catastrophic, but can be controlled with focal packing or even focal sacrifice depending on collateral circulation and a nonperforator-bearing segment.
- Venous bleeding is often best controlled with thrombogenic materials, tamponade, and time. Attempting to stop venous bleeding with cautery can worsen injuries and lead to increased blood loss.

- Injury to a bridging vein at the point where it attaches to the dura or bone can be challenging to repair. If cautery is not sufficient, often a gelatin sponge soaked in thrombin with some fibrin glue or other focal packing can be most useful.
- When the mastoid emissary vein is encountered during mastoid craniectomy, careful drilling around the vein can help expose it completely in order to cauterize or ligate it, prior to causing inadvertent injury to the transverse-sigmoid junction.

14.2 Introduction

Intraoperative vascular injuries are among the most feared complications encountered in both open and endoscopic skull base neurosurgery, placing the patient at risk of severe morbidity and potential mortality as well as testing the years of training and mental fortitude of the operating surgeon. Vascular injuries can occur instantaneously to arterial or venous structures and require surgeons to diagnose the source of bleeding and the severity of the injury to choose techniques from an armamentarium of hemostatic strategies. This must be accomplished while simultaneously working through a sea of red that hinders the ability to both precisely visualize the problem and repair it expeditiously.

When performing procedures on pathologies within the posterior fossa, vascular injury is more likely to occur prior to the intradural portion of the procedure. With retrosigmoid, far lateral or transcondylar approaches, vertebral artery (VA) injury can occur during the soft tissue dissection prior to removing any bone. Once bony removal begins, in particular with the retrosigmoid approach, the transverse and sigmoid sinuses are at risk. Preoperative planning, awareness of anatomical variants and dominant supply/drainage, and preparedness can prevent these accidental injuries from having disastrous consequences. During the intradural portion of the operation, the particularly small corridors of the posterior fossa combined with the delicate nature of the surrounding neural structures can make these events even more treacherous.

The techniques for achieving hemostasis and repairing arterial or venous bleeding can differ greatly. Small arterial and moderate venous injuries can often be alleviated with thrombogenic agents and tamponade or bipolar electrocautery while larger injuries may require temporary occlusion and direct repair with suture. Additionally, the types of pathologies being addressed by these approaches can greatly change the risk and likelihood of vascular injury and the surgeon's ability to repair damage, such as a chordoma encasing the basilar artery (BA) or a meningioma invading the dural venous sinus system. This chapter will review factors affecting the risk of major intraoperative vascular injuries, how to avoid such injuries, and techniques to address these events when they occur as well as examine subsequent effects and postoperative management.

14.3 Arterial Injury and Complications

14.3.1 Arterial Anatomy of the Posterior Fossa

The vertebrobasilar system, which supplies most of the blood to the structures within the posterior fossa, originates from the subclavian arteries bilaterally as the VAs and travels through the transverse foraminae of the cervical spine. After traversing the foramen at C1, the V3 segment of the VA courses posteromedially around the atlanto-occipital joint through the sulcus arteriosus of C1, deep to the muscles bounding the suboccipital triangle. Prior to piercing the dura at the lateral edge of the foramen magnum, the artery gives rise to the posterior meningeal and posterior spinal branches. Once intradural (V4), the VA courses anteromedially in front of or between the hypoglossal rootlets and joins the contralateral VA approximately at the level of the pontomedullary junction to become the BA.[1] Arising from the V4 segment is the paired anterior spinal artery and posterior inferior cerebellar artery (PICA), which courses posteriorly around the medulla and cerebellar tonsils between the lower cranial nerves (CN IX–XII).

As the BA runs across the anterior surface of the pons into the interpeduncular cistern, it gives off the anterior inferior cerebellar artery (AICA), numerous perforating arteries, and the superior cerebellar artery (SCA) within the infratentorial space (▶ Fig. 14.1). The AICA often arises from the lower half of the BA and courses within the subarachnoid space with relations to the pons, middle cerebellar peduncle, and petrosal surface of the cerebellum.[1] Also, it courses around CN VI–VIII and gives off a branch, the labyrinthine artery, which supplies the nerves within the internal auditory canal. The SCA arises near the basilar apex within the interpeduncular space and courses inferior to CN III and CN IV and posterolaterally around the pontomesencephalic junction near the tentorial edge.

14.3.2 Anatomical Variants

There are a number of anatomical variants in arterial anatomy of which skull base surgeons operating in the posterior fossa must be aware to avoid troublesome intraoperative situations. Careful review of preoperative imaging can often identify some of these variants and allow for greater care to be taken when this anatomy is encountered during the operation.

In the majority of cases, the VAs are of different calibers. The incidence of a hypoplastic VA, being defined as having smaller caliber than the contralateral VA but still terminating at the basilar junction, is approximately 20 to 40% and is most common on the left side.[2,3,4,5] As a result, preoperative vascular imaging to understand dominance is critical. Additionally, appropriate preoperative imaging should be obtained to study the course of the VA within the soft tissue as often it can have an ectatic course between C1 and C2 that can increase the risk of injury. The presence of an arcuate foramen, a bony bridge on the posterior arch of C1 that surrounds the VA, can be misleading when performing soft tissue dissection and should be noted on preoperative imaging. Presence of this variant can occasionally cause compression of the underlying VA, which may be notable prior to certain operations.[6] Another common variant that can be encountered during soft tissue dissection is the extracranial-extradural origin of PICA, which can occur in approximately 5 to 20% of cases (▶ Fig. 14.2).[7] Injury to this structure has the potential to cause lateral medullary and cerebellar infarcts resulting in significant swelling that can not only make the intracranial portion of the operation very challenging but also have severe neurological consequences.

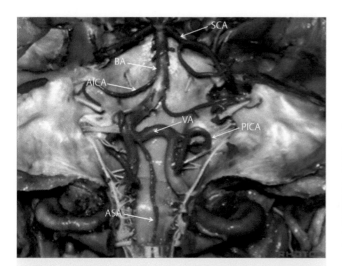

Fig. 14.1 Dorsal view of a cadaveric dissection detailing the anatomy of the posterior circulation arteries. Relationships between major vessels and other neural and bony anatomy are important, as they will be encountered in most of the approaches to the posterior fossa. AICA, anterior inferior cerebellar artery; ASA, anterior spinal artery; BA, basilar artery; PICA, posterior inferior cerebellar artery; SCA, superior cerebellar artery; VA, vertebral artery. (Courtesy of the Rhoton Collection, American Association of Neurological Surgeons [AANS]/Neurosurgical Research and Education Foundation [NREF].)

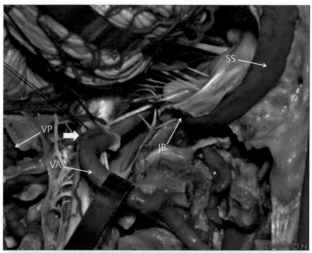

Fig. 14.2 Posterolateral cadaveric view (right side, similar to extreme lateral approach) showing extradural posterior inferior cerebellar artery (PICA) origin (Thick *arrow*) arising from the mobilized VA. Recognition of anatomical variants on preoperative imaging can prevent inadvertent sacrifice of critical vascular structures. JB, jugular bulb; SS, sigmoid sinus; VA, vertebral artery; VP, vertebral plexus. (Courtesy of the Rhoton Collection, American Association of Neurological Surgeons [AANS]/Neurosurgical Research and Education Foundation [NREF].)

14.3.3 Management Strategies for Arterial Injury

In skull base surgery, being prepared for a possible arterial injury can make a large difference in how well it is handled. As always, meticulously studying preoperative imaging for relationships between the targeted lesion and important arterial structures as well as the presence of collateral circulation, such as VA dominance or the presence of posterior communicating arteries, can help surgeons know when these structures will be encountered and provide clues regarding how to proceed at various stages of the operation. Available instrumentation including emergency suctions, temporary aneurysm clips, and fine suture and bypass instrumentation can help reduce time to action in case of an unexpected event. Other instruments that may prove useful during emergent situations, such as endoscopes or mirrors, could help in packing uncontrolled bleeding and give one time to plan an appropriate repair.

In addition to the appropriate tools, preparing the posterior fossa with appropriate brain relaxation can help improve success in the event of a vascular injury. In our practice, we routinely use mannitol during induction, as well as a lumbar drain to improve brain relaxation. More cerebrospinal fluid (CSF) can be drained, and quickly, by opening the cisterna magna early in the dissection or at any point necessary during the operation. All these measures can open the operative corridor to decrease the risk of injury and improve the surgeon's ability to have control if needed. If there is particular concern preoperatively based on the size or location of the lesion or involvement of vascular structures, a surgeon can pre-emptively prepare for an external ventricular drain at any of the posterior access locations, in particular Keen's or Frazier's point.[8] Finally, an adequate size cranial opening can aid in increasing the operative corridor. In an emergent situation, further removal of bone, especially near the foramen magnum, can help in increasing working space to repair injuries, provide proximal control, and aid in brain retraction; as a last resort, cerebellar resection can be performed to open space to achieve control of vascular injury or manage edema related to venous injury.

When arterial bleeding occurs during surgery, it is important to isolate the injury and determine the best way to control the bleeding (▶ Fig. 14.3). Initially, suction should be used to clear the field and specifically locate the injured vessel. This can be aided with the use of tamponade and cottonoids. For massive bleeding, a second suction in the field may be useful. Small injuries to major vessels or from perforating branches can often be controlled using targeted bipolar electrocautery. Larger injuries could require sacrifice of a vessel, which may not be possible depending on the vessel injured and the patient's collateral vasculature in which case repair of the vessel must be attempted. There are a couple considerations prior to large vessel sacrifice. First, the patient's collateral circulation must be studied. For instance, if the injury has occurred to a nondominant VA, the patient may tolerate sacrifice if the injury is proximal to PICA, as the vessel will likely adequately fill from the contralateral VA. The presence of sufficient posterior communicating vessels may allow for the sacrifice of a proximal BA injury, which will allow the perforators to continue to fill from the collateral anterior circulation. A second consideration is the effect of large vessel temporary occlusion. If intraoperative neuromonitoring is used, temporary occlusion of the injured vessel can demonstrate changes in signals helping to demonstrate whether or not the vessel can be sacrificed. Additionally, Doppler ultrasonography or indocyanine green (ICG) angiography may reveal if more distal critical vessels are filling after occlusion and hint that large vessel sacrifice can be performed safely.

In any large vessel injury, it is important to obtain proximal and distal control of the injured vessel. Placement of temporary clips can stop bleeding and allow better inspection of the injury to determine how it can be best repaired. When appropriate, primary closure can be attempted with 9–0 or 10–0 suture; however, within the small and deep confines of the posterior fossa, depending on the approach and injury, this can be quite challenging. If vessel sacrifice is necessary but contraindicated

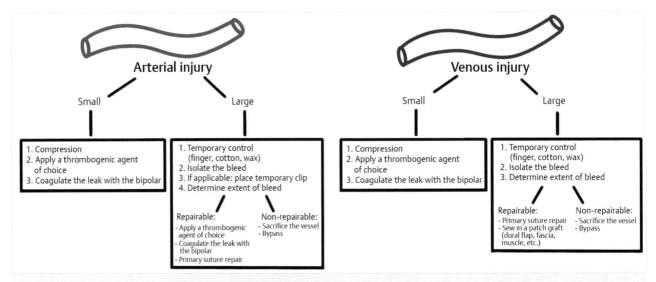

Fig. 14.3 Proposed management paradigm for managing vascular injury within the posterior fossa. Paramount to achieving control is identification of the injury usually through tamponade and inspecting the injury to determine the appropriate next steps. This flowchart proposes options for management of arterial and venous injury during open skull base surgery in the posterior fossa.

based on collateralization, bypass can be attempted via a number of possible techniques, such as removal of the injured segment and re-anastomosis of the vessel, anastomosis with local arterial supply (occipital artery or contralateral PICA), or possibly radial artery or saphenous vein grafts. Injuries to the BA can be particularly challenging because the depth of access to the vessel is long and the working space small. When injury occurs, sometimes bleeding can be controlled with packing of thrombogenic materials, cotton, and/or muscle. If the vessel cannot be sacrificed because of a lack of collateral circulation or the location of the injury in relation to perforators, then one can consider bringing the patient to angiography for repair/reconstruction with thrombectomy, if needed, and/or flow diversion. Unfortunately, this situation can be challenging to manage and often has dire consequences for the patient.

Avoidance of Arterial Injury

As always, preparation is paramount to avoiding intraoperative problems. Recognition of anatomical variants can be valuable to preventing intraoperative bleeding and subsequent devastating ischemia. Asymmetry in the VAs can be important for surgical planning by recognizing a dominant side. This knowledge can allow extra caution during the muscular dissection when approaching the posterior fossa as the artery can be encountered extracranially as it courses superolaterally between the transverse foramina of C1 and C2 and as it runs in the sulcus arteriosus. When possible, such as when approaching midline ventral lesions at the foramen magnum, consideration of the laterality of the approach should be made to avoid injury to the dominant VA. In addition, preoperative recognition of an extradural PICA origin can help prevent inadvertent sacrifice of a presumed muscular branch of the VA, which can help reduce the risk of potentially severe ischemia.

During the postoperative period, measures can be taken to avoid worsening of these complications. Strict blood pressure management, with avoidance of hypotension (systolic blood pressure [SBP] ≥ 120 mm Hg) to avoid watershed infarcts and permissive hypertension to preserve penumbra (SBP 140–180 mm Hg based on patient's baseline blood pressure), can prevent worsening of the initial ischemic effects of these injuries, helping to minimize neurological morbidity. Depending on the necessary techniques used to repair injuries (i.e., if primary repair of a vessel or bypass is necessary), early antiplatelet with Aspirin 81 mg daily may be necessary to prevent thrombus formation and embolization.

14.4 Venous Injury and Complications

14.4.1 Venous Anatomy of the Posterior Fossa

Venous structures are encountered throughout all stages of operations performed to approach the posterior fossa. While performing the soft tissue dissection, significant venous bleeding can be encountered from the venous plexus surrounding the VA. This extensive plexus is usually encountered deep to the muscles of the suboccipital triangle, in particular during the

muscular dissection for a far lateral approach and even with the inferior portion of a postauricular incision for a retrosigmoid or transmastoid approach.

The most treacherous venous anatomy encountered during open skull base operations, the dural venous sinus system, is often met at the beginning of the procedure prior to opening the dura. The dural venous sinuses are contained within the endosteal and meningeal dural layers with an inner lining of endothelium.[9,10] Unlike normal veins, they lack musculature and valves. The transverse sinus drains from the torcula into the sigmoid sinus and inevitably into the jugular vein (► Fig. 14.4). The transverse sinus begins near the inion and runs in a bony groove along the inner surface of the occipital bone entering the sigmoid sinus just medial to the petrous temporal bone. The sigmoid sinus then undergoes a tortuous course where it joins the jugular bulb within the mastoid portion of the temporal bone. Knowledge of surface and bony landmarks for identification of these structures prior to beginning drilling can help avoid injury. The inion can be used to approximate the location of the torcula, while the transverse-sigmoid junction can often be approximated as the midpoint of a line drawn from the root of the zygoma to the inion. Once soft tissue dissection has been completed, the transverse-sigmoid junction can be approximated by a point slightly inferior and medial to the asterion.[11] In addition, there is often a mastoid emissary vein that runs through the occipital bone in the retrosigmoid region that is encountered when exposing the transverse-sigmoid junction, which can bleed significantly.

The intradural venous system within the posterior fossa is divided into four groups based on their drainage and includes the superficial, deep, brainstem, and bridging veins (► Fig. 14.5).[12] The superficial veins drain and course along the three surfaces of the cerebellar hemispheres while the deep veins can be found within the fissures between the cerebellum, brainstem, and cerebellar peduncles. The veins draining the brainstem are named based on their drainage and course along the three segments of

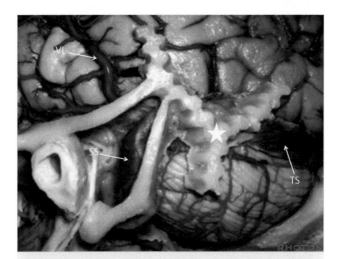

Fig. 14.4 Posterolateral cadaveric dissection (left side) demonstrating dural venous sinus anatomy in relation to superficial cranial landmarks. SS, sigmoid sinus; star, asterion; TS, transverse sinus; VL, vein of Labbe. (Courtesy of the Rhoton Collection, American Association of Neurological Surgeons [AANS]/Neurosurgical Research and Education Foundation [NREF].)

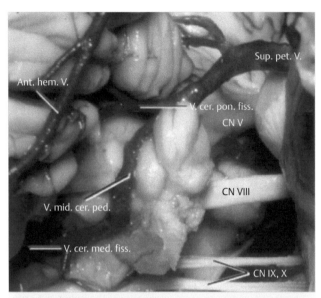

Fig. 14.5 Cadaveric dissection (right side) demonstrating the intradural venous anatomy along the petrosal surface of the cerebellum and brainstem from a lateral approach, particularly the superior petrosal vein's relationship with CN V and the petrosal surface of the temporal bone. This vessel can be injured in most lateral approaches to the posterior fossa but it often can be sacrificed without consequence. (Reproduced with permission of Oxford University Press from Rhoton.[12])

the brainstem. Finally, the bridging veins that collect drainage from the rest of the posterior fossa are named after their inevitable drainage site and include the galenic group, the petrosal group, and the tentorial group.

Sequelae from injury or sacrifice of the veins of the posterior fossa is uncommon, largely because of extensive anastomosis; however, knowledge of the anatomy can prevent inadvertent bleeding or can aid in finding likely sources of venous bleeding to obtain hemostasis.[12] The bridging veins are among the more relevant veins encountered during open skull base surgery in the posterior fossa. In particular, the superior petrosal veins that course in the rostral aspect of the cerebellopontine angle can be encountered when targeting lesions of the cerebellopontine angle, petrous dura, or trigeminal nerve and can even be inadvertently damaged when operating on other lesions along the petrosal surface of the cerebellum, brainstem, and cranial nerves. In addition, when performing supracerebellar infratentorial approaches, one will encounter the precerebellar vein on the way to the quadrageminal cistern, which can often be sacrificed without consequence, as well as deep venous structures within the cistern, including the vein of Galen and internal cerebral veins as well as the paired basal veins of Rosenthal within the ambient cisterns, laterally, which must be preserved. Although located in the supratentorial space, it is worth noting that the vein of Labbe drains into the dural venous sinuses approximately near the transverse-sigmoid junction. Care must be taken to preserve this vein, particularly when performing transpetrosal approaches for pathologies that may involve both compartments. Injury to this vein can result in venous infarction of the posterior temporal lobe with severe neurologic consequences.

14.4.2 Anatomical Variants

Similar to arterial anatomy, there exist normal anatomic venous variants that skull base surgeons must be able to recognize on preoperative studies. One of the most prevalent is asymmetry or dominance of the dural venous sinus system. A number of observational studies have demonstrated asymmetry of the transverse sinuses in approximately 10.0 to 66.9% of patients, with hypo- or aplasia of the left transverse sinus being more common, with an incidence ranging from 25.4 to 59%.[13,14,15] This disparity is thought to be explained by the fact that the right-sided transverse sinus drains the cerebral hemispheres through the superior sagittal sinus while the left transverse sinus drains the straight sinus and the deep cerebral venous system.

Another variant of the dural venous sinuses is the presence of the occipital sinus, which runs vertically or obliquely underneath the occipital bone. When present, this is usually the smallest of the dural venous sinuses that connect the marginal sinus and vertebral venous plexus to the torcula, inevitably draining into the jugular venous system. Most commonly, the occipital sinus is singular but it can be duplicated bilaterally and rarely triplicated.[16] The presence of the occipital sinus is considered a persistence of a venous channel expected to regress with age as early as in the 6th and 7th months of gestation.[17] One study using magnetic resonance venography (MRV) to examine venous sinus anatomy as it relates to age demonstrated incidence of an occipital sinus in 24% of the population less than 1 year of age trending downward to an incidence of 2.8% in age groups of 16 to 20 years.[18] Other studies have demonstrated similar findings of age-related decreased incidence.[19,20]

The most clinically relevant of the bridging veins, the superior petrosal or Dandy's vein, can vary based on its entry point to the superior petrosal sinus relative to the internal acoustic meatus (i.e., medial, intermediate, and lateral) as well as based on the number of tributaries.[12] In cadaveric studies, the medial position was found to be most common (64.7%), followed by the lateral type (26.5%) and intermediate type (8.8%). With regard to the number of tributaries, most commonly the superior petrosal vein was found to have two (50%), followed by one (40%) and three (10%).[21]

14.4.3 Management Strategies for Venous Injury

For a surgeon not comfortable managing venous bleeding, skull base neurosurgery is not an ideal subspecialty. Venous bleeding, although of lower pressure than arterial bleeding, can be torrential and rapidly obscure the surgical field, which can present challenges in regaining control. Beyond significant blood loss, venous bleeding can also result in life-threatening complications including air embolism, venous sinus thrombosis and occlusion, embolization, and formation of secondary dural arteriovenous malformations.

The mainstay in controlling venous bleeding is often the use of hemostatic agents, tamponade, and time (▶ Fig. 14.3). Often collagen or gelatin sponges soaked in fibrinogen or thrombin, flowable gelatin matrices, or oxidized cellulose can be successful in controlling small injuries, even in the dural venous sinuses; however, one downside to these products is that they can induce cascades causing clotting and potentially turn a small injury into an occlusive thrombus.[22] Bolstering these products with fibrin glue can be effective in not only achieving hemostasis but to more reliably keep these materials in place.

Many of the techniques for repair of dural venous sinuses have been developed from work done with traumatic injuries and resection of meningiomas invading the superior sagittal sinus. Techniques for direct repair of dural venous sinuses can be more involved and complex, including directly suturing the injury, use of autologous venous or arterial graft with the use of shunts, dural or fascial or muscle grafts, pericranial patching, or allograft or synthetic patch grafts.[23,24,25,26,27,28,29] There are a number of disadvantages to some of these techniques. Direct repair can be problematic when the dura is very fragile and placement of even a single suture can result in further tears, creating a larger problem. Although vessel grafts can restore appropriate sinus flow, the major disadvantage is the requirement for temporary occlusion of the already injured sinus and the time-consuming nature of the repair to both harvest a graft and create an anastomosis. In addition, graft patency rates are generally quite low. Other types of patch grafts can be useful in controlling bleeding; however, the site of harvest must be a consideration. In particular, with operations in the posterior fossa, using a dural graft could increase the risk of CSF leak by making primary dural repair more difficult and leaving larger gaps. In our practice, we often repair large sinus injuries using dural grafts bolstered with thrombin-soaked, hemostatic gelatin sponges. Hemostatic sponges are placed directly over the injury and the dura is then flapped over the sponge and tacked to the edge of the craniotomy through small tack-up holes. This technique balances the need to be efficient and often effectively repairs the injury without requiring sinus occlusion or sacrifice.

Avoidance of Venous Injury

Most important to avoiding intraoperative catastrophe is preparation. Thoroughly studying the preoperative imaging for variant anatomy and prominent venous structures, having all necessary materials and tools needed to manage excessive bleeding readily available, and having a checklist of techniques to regain control when an injury occurs can turn a near-fatal event into a routine episode. There are some common points during a procedure where venous bleeding can occur, and knowing these points and how to pre-emptively control them can be helpful. When sinus injury occurs, it is important to take precautions to prevent air embolism, which may include copious irrigation and lowering the head of bed. When there is particular concern for sinus injury, precordial Doppler is recommended to help identify air emboli and appropriately treat them expeditiously.

As previously discussed, soft tissue dissection of the suboccipital musculature at the level of the foramen magnum can result in bleeding from the vertebral venous plexus. Careful, subperiosteal dissection of this tissue can help minimize this bleeding and often the veins of the plexus can be identified without injury, if particular caution is taken. However, when bleeding is encountered, often the best way to control it is through the use of hemostatic materials (we prefer flowable gelatin matrices and gelatin sponges soaked in thrombin), tamponade, and time. Attempting to use electrocautery on

this fragile venous system can sometimes result in larger injuries, especially if the walls of the veins become stuck to instruments.

When performing a midline, suboccipital approach, the presence of an occipital sinus can be disastrous. The presence of this structure should be noted on preoperative imaging. When present, the dural opening must be performed carefully and, when approaching the midline, use of bipolar cauterization and/or clips can help coagulate or ligate the sinus prior to incising this structure.

Often sinus injury can occur at the transverse-sigmoid junction when the mastoid emissary vein is encountered during the mastoid craniectomy portion of a retrosigmoid approach. Furthermore, this vein can even travel through the bone and can cause significant venous bleeding when clearing the soft tissue. When encountered at this point, it is important to clear the soft tissue fully from around the exit site of the vein at which point bone wax can be effective in stopping bleeding. While drilling, it is sometimes possible to clear the bone around the vein in a controlled fashion so that the vein can be ligated or cauterized prior to being torn from the sinus.

Additionally, the sigmoid sinus can be directly injured during mastoid drilling. This can occur via direct injury from a drill or rongeur or potentially from heat created by the drill. The risk of direct injury can increase if the sinus is particularly protuberant into the mastoid bone. When drilling, care should be taken to adequately thin the bone and dissect in from the sinus in a controlled fashion.

Once intradural, the highest risk of injury can be to the bridging veins of the posterior fossa, in particular, the superior petrosal vein through a retrosigmoid approach. When CSF has been significantly drained and the cerebellum begins to sag, tension can be placed on this vein. In combination with drying out, injury can occur inadvertently, even when working some distance away. Often this vein can be sacrificed in a controlled fashion, without consequence, which can prevent unexpected injury and is reported in many large case series as being safe; however, there exist reports of complications associated with its sacrifice ranging from auditory hallucinations to venous infarction and cerebellar hemorrhage.[30,31,32,33,34,35,36,37] In our practice, we routinely preserve this vein and rarely sacrifice it intentionally. For the majority of pathologies within the posterior fossa, this goal can be achieved because most pathology is inferior to the vein. Situations in which we would consider sacrificing this vessel would be when the vein is in the way of accomplishing the goal of surgery; for example, resection of a trigeminal schwannoma from a posterior approach, or occasionally with very large tumors where increasing the working space by sacrificing the vein can prevent inadvertent injury and bleeding and aid in tumor resection and preservation of neurologic function.

When sacrificing the vein it is best to coagulate with bipolar electrocautery and then cut the vessel half way to ensure it has been fully cauterized. If necessary, further cautery can be used prior to finishing dividing the vessel. This technique can help minimize bleeding if the vessel has not been fully cauterized. If a bridging vein is injured at the point where it attaches to the dura or bone, this can be challenging to repair. In some instances cautery can be sufficient; however, often gelatin sponge soaked in thrombin with some fibrin glue can be most useful.

The fibrin glue can help hold the sponge in place if gravity is working against keeping the material in place.

14.4.4 Dural Venous Sinus Thrombosis and Postoperative Management

Following a venous sinus injury, other than the necessary maneuvers required to control the bleeding, thrombogenic cascades are initiated that can lead to propagation of clot and potential occlusion of major draining sinuses. Some studies have shown that translabyrinthine exposures, which involve early skeletonization and retraction of the sigmoid sinus, without injury can result in an incidence of dural venous sinus thrombosis ranging from 2.1 to 9.6%, regardless of pathology.[38,39,40,41] Furthermore, the rate of postoperative dural venous sinus thrombosis found in patients undergoing operations for cerebellopontine angle masses ranges from 11.6 to 15.9%.[42,43] In our own series of patients undergoing translabyrinthine approaches for vestibular schwannomas, we found an incidence of thrombosis in 16.4% on routine perioperative magnetic resonance imaging (MRI). Only four of these patients had symptoms attributable to thrombosis. This finding was consistent with the rate of thrombosis in patients with vestibular schwannomas, which ranges from 6.0 to 38.9%, regardless of approach.[44,45] Risk factors shown to be associated with development of postoperative thrombosis include length of operation, amount of exposure of the sinus and necessary manipulation, fixed retraction, mechanical injury as well as dehydration, pregnancy, use of oral contraceptives, infection, and hematologic disease.[22,39,43]

Although often asymptomatic, continued clot progression can potentially result in venous infarction and devastating neurologic consequences, including seizures, coma, and death, in the early postoperative period.[46] The effects of thrombosis can be even seen weeks to months postoperatively, with patients presenting with an increased risk of CSF or pseudotumor cerebri.[39,47] Although rare, Keiper and colleagues examined a large series of patients with symptomatic postoperative sinus thrombosis revealing an incidence of 4.6% ($n = 5/107$) developing pseudotumor cerebri following suboccipital or translabyrinthine approaches for cerebellopontine angle lesions, necessitating both medical and/or surgical CSF diversion.[39]

Management of postoperative dural venous sinus thrombosis can range from hydration alone to full therapeutic anticoagulation. Because of the nonbenign associated effects, some authors recommend aggressive treatment. A Cochrane review of patients with nonoperative venous sinus thromboses revealed an absolute risk reduction of 13% for death and dependency associated with the use of anticoagulation with zero patients experiencing intracranial hemorrhage after initiation of anticoagulation.[48] Although the use of anticoagulation for nonoperative thrombosis is less controversial, its use in the immediate postoperative period can be concerning, especially given the 40% risk of intracerebral hemorrhage among nonoperative patients.[46,49,50] Despite this risk, one series of five patients that had developed postoperative sinus thrombosis following resection of vestibular schwannoma underwent anticoagulation with heparin-bridge to warfarin, within approximately 24 hours from surgery, with resolution of thrombosis at 6-month follow-up and no neurologic complications.[43] Conversely, a series of 24 patients with asymptomatic thromboses that had undergone surgical resection of lesions involving the dural venous sinuses in both the supratentorial and infratentorial spaces were managed conservatively with 23 patients going untreated and one patient receiving hydration.[47] No neurological consequences were observed in this study; however, there was a statistically significant increased rate of CSF leakage found when compared to patients who did not develop thrombosis. Given these data, it may be reasonable to treat thrombosis to prevent delayed postoperative CSF associated complications, taking into account the degree of occlusion and individual patient risk factors. In our practice, we often treat incidental postoperative dural venous sinus thrombosis with Aspirin 81 mg, after postoperative day 5. The determination of when to treat an incidental thrombus is determined subjectively based on size, symptomatology, and perceived degree of occlusion.

14.5 Conclusion

Although major vascular injury during open skull base surgery in the posterior fossa can be an overwhelming complication, preparation regarding the anatomy to be encountered and the techniques to rapidly control bleeding can help surgeons avoid these events and prevent morbidity and potential mortality of their patients when they occur. Attentive postoperative management following an injury can prevent worsening of these events and long-term complications that may occur.

References

[1] Rhoton AL, Jr. The cerebellar arteries. Neurosurgery. 2000; 47(3) Suppl:S29–S68

[2] Bruneau M, Cornelius JF, George B. Anterolateral approach to the V1 segment of the vertebral artery. Neurosurgery. 2006; 58(4) Suppl 2:ONS-215–ONS-219, discussion ONS-219

[3] Bruneau M, Cornelius JF, George B. Antero-lateral approach to the V3 segment of the vertebral artery. Neurosurgery. 2006; 58(1) Suppl:ONS29–ONS35, discussion ONS29–ONS35

[4] Jeng JS, Yip PK. Evaluation of vertebral artery hypoplasia and asymmetry by color-coded duplex ultrasonography. Ultrasound Med Biol. 2004; 30 (5):605–609

[5] Bruneau M, De Witte O, Regli L, George B. Anatomical variations. In: George B, Bruneau M, Spetzler RF, eds. Pathology and Surgery Around the Vertebral Artery. Paris, France: Springer-Verlag France; 2011:53–74

[6] Ahn J, Duran M, Syldort S, et al. Arcuate foramen: anatomy, embryology, nomenclature, pathology, and surgical considerations. World Neurosurg. 2018; 118:197–202

[7] Fine AD, Cardoso A, Rhoton AL, Jr. Microsurgical anatomy of the extracranial-extradural origin of the posterior inferior cerebellar artery. J Neurosurg. 1999; 91(4):645–652

[8] Morone PJ, Dewan MC, Zuckerman SL, Tubbs RS, Singer RJ. Craniometrics and ventricular access: a review of Kocher's, Kaufman's, Paine's, Menovksy's, Tubbs', Keen's, Frazier's, Dandy's, and Sanchez's points. Oper Neurosurg (Hagerstown). 2020; 18(5):461–469

[9] Kiliç T, Akakin A. Anatomy of cerebral veins and sinuses. Front Neurol Neurosci. 2008; 23:4–15

[10] Massrey C, Altafulla JJ, Iwanaga J, et al. Variations of the transverse sinus: review with an unusual case report. Cureus. 2018; 10(9):e3248

[11] Hall S, Peter Gan YC. Anatomical localization of the transverse-sigmoid sinus junction: comparison of existing techniques. Surg Neurol Int. 2019; 10:186

[12] Rhoton AL, Jr. The posterior fossa veins. Neurosurgery. 2000; 47(3) Suppl: S69–S92

[13] Alper F, Kantarci M, Dane S, Gumustekin K, Onbas O, Durur I. Importance of anatomical asymmetries of transverse sinuses: an MR venographic study. Cerebrovasc Dis. 2004; 18(3):236–239

[14] Goyal G, Singh R, Bansal N, Paliwal VK. Anatomical variations of cerebral MR venography: is gender matter? Neurointervention. 2016; 11(2):92–98

[15] Surendrababu NR, Subathira, Livingstone RS. Variations in the cerebral venous anatomy and pitfalls in the diagnosis of cerebral venous sinus thrombosis: low field MR experience. Indian J Med Sci. 2006; 60(4):135–142

[16] Das AC, Hasan M. The occipital sinus. J Neurosurg. 1970; 33(3):307–311

[17] Okudera T, Huang YP, Ohta T, et al. Development of posterior fossa dural sinuses, emissary veins, and jugular bulb: morphological and radiologic study. AJNR Am J Neuroradiol. 1994; 15(10):1871–1883

[18] Larson AS, Lanzino G, Brinjikji W. Variations of intracranial dural venous sinus diameters from birth to 20 years of age: an MRV-based study. AJNR Am J Neuroradiol. 2020; 41(12):2351–2357

[19] Mizutani K, Miwa T, Akiyama T, Sakamoto Y, Fujiwara H, Yoshida K. Fate of the three embryonic dural sinuses in infants: the primitive tentorial sinus, occipital sinus, and falcine sinus. Neuroradiology. 2018; 60(3):325–333

[20] Widjaja E, Griffiths PD. Intracranial MR venography in children: normal anatomy and variations. AJNR Am J Neuroradiol. 2004; 25(9):1557–1562

[21] Matsushima T, Rhoton AL, Jr, de Oliveira E, Peace D. Microsurgical anatomy of the veins of the posterior fossa. J Neurosurg. 1983; 59(1):63–105

[22] Ohata K, Haque M, Morino M, et al. Occlusion of the sigmoid sinus after surgery via the presigmoidal-transpetrosal approach. J Neurosurg. 1998; 89(4):575–584

[23] Donaghy RM, Wallman LJ, Flanagan MJ, Numoto M. Saggital sinus repair. Technical note. J Neurosurg. 1973; 38(2):244–248

[24] Hakuba A, Huh CW, Tsujikawa S, Nishimura S. Total removal of a parasagittal meningioma of the posterior third of the sagittal sinus and its repair by autogenous vein graft. Case report. J Neurosurg. 1979; 51(3):379–382

[25] Kapp JP, Gielchinsky I, Petty C, McClure C. An internal shunt for use in the reconstruction of dural venous sinuses. Technical note. J Neurosurg. 1971; 35(3):351–354

[26] Rish BL. The repair of dural venous sinus wounds by autogenous venorrhaphy. J Neurosurg. 1971; 35(4):392–395

[27] Sindou M, Hallacq P. Venous reconstruction in surgery of meningiomas invading the sagittal and transverse sinuses. Skull Base Surg. 1998; 8(2):57–64

[28] Sindou MP, Alvernia JE. Results of attempted radical tumor removal and venous repair in 100 consecutive meningiomas involving the major dural sinuses. J Neurosurg. 2006; 105(4):514–525

[29] Matsushima K, Kohno M, Tanaka Y, Nakajima N, Ichimasu N. Management of sigmoid sinus injury: retrospective study of 450 consecutive surgeries in the cerebellopontine angle and intrapetrous region. Oper Neurosurg (Hagerstown). 2020 (Online ahead of print)

[30] Anichini G, Iqbal M, Rafiq NM, Ironside JW, Kamel M. Sacrificing the superior petrosal vein during microvascular decompression. Is it safe? Learning the hard way. Case report and review of literature. Surg Neurol Int. 2016; 7 Suppl 14:S415–S420

[31] Gharabaghi A, Koerbel A, Löwenheim H, Kaminsky J, Samii M, Tatagiba M. The impact of petrosal vein preservation on postoperative auditory function in surgery of petrous apex meningiomas. Neurosurgery. 2006; 59(1) Suppl 1:ONS68–ONS74, discussion ONS68–ONS74

[32] Liebelt BD, Barber SM, Desai VR, et al. Superior petrosal vein sacrifice during microvascular decompression: perioperative complication rates and comparison with venous preservation. World Neurosurg. 2017; 104:788–794

[33] Masuoka J, Matsushima T, Hikita T, Inoue E. Cerebellar swelling after sacrifice of the superior petrosal vein during microvascular decompression for trigeminal neuralgia. J Clin Neurosci. 2009; 16(10):1342–1344

[34] McLaughlin MR, Jannetta PJ, Clyde BL, Subach BR, Comey CH, Resnick DK. Microvascular decompression of cranial nerves: lessons learned after 4400 operations. J Neurosurg. 1999; 90(1):1–8

[35] Narayan V, Savardekar AR, Patra DP, et al. Safety profile of superior petrosal vein (the vein of Dandy) sacrifice in neurosurgical procedures: a systematic review. Neurosurg Focus. 2018; 45(1):E3

[36] Sakata K, Al-Mefty O, Yamamoto I. Venous consideration in petrosal approach: microsurgical anatomy of the temporal bridging vein. Neurosurgery. 2000; 47(1):153–160, discussion 160–161

[37] Samii M, Tatagiba M, Carvalho GA. Retrosigmoid intradural suprameatal approach to Meckel's cave and the middle fossa: surgical technique and outcome. J Neurosurg. 2000; 92(2):235–241

[38] Jean WC, Felbaum DR, Stemer AB, Hoa M, Kim HJ. Venous sinus compromise after pre-sigmoid, transpetrosal approach for skull base tumors: a study on the asymptomatic incidence and report of a rare dural arteriovenous fistula as symptomatic manifestation. J Clin Neurosci. 2017; 39:114–117

[39] Keiper GL, Jr, Sherman JD, Tomsick TA, Tew JM, Jr. Dural sinus thrombosis and pseudotumor cerebri: unexpected complications of suboccipital craniotomy and translabyrinthine craniectomy. J Neurosurg. 1999; 91(2):192–197

[40] Leonetti JP, Reichman OH, Silberman SJ, Gruener G. Venous infarction following translabyrinthine access to the cerebellopontine angle. Am J Otol. 1994; 15(6):723–727

[41] Sade B, Mohr G, Dufour JJ. Vascular complications of vestibular schwannoma surgery: a comparison of the suboccipital retrosigmoid and translabyrinthine approaches. J Neurosurg. 2006; 105(2):200–204

[42] Kow CY, Caldwell J, Mchugh F, Sillars H, Bok A. Dural venous sinus thrombosis after cerebellopontine angle surgery: should it be treated? J Clin Neurosci. 2020; 75:157–162

[43] Moore J, Thomas P, Cousins V, Rosenfeld JV. Diagnosis and management of dural sinus thrombosis following resection of cerebellopontine angle tumors. J Neurol Surg B Skull Base. 2014; 75(6):402–408

[44] Abou-Al-Shaar H, Gozal YM, Alzhrani G, Karsy M, Shelton C, Couldwell WT. Cerebral venous sinus thrombosis after vestibular schwannoma surgery: a call for evidence-based management guidelines. Neurosurg Focus. 2018; 45(1):E4

[45] Guazzo E, Panizza B, Lomas A, et al. Cerebral venous sinus thrombosis after translabyrinthine vestibular schwannoma—a prospective study and suggested management paradigm. Otol Neurotol. 2020; 41(2):e273–e279

[46] Medel R, Monteith SJ, Crowley RW, Dumont AS. A review of therapeutic strategies for the management of cerebral venous sinus thrombosis. Neurosurg Focus. 2009; 27(5):E6

[47] Benjamin CG, Sen RD, Golfinos JG, et al. Postoperative cerebral venous sinus thrombosis in the setting of surgery adjacent to the major dural venous sinuses. J Neurosurg. 2018:1–7 (Online ahead of print)

[48] Coutinho JM, de Bruijn SF, deVeber G, Stam J. Anticoagulation for cerebral venous sinus thrombosis. Stroke. 2012; 43(4):e41–e42

[49] Einhäupl KM, Villringer A, Meister W, et al. Heparin treatment in sinus venous thrombosis. Lancet. 1991; 338(8767):597–600

[50] Saposnik G, Barinagarrementeria F, Brown RD, Jr, et al. American Heart Association Stroke Council and the Council on Epidemiology and Prevention. Diagnosis and management of cerebral venous thrombosis: a statement for healthcare professionals from the American Heart Association/American Stroke Association. Stroke. 2011; 42(4):1158–1192

15 Perforator Injury During Endoscopic Endonasal Skull Base Surgery

João Mangussi-Gomes, Matheus F. de Oliveira, Eduardo A. S. Vellutini, and Aldo C. Stamm

Summary

Perforators are especially prone to injury during endoscopic endonasal approaches (EEAs) due to their small caliber, long trajectories, and often close relationship with skull base tumors. Injury to such vessels may result in ischemia or hemorrhage in important areas of the brain, causing severe disabilities or even death. In this chapter, the anatomy of perforators is presented in a way that is logical for endoscopic skull base surgeons. Ways to prevent their injuries, measures to take when injuries happen, and a clinical example are also discussed.

Keywords: Arterioles, perforators, ischemia, endoscopic endonasal approaches, skull base

15.1 Key Learning Points

- Any vessel injury during endoscopic endonasal approaches (EEAs) may result in high morbidity or even mortality.
- Perforators are particularly vulnerable during EEA due to their small caliber, long trajectories, close relationship to other important neurovascular structures, and altered anatomy in the context of skull base diseases.
- Clinical consequences deriving from injuries to perforators may range from no deficit to death, depending on the brain areas nourished by these perforators, and the collateral blood supply to such areas.
- Knowing the detailed anatomy of perforators from an endoscopic endonasal point of view, correctly identifying perforators during surgery, and employing microdissection techniques are all important measures to prevent vascular injuries during EEA.
- The best treatment strategy for injured perforators is prevention; once perforators are injured, they cannot be sutured, repaired, or bypassed; delicate bipolar cauterization of the injured vessel is usually sufficient to avoid hemorrhage and worse consequences.

15.2 Introduction

The development of EEAs is recognized as one of the most important recent advances in the field of skull base surgery. The EEA has allowed access to lesions in the ventral skull base through a natural and minimally invasive pathway, avoiding brain retraction.[1] In spite of this, the EEA has also brought new challenges. Relevant vessels of different sizes are all in close relationship with the skull base, and, in some cases, present in the pathway to areas of surgical interest.

Injuries to large vessels like the internal carotid artery (ICA) during EEA present as surgical accidents that must be rapidly dealt with. Because this is such a feared complication, it is highly discussed worldwide and different groups have already suggested standardized management protocols for this type of injury.[2,3,4] However, the literature is scarce on injuries to perforators during EEA. Perforators are tiny arteries that penetrate the brain and some cranial nerves or nuclei, and are highly variable in number, size, and distribution. They can often be encroached or encased by tumors, making identification and preservation extremely difficult in some cases. Regardless of their caliber, injuries to such vessels can have little or no consequence or can be similarly catastrophic, resulting in severe disabilities or even death.

Compartmentalization of skull base perforators from an endonasal perspective is proposed in this chapter. Ways to prevent injuries, measures to take when inadvertent lesions happen, and a clinical example are also discussed.

15.3 Compartmentalization of Skull Base Perforators—Related Pathologies and Potential Complications

For ease of comprehension, perforators related to EEA can be localized into three different compartments: anterior, posterior, and inferior. The anterior compartment consists of small arteries branching from the ICAs and anterior cerebral arteries (ACAs). The posterior perforating system consists of perforators arising from the posterior communicating artery (PComA), posterior cerebral artery (PCA), superior cerebellar artery (SCA), and upper basilar artery (UBA). The inferior perforating system consists of perforators from the lower basilar artery (LBA), vertebral arteries (VAs), anterior inferior cerebellar artery (AICA), and posterior inferior cerebellar artery (PICA).

The diseases related to these perforators are those most often encountered in each specific skull base compartments. Likewise, the potential complications resulting from injury of such perforators are closely linked to the specific area of the brain or cranial nerves nourished by these perforators, as discussed below.

15.3.1 The Anterior Compartment

Perforators in the anterior compartment are mostly related to anterior fossa, sellar, and suprasellar diseases, such as olfactory groove and *tuberculum sellae* meningiomas, craniopharyngiomas, pituitary adenomas, Rathke's cleft cysts, and others. Such arteries are often seen during transcribriform and/or transplanum-transtuberculum approaches (**Video 15.1**)

Anterior Cerebral Artery (ACA)

The ACA has five segments, numbered from A1 to A5. The A1 segment, extending from the ICA bifurcation to the anterior communicating artery (AComA), is the most basal segment from where most perforating branches originate.[5,6,7]

The medial lenticulostriate perforators, ranging from 1 to 11 branches (average of 6), arise from the posterosuperior aspect of the proximal half of A1 segment and follow a direct posterior and superior course to enter the medial half of the anterior perforated substance (APS).

Perforators from AComA, ranging from 0 to 4 (average of 1.6), usually arise from its posterior aspect, and supply the APS, the infundibulum, the optic chiasm, the subcallosal area, and the preoptic areas of the hypothalamus.

Heubner's recurrent artery arises in approximately 80% of individuals from the proximal A2 segment, bends backward above its parent vessel, and courses posterior to the A1 segment in 60% of individuals; it is the largest and longest branch directed to the APS. It passes above the carotid bifurcation and accompanies the M1 segment into the medial part of the sylvian fissure before entering the anterior and middle portions of the full mediolateral extent of the APS.

Ischemic events in this compartment, most often due to injuries to A1 or AComA perforators, may result in personality disorders, intellectual deficits, and altered level of consciousness. Occlusion of A2 branches, especially Heubner's recurrent artery, may cause hemiparesis with brachial predominance or dysphasia due to caudate, putamen, and internal capsule infarcts. Emotional changes, personality disorders, and intellectual deficits may also be ascribed to ischemia in this area.[6]

Internal Carotid Artery (ICA)

The supraclinoid portion of ICA is usually divided into three segments based on the origin of its major branches: the ophthalmic segment extends from the ophthalmic artery origin to the posterior communicating artery (PComA), the communicating segment extends from the PComA origin to the anterior choroidal artery (AChA), and the choroidal segment extends from the AChA origin to the ICA bifurcation. The first two segments are more related to EEA as the choroidal segment has a posterolateral course. The PComA has a posteroinferior course and will be discussed later in this chapter.[7,8]

Perforators from the ophthalmic segment usually comprise four rami (ranging from 1 to 7) arising from the posteromedial aspect of the ICA and are distributed to the pituitary gland, stalk, optic chiasm, and, less commonly, optic nerve, premamillary bodies, third ventricle floor, and optic tract. The superior hypophyseal arteries, which can range from 1 to 5 in number and can be either uni- or bilateral, run medially to supply the optic chiasm, pituitary stalk, and anterior lobe of the pituitary gland (▸ Fig. 15.1). Bilateral injury of superior hypophyseal arteries may increase the risk of stalk and pituitary dysfunction. Chiasmal dysfunction (visual field defects), in turn, may occur with even a unilateral superior hypophyseal artery lesion.[9]

15.3.2 The Posterior Compartment

Perforators in the posterior compartment are more related to the transsphenoidal-transclival approaches for removal of upper clival chordomas and meningiomas, and some pituitary adenomas or large craniopharyngiomas with inferior extension.[10]

The posterior compartment has perforators arising from the PComA, UBA, PCA, and SCA. In the posterior compartment, perforators comprise a less intricate vascular network, which supplies the posterior perforated substance (PPS) to irrigate the upper brainstem and the posterior diencephalon (thalamoperforating arteries). Although these perforators are smaller in number when compared to the anterior compartment, ischemic injuries resulting from their lesions may cause much more severe neurological impairment due to the involvement of white matter tracts and nuclei within the brainstem and diencephalon.

Posterior Cerebral Artery (PCA)

The PCA is divided into four segments, from P1 to P4, with P1 and P2 being the most important sites for perforators, and P1 being the most common site of perforators seen during EEA. P1 extends from the basilar bifurcation to the site where the PComA joins the PCA.[11,12]

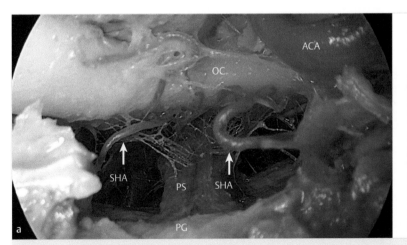
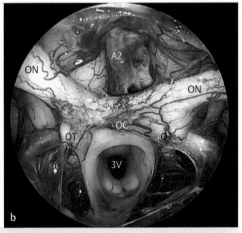

Fig. 15.1 (a) Endoscopic endonasal anatomical view of small arteries and perforators in the anterior compartment. Superior hypophyseal arteries (SHAs) usually nourish optic chiasm (OC), pituitary stalk (PS), and pituitary gland (PG). (b) Endoscopic endonasal surgical view after removal of a craniopharyngioma—note the dense network of perforators that nourishes the optic apparatus. ACA, anterior cerebral artery; A2, A2 segment of anterior cerebral artery; 3V, third ventricle; ON, optic nerve; OT, optic tract.

The main branches arising from the PCA that are relevant to EEA are the posterior thalamoperforating arteries, and the short and long circumflex arteries. The posterior thalamoperforating arteries, which arise from P1 and enter the brain through the PPS, interpeduncular fossa, and medial crus cerebri, supply the anterior and part of the posterior thalamus, hypothalamus, subthalamus, substantia nigra, red nucleus, oculomotor and trochlear nuclei, oculomotor nerve, mesencephalic reticular formation, pretectum, rostromedial floor of the third ventricle, and the posterior portion of the internal capsule (▶ Fig. 15.2). The short and long circumflex arteries often arise from P1 and less frequently from P2; the short circumflex artery courses around the midbrain and terminates at the geniculate bodies, whereas the long circumflex artery courses around the midbrain and reaches the colliculi.

Interruption of these arteries, especially the thalamoperforating pedicle, may lead to a paramedian thalamic infarct, which results in cognitive impairment, executive dysfunction, memory impairment, aphasia, decreased vigilance, and vertical gaze paresis. The symptoms can be more severe if the left and right paramedian arteries originate from a single pedicle (artery of Percheron), leading to bilateral ischemia (▶ Fig. 15.3).[13]

Posterior Communicating Artery (PComA)

Perforators do not arise from the communicating segment of the ICA in 60% of individuals.[7,8] Perforators arise mainly from the PComA and range from 1 to 14 in number, predominantly from the proximal half of the artery. They course superiorly and terminate on the third ventricle floor. The largest branch from the PComA is the premammillary artery, also called anterior thalamoperforating artery. Its interruption may cause anterior thalamic ischemia with cognitive and consciousness impairment and vertical gaze paresis (▶ Fig. 15.2 and ▶ Fig. 15.4). The

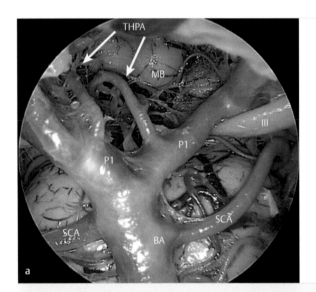
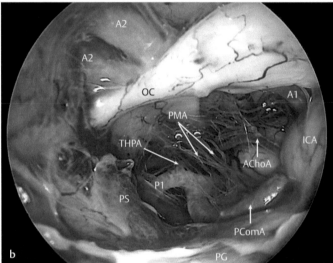

Fig. 15.2 (a) Endoscopic endonasal anatomical view of the thalamoperforating arteries (THPA) from the P1 segment of the posterior cerebral artery (P1). **(b)** Endoscopic endonasal surgical view after removal of a craniopharyngioma. A1, A1 segment of anterior cerebral artery; A2, A2 segment of anterior cerebral artery; AChoA, anterior choroidal artery; BA, basilar artery; ICA, internal carotid artery; III, oculomotor nerve; MB, mammillary bodies; OC, optic chiasm; PComA, posterior communicating artery; PG, pituitary gland; PMA, premammillary arteries; PS, pituitary stalk; SCA, superior cerebellar artery.

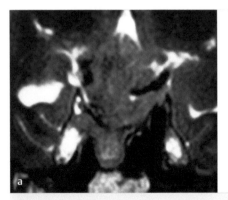
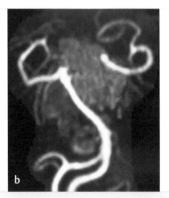
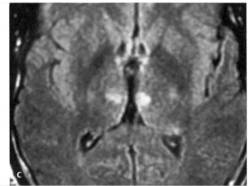

Fig. 15.3 (a, b) T2-weighted coronal magnetic resonance (MR) images of a recurrent pituitary adenoma with extensive vascular proximity (magnetic resonance angiography [MRA] reconstruction). Bilateral thalamic infarcts seen on fluid-attenuated inversion recovery (FLAIR) MRI after surgery **(c)** due to occlusion of a single thalamoperforating pedicle (artery of Percheron).

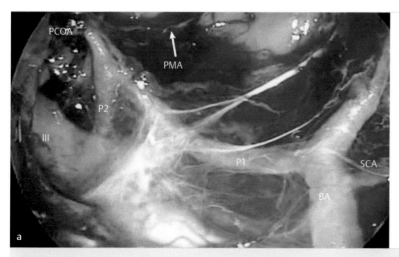
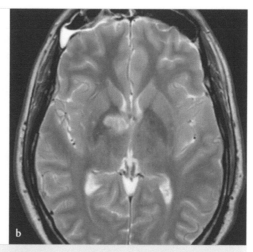

Fig. 15.4 (a) Endoscopic endonasal surgical view of the right premammillary (PMA) during resection of a posterior fossa chordoma. (b) Anterior thalamic infarct developed after surgery due to lesion of this artery, seen on axial T2-weighted magnetic resonance imaging (MRI). BA, basilar artery; III, right oculomotor nerve; P1 and P2, P1 and P2 segments of right posterior cerebral artery; PCOA, posterior communicating artery; SCA, superior cerebellar artery.

infundibular arteries are another group of arteries that arise from the PComA and supply the same area as the superior hypophyseal artery.[11,12]

Basilar Artery (BA)

A mean of eight branches usually arise from the lateral and dorsal aspect of the BA (▶ Fig. 15.5). There are no perforators on the ventral aspect of the vessel. Perforators irrigate the lateral pons, mesencephalon, and PPS. Those arising close to the origin of the SCA intermingle with the direct perforating branches arising from the proximal SCA. Those arising above the origin of the SCA enter the interpeduncular fossa. Their interruption will cause motor deficits due to cerebral peduncle ischemia.

Superior Cerebellar Artery (SCA)

The SCA is the most rostral of all infratentorial vessels; it arises close to the BA apex and encircles the pons and the lower midbrain. It supplies the tentorial surface of the cerebellum, the upper brainstem, the deep cerebellar nuclei, and the inferior colliculi.

Perforators arising from the SCA are divided into direct and circumflex types. The direct type follows a straight course to enter the brainstem while the circumflex type winds around the brainstem before perforating it. The circumflex perforating arteries are subdivided into short and long types. The short circumflex type travels up to 90 degrees around the circumference of the brainstem. The long circumflex type travels a greater distance to reach the dorsal surface. Both types of circumflex arteries send branches into the brainstem along their course. Inferolateral territory ischemia may present with hypoesthesia, ataxia, hemiparesis, cognitive impairment, executive dysfunction, and aphasia.[13]

15.3.3 The Inferior Compartment

Inferior compartment perforators are at risk of injury during EEA to the lower clivus and craniocervical junction, such as for chordomas, meningiomas, and metastases.[10]

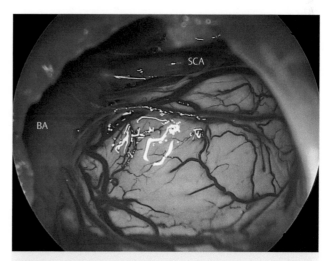

Fig. 15.5 Endoscopic endonasal surgical view of the basilar artery (BA) and its perforators. SCA, superior cerebellar artery.

Most of them arise from the intradural segment of VAs, lower BA, and posterior fossa arteries (PICA, AICA). Such vessels usually irrigate the pons, medulla, cerebellum, and spinal cord. Perforators in the inferior compartment are smaller in number when compared to the anterior compartment, although ischemic injuries resulting from their lesions may have terrible consequences due to the involvement of white matter tracts and nuclei in the brainstem and spinal cord.[14]

Vertebral Artery (VA)

Perforators from the VA supply the paramedian region of the upper medulla, including the pyramidal bundles, medial lemniscus, medial longitudinal fasciculus, cranial part of the hypoglossal nucleus, and paramedian reticular formation (▶ Fig. 15.6). Hence, occlusion of these perforators leads to a medial medullary syndrome, with contralateral hemiplegia, loss of touch and proprioception, and ipsilateral paralysis of the tongue.

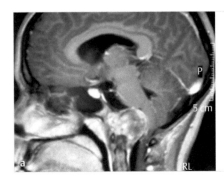
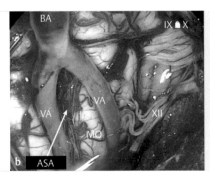

Fig. 15.6 (a, b) Magnetic resonance (MR) image of a lower clival chordoma. Endoscopic endonasal surgical view of the same patient, after removal of the tumor. ASA, anterior spinal artery; BA, basilar artery; MO, medulla oblongata; VA, vertebral artery; XII, hypoglossal nerve; IX, glossopharyngeal nerve; X, vagus nerve.

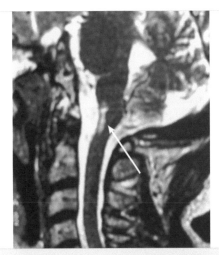

Fig. 15.7 Magnetic resonance (MR) image of a patient with ischemic event in the medulla oblongata (*arrow*) after the removal of a foramen magnum meningioma.

The anterior spinal artery is an important branch, arising directly from the V4 segment. It can have a unilateral origin in 15 to 40% of patients and irrigate the anterior two-thirds of the spinal cord. Its injury may lead to severe spastic tetraplegia and loss of pain and temperature sensation, albeit with preservation of proprioception (▶ Fig. 15.7).[15]

Anterior Inferior Cerebellar Artery (AICA)

The AICA and PICA are defined according to their origin, rather than by the portions of the cerebellum supplied by them. The AICA arises more frequently from the lower third and less frequently from the middle third of the BA. It courses posteriorly, laterally, and usually inferiorly relative to the belly of the pons, in contact with either the superior or inferior aspect of the abducens nerve. Along its course, it supplies the lateral aspect of the lower two-thirds of the pons and the upper medulla.

Perforators arise from the nerve-related vessels and irrigate nerve-related zones and the adjacent part of the pons, the pons around the entry zone of the trigeminal nerve, the superolateral medulla, and the glossopharyngeal and vagus nerves. Their occlusion may cause hemiparesis, ataxia, facial paralysis, hearing loss, and strabismus.

Posterior Inferior Cerebellar Artery (PICA)

The PICA arises from the VA and supplies the medulla, the inferior *vermis*, the inferior portion of the fourth ventricle, the tonsils, and the inferior aspect of the cerebellum.

The perforating branches of the PICA overlap with those arising from the vertebral artery. The vertebral artery segment distal to the PICA origin more frequently gives rise to perforating arteries, rather than the segment proximal to the PICA origin. The perforating branches arising between the entry of the vertebral artery in the dura mater and the PICA origin are most commonly of the short circumflex or direct type and terminate predominantly on the lateral side of the medulla.

Those arising between the PICA origin and the vertebrobasilar junction are predominantly of the short circumflex type and terminate on the anterior and lateral surfaces of the medulla. The vertebral artery segment distal to the PICA origin also gives rise to a few branches that enter the choroid plexus, protruding from the foramen of Luschka.

Contralateral hemiparesis, ataxia, tremors, dysesthesia, and dysphagia are classic symptoms in lateral medullary syndrome following proximal occlusion of PICA, also known as Wallenberg syndrome. The isolated occlusion of its branches may also cause some of the above symptoms in variable degrees.[15]

15.4 Injury Avoidance and Management Strategies

An inadvertent injury to a perforator might have no consequences at all or can result in catastrophic complications, regardless of how it is managed. Therefore, the best treatment for perforator injury during EEA is prevention and the best way to prevent their injury is to keep their existence, anatomic location, and relationship to the tumor in mind while operating.

Because of their small caliber, variable anatomy, and frequent encroachment by tumors, perforators may not be clearly identifiable before or during surgery and are highly vulnerable. There are basically two strategies to employ to avoid perforator during EEA: correctly identifying them and applying microdissection techniques.

Correctly identifying perforators during EEA is a challenging task. First of all, surgeons must be well aware of the possible nature of the disease they are dealing with and anatomical peculiarities of the region involved by each disease. Whenever involvement of perforators by tumor is suspected, specific vascular examinations (CT or MR angiography) should be ordered before surgery. Confirmation of vascular encroachment by tumor enables the surgeons to frankly discuss risks and benefits of surgery with patients, and to prepare for possible surgical challenges.

During surgery, anatomical knowledge and gentle microdissection of intracranial contents are key to prevent injury to perforators. Although neuronavigation tools (CT and/or MR) are very helpful in identifying fixed anatomical landmarks, like bony limits, there is usually a shift between the surgical view and neuronavigation images for soft tissues, including tumors and vessels. The margin of error increases as the skull base is dissected and tumors are removed, causing an anatomical distortion of tissues. Therefore, surgeons should not rely exclusively on neuronavigation to localize small arteries within or close to tumors during surgery. Intraoperative neurophysiological monitoring may be used in cases with potential manipulation of perforators. This allows real-time assessment of cortical and long tract functions, including somatosensitive and motor pathways. Motor evoked potentials (MEPs) or brainstem auditory evoked responses (BSERs) may be necessary in addition to somatosensory evoked potentials (SSEPs) to detect a perforator injury or spasm. Nevertheless, the applicability of monitoring is rather to identify established lesions than to prevent them from occurring. On the other hand, in surgeries with documented decreased neurophysiological response, the surgical strategy might be changed toward partial resection of tumor in order to avoid further vascular and brain tissue damage.

Although not routinely used, microvascular Doppler probes specifically built for EEA procedures can be employed.[16] In addition, endoscopes with near-infrared filters allowing for indocyanine green (ICG) and other fluorescence angiography techniques are becoming available to help identify these vessels intraoperatively.[17]

Once a perforator is correctly identified, wide and clear visualization of the surgical field is paramount. Hemostasis of mucosal edges and other nasal structures, and the surgical site itself, must be achieved. Blind curettage of tumors from regions that are not widely exposed must be always avoided. Whenever possible, the proximal and distal segments of the perforator should be exposed. Saline-soaked neuropatties are used to protect and dissect the vessels from surrounding neurovascular structures. Microdissection techniques are employed, and perforators are preferentially dissected from proximal to distal, which permits early identification of the plane of dissection and avoids over-manipulation of the perforator's thinner and more delicate distal end. Long and delicate instruments are used to carefully and gently dissect perforators off tumors. Blunt instruments are preferred over sharp instruments and care must be taken when manipulating bipolar cautery forceps close to small vessels. The importance of bimanual dissection at this surgical step cannot be overemphasized—suction, traction, counter-traction, and protection techniques can all be employed by the operating surgeon. When perforators are completely dissected or freed from tumor, they must be protected with saline-soaked neuropatties, and further manipulation should be avoided until the end of surgery. Although not routinely used by

the authors of this chapter, topical vasodilators like papaverine may be useful to prevent spasm or occlusion of recently dissected vessels.

The decision to completely dissect perforators off a tumor and try to achieve gross total removal is often challenging. Surgical goals should be clear in advance and members of the surgical team should maintain constant dialogue during the procedure and periodically reassess the feasibility of continuing microvascular dissection. For example, if there is no dissection plane between perforators and the tumor, or if the tumor completely encases vessels, continuing the dissection becomes too risky and some residual tumor might be wisely left behind. This becomes particularly true if the lesion is benign, the residue is small, and the perforator is truly important. The greatest prize for a surgeon should always be the patient, not the postoperative MR.

When a perforator is accidently injured, bleeding is usually minor. For minor bleeding, application of hemostatic materials on the surgical bed such as gelfoam® or Surgicel®, soaked or not in thrombin, or merely warm irrigation is usually effective. For larger bleedings, however, there is no other way of controlling bleeding other than completely sealing the vessel with delicate bipolar cauterization. Suturing, reconstructing, or bypassing the vessel is virtually impossible. As a result, ischemia of certain brain areas and/or cranial nerves might happen, and clinical consequences largely depend on the importance of the injured vessel to that particular brain area and/or cranial nerve. If collateral circulation is enough, patients might avoid clinical symptoms after surgery.

If bleeding from an injured perforator or small artery goes unnoticed, postoperative subarachnoid hemorrhage might occur. As a consequence, cerebral vasospasm and delayed cerebral ischemia might develop. In this case, ischemic consequences for the brain are clinically much more significant than an isolated perforator injury, as depicted in the following section.[18]

15.5 Case Example

15.5.1 Case Vignette

A 66-year-old male patient presented with a 6-month history of progressive bitemporal visual loss, fatigue, and decreased libido. Visual field testing revealed bitemporal hemianopsia and hormonal testing revealed hypogonadotrophic hypogonadism with normal prolactin. A sellar MR revealed a large pituitary adenoma with suprasellar extension and compression of the optic chiasm (▶ Fig. 15.8).

The patient underwent EEA for removal of the tumor. After adequately exposing the sella and opening the dura, the tumor

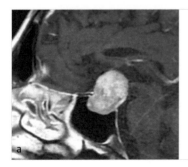
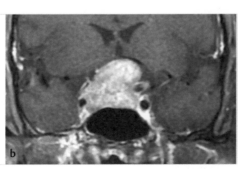

Fig. 15.8 Sagittal (a) and coronal (b) postcontrast, T1-weighted magnetic resonance (MR) images demonstrating a pituitary macroadenoma with suprasellar extension.

was completely dissected and aspirated. Normal pituitary gland was identified and preserved. There were no signs of injury to the arachnoid tissue or any intraoperative cerebrospinal fluid (CSF) leak (▶ Fig. 15.9).

After 2 days of surgery, the patient developed visual deterioration and intense headache. A CT scan showed signs of subarachnoid hemorrhage within the suprasellar region, extending to the interpeduncular cistern. A cerebral angiography showed no signs of vessel injury or ruptured aneurysms (▶ Fig. 15.10).

The patient was brought back to the operating room, and revision surgery was undertaken. The arachnoid was still intact but was bulging through the sellar defect. The arachnoid was incised and blood clot was removed from the sellar and suprasellar region. The optic nerves and chiasm were decompressed, and the skull base defect was reconstructed (▶ Fig. 15.11). The patient had immediate visual improvement after recovering

from general anesthesia and nimodipine was initiated for prevention of cerebral vasospasm.

The patient then began developing recurrent episodes of altered mental status (decreased levels of consciousness, confusion, hypersomnia, and short- and long-term memory problems) and dysautonomia (hypotension, diaphoresis, and tachycardia). CT and MR scans revealed areas of cerebral ischemia in the frontal and temporal lobes, thalamus, and hypothalamus (▶ Fig. 15.12a, b). Angio-MR images disclosed right middle cerebral artery vasospasm and transcranial Doppler ultrasonography demonstrated loss of cerebral autoregulatory capacity (▶ Fig. 15.12c). Cerebral vasospasm and delayed cerebral ischemia were suspected, nimodipine was maintained, and isolated hypertension was initiated.

On clinical follow-up, the patient clinically improved and was discharged from hospital 45 days after his first surgery. He still has occasional mild confusion and short- and long-term memory problems, even after 2 years of follow-up.

15.5.2 Discussion

It is intriguing in this case that gross total removal of a pituitary adenoma was performed through an EEA, arachnoid tissue was completely preserved during surgery, and the subarachnoid space was not violated. Postoperative angiogram was normal and, therefore, the origin of the subarachnoid bleeding was not obvious.

Nonaneurysmal subarachnoid hemorrhage following transnasal pituitary surgery is quite rare.[19,20] In the case presented, we believe that a perforator, such as the superior hypophyseal artery or its branches, may have adhered to the arachnoid membrane lying over the tumor capsule during its growth. When the adenoma was removed, and arachnoid membrane herniated into the sellar region, some of these perforators stretched out and ruptured.

Another complication presented by the patient was cerebral vasospasm and delayed cerebral ischemia. It is known that both conditions might occur as a consequence of intracranial vessel injury and subarachnoid haemorrhage.[18,19] As soon as subarachnoid hemorrhage was diagnosed, and vascular injury and cerebral vasospasm were suspected, the patient was given nimodipine, a calcium channel blocker. Although this drug does not prevent or improve angiographic cerebral vasospasm, it has been shown that it can reduce the risk of poor neurological

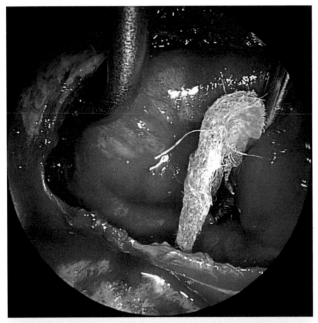

Fig. 15.9 Endoscopic endonasal surgical view after gross total resection of the pituitary macroadenoma was achieved. Note the intact arachnoid membrane with thin gland covering herniating into the sellar region.

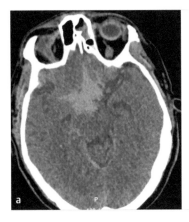
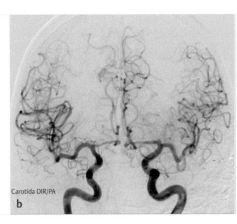

Carotida DIR/PA

Fig. 15.10 **(a)** Axial computed tomography (CT) scan showing subarachnoid hemorrhage in the suprasellar region extending to the interpeduncular cistern. **(b)** A cerebral angiogram disclosed no abnormalities.

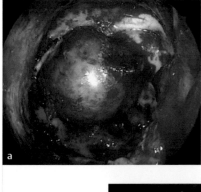
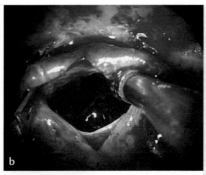
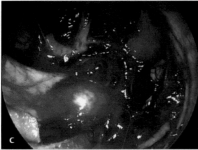

Fig. 15.11 (a) Endoscopic endonasal surgical view demonstrating an intact arachnoid membrane herniating through the sellar defect. (b) The arachnoid was incised and significant blood clot was removed from within the sellar and suprasellar region. (c) The optic apparatus was decompressed, and no bleeding vessel was identified.

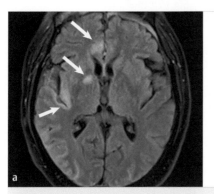
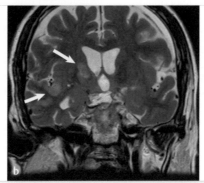
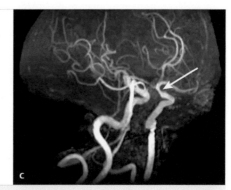

Fig. 15.12 Axial fluid-attenuated inversion recovery (FLAIR) (a) and coronal T2 (b) magnetic resonance (MR) images showing various areas of brain ischemia (arrows) in the frontal and temporal lobes, thalamus, and hypothalamus. (c) Angio-MR image revealing right cerebral artery vasospasm (arrow).

outcomes in patients with risk of delayed cerebral ischemia.[19] In spite of the treatment, the patient still presented dysautonomia and fluctuations in his mental status, hypersomnia, and short- and long-term memory problems.

15.5.3 Root Cause Analysis

It is unknown what could have prevented all complications featured in this vignette. The initiating factor was probably the rupture of a small arterial branch (a perforator) in the subarachnoid space, just above the sellar region. In this area lie the superior hypophyseal arteries and its rami, which were not seen during surgery due to complete preservation of the arachnoid membrane.[9] Although any recommendation derived from this particular experience is merely anecdotal, preventing overherniation of the arachnoid tissue into the sellar region could have prevented over-stretching of small arteries and their

consequent rupture. This could be achieved by filling the sellar region with small amounts of abdominal fat before closing the skull base defect. Besides that, other microdissection techniques applied in this case were key to prevent further inadvertent injuries, like avoiding blind curettage of tumor in the suprasellar region.

15.6 Conclusion

Injury to perforators should be always prevented during skull base surgery. Correctly identifying such small vessel and applying microdissection techniques are key to avoid catastrophic postoperative complications. If any perforator is injured, bleeding must be controlled immediately, and further ischemic complications should be suspected, including cerebral vasospasm and delayed ischemia.

References

[1] Kassam AB, Prevedello DM, Carrau RL, et al. Endoscopic endonasal skull base surgery: analysis of complications in the authors' initial 800 patients. J Neurosurg. 2011; 114(6):1544–1568

[2] Muto J, Carrau RL, Oyama K, Otto BA, Prevedello DM. Training model for control of an internal carotid artery injury during transsphenoidal surgery. Laryngoscope. 2017; 127(1):38–43

[3] Pacca P, Jhawar SS, Seclen DV, et al. "Live cadaver" model for internal carotid artery injury simulation in endoscopic endonasal skull base surgery. Oper Neurosurg (Hagerstown). 2017; 13(6):732–738

[4] Gardner PA, Tormenti MJ, Pant H, Fernandez-Miranda JC, Snyderman CH, Horowitz MB. Carotid artery injury during endoscopic endonasal skull base surgery: incidence and outcomes. Neurosurgery. 2013; 73(2) Suppl Operative: ons261–ons269, discussion ons269–ons270

[5] Rosner SS, Rhoton AL, Jr, Ono M, Barry M. Microsurgical anatomy of the anterior perforating arteries. J Neurosurg. 1984; 61(3):468–485

[6] Serizawa T, Saeki N, Yamaura A. Microsurgical anatomy and clinical significance of the anterior communicating artery and its perforating branches. Neurosurgery. 1997; 40(6):1211–1216, discussion 1216–1218

[7] Rhoton AL, Jr. The supratentorial arteries. Neurosurgery. 2002; 51(4) Suppl: S53–S120

[8] Rhoton AL, Jr. The cerebrum. Anatomy. Neurosurgery. 2007; 61(1) Suppl:37–118, discussion 118–119

[9] Truong HQ, Najera E, Zanabria-Ortiz R, et al. Surgical anatomy of the superior hypophyseal artery and its relevance for endoscopic endonasal surgery. J Neurosurg. 2018; 131(1):154–162

[10] Kassam A, Snyderman CH, Mintz A, Gardner P, Carrau RL. Expanded endonasal approach: the rostrocaudal axis. Part II. Posterior clinoids to the foramen magnum. Neurosurg Focus. 2005; 19(1):E4

[11] Hardy DG, Peace DA, Rhoton AL, Jr. Microsurgical anatomy of the superior cerebellar artery. Neurosurgery. 1980; 6(1):10–28

[12] Párraga RG, Ribas GC, Andrade SEGL, de Oliveira E. Microsurgical anatomy of the posterior cerebral artery in three-dimensional images. World Neurosurg. 2011; 75(2):233–257

[13] Carrera E, Michel P, Bogousslavsky J. Anteromedian, central, and posterolateral infarcts of the thalamus: three variant types. Stroke. 2004; 35(12):2826–2831

[14] Marinković SV, Gibo H. The surgical anatomy of the perforating branches of the basilar artery. Neurosurgery. 1993; 33(1):80–87

[15] Lister JR, Rhoton AL, Jr, Matsushima T, Peace DA. Microsurgical anatomy of the posterior inferior cerebellar artery. Neurosurgery. 1982; 10(2): 170–199

[16] Enseñat J, Alobid I, de Notaris M, et al. Endoscopic endonasal clipping of a ruptured vertebral-posterior inferior cerebellar artery aneurysm: technical case report. Neurosurgery. 2011; 69(1) Suppl Operative:E121–E127, discussion E127–E128

[17] Catapano G, Sgulò F, Laleva L, Columbano L, Dallan I, de Notaris M. Multimodal use of indocyanine green endoscopy in neurosurgery: a single-center experience and review of the literature. Neurosurg Rev. 2018; 41(4): 985–998

[18] Eseonu CI, ReFaey K, Geocadin RG, Quinones-Hinojosa A. Postoperative cerebral vasospasm following transsphenoidal pituitary adenoma surgery. World Neurosurg. 2016; 92:7–14

[19] Veldeman M, Höllig A, Clusmann H, Stevanovic A, Rossaint R, Coburn M. Delayed cerebral ischaemia prevention and treatment after aneurysmal subarachnoid haemorrhage: a systematic review. Br J Anaesth. 2016; 117(1): 17–40

[20] Shu H, Tian X, Wang H, Zhang H, Zhang Q, Guo L. Nonaneurysmal subarachnoid hemorrhage secondary to transsphenoidal surgery for pituitary adenomas. J Craniofac Surg. 2015; 26(2):e166–e168

16 Perforator Injury During Open Skull Base Surgery

Nicholas T. Gamboa and William T. Couldwell

Summary

The basal perforators comprise small direct arterial branches of the main cerebral vessels and supply the paramedian regions of the brainstem, diencephalon, and deep regions of the cerebrum. These delicate perforator vessels must be preserved during open skull base surgery to prevent significant postoperative neurological sequelae. An in-depth knowledge of perforator anatomy is essential when planning a surgical approach to complex skull base disease. Although microsurgical techniques and other intraoperative technologies have decreased the risk of perforator injury, it is imperative for the skull base neurosurgeon to thoughtfully plan out an individualized surgical approach for each patient based on the preoperative vascular imaging and specific pathology. Intraoperatively, the perforator arteries that are at risk of inadvertent injury must be meticulously identified, dissected, and displaced. Although injury to cerebral perforators is not entirely preventable, it can be greatly minimized through a combination of thoughtful planning, careful attention intraoperatively, and through the utilization of intraoperative technologies to assess perforator flow dynamics.

Keywords: Basal perforators, choroidal arteries, lateral lenticulostriate arteries, medial striate arteries, microvascular anatomy, perforator injury, skull base surgery, thalamic arteries, vascular neurosurgery

16.1 Key Learning Points

- Knowledge of perforator microanatomy, its common variations, and the relationship of perforators to skull base pathology is essential for reducing morbidity and mortality in skull base neurosurgery.
- Extensive preoperative planning using available vascular imaging is critical to understand each patient's parent and perforator arterial anatomy and develop an appropriate individualized microsurgical approach to pathology of the skull base.
- The skull base neurosurgeon must remain mindful that microvascular anatomy can be significantly altered in the setting of disease.
- Various technologies can be used intraoperatively to assess perforator patency. These include micromirrors and endoscopes for visualization, microvascular Doppler ultrasonography, electrophysiological monitoring with evoked potentials (both motor and somatosensory), fluorescein or indocyanine green video angiography, and intraoperative digital subtraction angiography.
- Optimal patient positioning and intraoperative brain relaxation can assist the neurosurgeon by minimizing the need for fixed and dynamic retraction, thereby decreasing the risk of inadvertent perforator flow disruption during skull base surgery.

- The senior author commonly uses a dilute solution of papaverine (3 mg/mL) directly on the visualized perforating vessels during and after dissection to reduce manipulation-induced vasospasm, which may result in infarction.

16.2 Introduction

The basal perforating vessels (perforators) of the brain represent small direct arterial branches of the vertebrobasilar, internal carotid, and main cerebral arteries that supply the paramedian regions of the brainstem, diencephalon, and deep regions of the cerebral hemispheres (notably, the basal ganglia and internal capsules) (▶ Fig. 16.1). These often-delicate perforator vessels serve the critical role of perfusing key areas of the cerebrum and brainstem and therefore must be preserved during open skull base surgery to prevent significant postoperative neurological sequelae. Despite significant advancements in neurosurgical techniques and intraoperative technologies, these small and tenuous vessels, which often measure less than 1 mm in diameter, remain at significant risk of damage during neurosurgical procedures, particularly during manipulation of and dissection around the delicate neurovascular structures of the skull base. An in-depth knowledge of perforator anatomy serves an indispensable role in skull base neurosurgery—because great care must be taken by the surgeon to navigate around and avoid damage of these critical structures. A comprehensive understanding of the microvascular anatomy of the cerebral circulation, including the origins of perforator arteries, their takeoff trajectories, subarachnoid course, anastomoses, and subsequent branching patterns and parenchymal distributions, is essential for selection of appropriate microsurgical or endovascular treatment modalities, particularly when the anatomy of the skull base is distorted by complex vascular or neoplastic disease. This chapter will discuss basal perforator anatomy, relevant skull base pathology, and complication avoidance when planning and performing an open surgical approach to complex pathology of the skull base.

16.3 Vascular Challenges

The vascular challenges related to perforator injury during open skull base surgery stem from the delicate nature of the basal perforator vessels, their complex and highly variable anatomy, the abundance of numerous ramifying extracerebral branches, and the often close association with skull base pathology. These vascular challenges of skull base surgery can be further complicated by multiple reoperations, radiation therapy, and chemotherapy—distorting normal anatomical planes and obscuring skull base anatomy. ▶ Table 16.1 outlines the basal perforator vessels derived from each of the major cerebral arteries and summarizes the literature regarding their parent segments, numbers (mean and range), vessel diameters (mean and range), takeoff trajectories, and structures supplied.

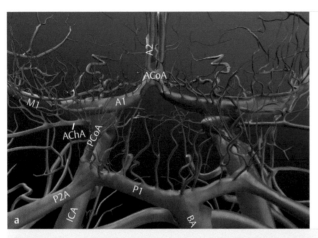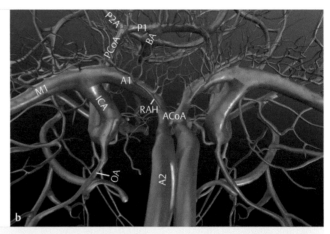

Fig. 16.1 Three-dimensional rendering of the circle of Willis, its branches, and the numerous perforating branches of the main cerebral arteries. **(a)** Posterior and superior view demonstrating the posterior circulation: basilar artery (BA), precommunicating segment of the posterior cerebral artery (P1), anterior postcommunicating segment of the posterior cerebral artery (P2A), and its connection with the anterior circulation via the posterior communicating artery (PComA). The anterior circulation is denoted by the internal carotid artery (ICA), anterior choroidal artery (AChA), horizontal segment of the middle cerebral artery (M1), precommunicating segment of the anterior cerebral artery (A1), anterior communicating artery (AComA), and postcommunicating segment of the anterior cerebral artery (A2). **(b)** Anterior and superior view of the circle of Willis. The ophthalmic artery (OA) can be seen branching and coursing anteriorly from the ophthalmic segment of the ICA. (Modified with permission from *The Neurosurgical Atlas* by Aaron Cohen-Gadol, MD.)

Table 16.1 Overview of basal perforator vessels derived from each of the major cerebral arteries, their parent segments, numbers, vessel diameters, takeoff trajectories, and structures supplied

Parent artery, segment	Perforator	Number		Vessel diameter (µm)		Takeoff direction	Structures supplied	References
		Mean	Range	Mean	Range			
ACA, A1	MSA	6.6	1–12	276	80–710	PS	Anterior commissure, anterior hypothalamus, anteroinferior striatum, optic chiasm, pillars of fornix, septum pellucidum	Marinković et al, 1986[1] Perlmutter and Rhoton, 1976[2]
	RAH	1	0–2	462	180–850	PS	Anterior limb of internal capsule, anterior putamen and globus pallidus, head of caudate	Marinković et al, 1986[1] Perlmutter and Rhoton, 1976[2]
MCA, M1	LSA	10.4	1–21	350	100–2,200	PS	Head and body of caudate nucleus, internal capsule, lateral anterior commissure, lateral globus pallidus, putamen, substantia innominata	Rosner et al, 1984[3] Umansky et al, 1985[4]
Choroidal ICA	AChA C	4.6	2–9	317	90–600	PM	Anterior hippocampus, anterolateral midbrain, amygdaloid nucleus, globus pallidus internus, lateral geniculate body, optic tract, posterior limb and genu of internal capsule, subthalamic nucleus, tail of caudate nucleus	Marinković et al, 1999[5] Rhoton et al, 1979[6]
	AChA P	1.7	0–6	700	400–1,100	PM		
	ICA perforators	3.9	1–9	243	70–470	PS	Anterior perforated substance, optic tract, uncus	Marinković et al, 1990[7] Rosner et al, 1984[3]
PComA	TTA	1.3	1–2	493	280–780	PS	Anterior thalamus, cerebral peduncle, mammillary body and mammillothalamic tract, medial subthalamus, pillars of fornix, posterior hypothalamus, posterior limb of internal capsule	Gibo et al, 2001[8] Saeki and Rhoton, 1977[9]

(Continued)

Table 16.1 (*Continued*) Overview of basal perforator vessels derived from each of the major cerebral arteries, their parent segments, numbers, vessel diameters, takeoff trajectories, and structures supplied

Parent artery, segment	Perforator	Number		Vessel diameter (μm)		Takeoff direction	Structures supplied	References
		Mean	Range	Mean	Range			
PCA, P1	TPA	2	1–10	321	100–750	PS	Midbrain, medial thalamus, posterior hypothalamus, subthalamus	Marinković et al, 1986[10] Saeki and Rhoton, 1977[9]
PCA, P2A/P2P	TGA	5.7	2–12	346	70–580	PS	Brachium of superior colliculus, medial and lateral geniculate bodies, pulvinar of thalamus	Milisavljević et al, 1991[11] Zeal and Rhoton, 2009[12]

Abbreviations: ACA, anterior cerebral artery; AChA C, cisternal segment of anterior choroidal artery; AChA P, plexal segment of anterior choroidal artery; ICA, internal carotid artery; LSA, lenticulostriate arteries; MCA, middle cerebral artery; MSA, medial striate arteries; PCA, posterior cerebral artery; PComA, posterior communicating artery; PM, posteromedial; PS, posterosuperior; RAH, recurrent artery of Heubner; TGA, thalamogeniculate arteries; TPA, thalamoperforate arteries; TTA, thalamotuberal arteries.

16.4 Perforator Injury Avoidance

16.4.1 Fundamentals of Perforator Flow Monitoring and Injury Avoidance

To avoid inadvertent injury to perforator arteries, numerous intraoperative technologies have been developed to either visualize hidden perforator branches or evaluate perforator vessel patency intraoperatively. These modalities include micromirrors or endoscopes, intraoperative digital subtraction angiography (DSA), microvascular Doppler ultrasonography, electrophysiological monitoring of motor and somatosensory evoked potentials, and fluorescein or indocyanine green (ICG) video angiography. Although these technologies have significant utility, particularly when there is concern for possible parent or perforator artery occlusion, they each have relative advantages and disadvantages and cannot always perfectly monitor for blood flow disturbance in all neighboring perforating arteries during skull base surgery.

Micromirrors and endoscopes prove particularly useful for direct visualization of critical neurovascular structures, such as perforator vessels that remain out of view when using the operating microscope (e.g., perforators located behind the dome of an aneurysm or on the deep aspect of a tumor).[13] These modalities prove particularly useful after placement of a microsurgical clip, as they allow the surgeon to visualize the backside of the aneurysm, evaluate the aneurysm's hidden anatomical features, and ensure optimal clip placement that does not incorporate any perforators or other critical neurovascular structures into the clip construct. In addition, angled endoscopes can be useful when attempting to visualize vasculature displaced or hidden by tumors near the skull base, which can parasitize branches from the main cerebral arteries and perforators that surround them.

Microvascular Doppler ultrasonography is a valuable tool for real-time assessment of blood flow through vessels in a noninvasive manner based upon their flow velocity.[14] Although the probe can measure as small as 1 mm, it can prove to be difficult to accurately assess perforator vessel flow dynamics when placing the probe on target perforator vessels in a deep surgical field without also detecting the flow of nearby vessels, thereby confounding intraoperative assessment of vessel patency.[15,16] Further, microvascular Doppler ultrasonography cannot always reliably discern whether blood flow within a perforator vessel is sufficient to avoid infarction and cannot reliably assess flow within vessels smaller than 0.5 mm in diameter.[17] In contrast to the conventional microvascular Doppler ultrasonography probe, a microvascular ultrasonic flow probe (Microvascular Flowprobe, Transonics Systems Inc., Ithaca, NY) has been shown in both in vitro and in vivo studies to provide the operator with both a quantitative and a qualitative assessment of vessel flow dynamics that is not confounded by factors such as hematocrit or vessel wall thickness.[18,19]

Electrophysiological monitoring with motor evoked potentials can detect decreased blood flow through the anterior choroidal artery (AChA), medial striate artery (MSA), or lenticulostriate artery (LSA) perforator branches within 60 seconds,[20,21,22] but detection of flow disturbance within perforators of the posterior communicating artery (PComA) or posterior thalamic arteries cannot be monitored in this fashion, as they may not supply the pyramidal tract. Furthermore, variant anatomy, collateralization, and certain highly variable perforating vessels (e.g., recurrent artery of Huebner [RAH]) can defy consistent localization, and therefore, disturbance of their flow cannot always be reliably detected via electrophysiological monitoring. The use of motor and somatosensory evoked potentials allows the operator to intraoperatively assess for compromised cerebral blood flow and infarction by observing either a decrease or a loss of evoked potentials. It should be noted, however, that electrophysiological monitoring can be influenced by anesthetic technique and in some instances can have either false-negative or false-positive evoked potential changes in the setting of ischemic and no ischemic injury, respectively.[23,24]

Traditionally, intraoperative DSA has been used in combination with direct visualization to assess for patency of nearby parent or branching vessels and remains widely used in vascular and skull base neurosurgery.[25,26] Its advantages include evaluation of the entire cerebral circulation, and it can reveal adequacy of aneurysmal clip placement or residual arteriovenous malformations and fistulas. However, this method can be logistically difficult, invasive, time-consuming, and costly and can have limited resolution—making confirmation of perforator vessel patency difficult or impossible.

Fluorescein or ICG angiography has proven to be a particularly useful tool in many tumor and vascular neurosurgical cases. Fluorescein and ICG video angiography are rapid and repeatable modalities (after 20- to 30-minute washout delay) that are readily incorporated into the operating microscope and use intravascular fluorescence that enables visualization of small perforator vessels that can be difficult to discern with conventional intraoperative DSA. However, appreciable fluorescence of perforators can be restricted to the operative field and can be obscured by blood, pathology, or normal brain parenchyma. Moreover, fluorescein or ICG video angiography does not provide a quantitative assessment of perforator flow. Despite this, Raabe et al[27] demonstrated that ICG video angiography was comparable with intra- and postoperative DSA in 90% of cases and provided neurosurgeons with clinically significant intraoperative information leading to aneurysmal clip correction in 9% of cases.

Intraoperative assessment of perforator flow dynamics with the abovementioned modalities can provide critical information to the skull base neurosurgeon and can help with complication avoidance. However, it is our experience that these technologies must be combined with clinical judgment, adequate perforator dissection, and careful intraoperative inspection of the perforator branches to minimize the risk of postoperative perforator artery distribution infarctions.

16.4.2 Technical Nuances

The ideal neurosurgical skull base approach is one that allows the surgeon to successfully access and treat the underlying disease while leaving surrounding brain tissue and vessels completely undisturbed. Accordingly, preoperative planning regarding the optimal surgical approach, patient positioning, and use of gravity retraction and natural anatomical planes must be carefully thought out beforehand.

Brain relaxation can be particularly important with respect to skull base surgery and perforator artery injury avoidance, especially in cases of intracranial aneurysm rupture with elevated intracranial pressure, hyperemia, and hydrocephalus. This can be accomplished through judicious intraoperative drainage of cerebrospinal fluid via an external ventricular drain or lumbar drain, administration of intravenous hypertonic saline or mannitol at a dose of 1 to 2 g/kg body weight, preoperative administration of 10 mg of dexamethasone intravenously, mild intraoperative hyperventilation (PaCO$_2$ 30–35 mm Hg), and optimal positioning with the head elevated slightly above the heart and without excessive flexion or lateral rotation of the neck to minimize venous engorgement. Collectively, these modalities minimize cerebral volume and lessen the need for dynamic and fixed retraction by improving visualization and exposure using normal anatomical planes—thereby decreasing the risk for inadvertent flow disruption within the delicate perforator vessels by inadvertent or excessive manual brain retraction. It is also important for mean arterial pressure to be monitored closely during surgery, as manipulation of the vessels may induce local vasospasm. The deleterious resultant ischemia and ischemic penumbra may be reduced with permissive hypertension when vasospasm is encountered. It is the senior neurosurgeon's preference to maintain or increase mean arterial pressure during dissection of vascular structures, with routine use of dilute papaverine solution (3 mg/mL in 1-mL aliquots) applied in the presence of visualized spasm of the vessels.

16.5 Related Pathologies

16.5.1 Open Skull Base Surgery for Pathology Near the Anterior Circulation

The anterior communicating artery (AComA) complex constitutes the most common site of intracranial aneurysms and is associated with approximately 30% of ruptured aneurysms.[28,29] Given the frequent heterogeneity of the vascular anatomy in this area (with anomalies present in up to 60% of cases), the high degree of variability in angioarchitecture of aneurysms of this region (i.e., aneurysm neck, dome size, sac morphology, and projection orientation), and the proximity of these aneurysms to neighboring perforator vessels and other critical neurovascular structures of the skull base, they prove to be some of the most challenging cases to treat surgically.[29]

Aneurysms of the AComA can be approached from interhemispheric, supraorbital, orbitozygomatic, subfrontal, pterional, or extended skull base approaches. The laterality of the approach to this region often depends on symmetry of the A1 segments. If the A1 segments are symmetric, a right-sided approach is often favored to avoid involvement of the speech-dominant hemisphere. However, if one of the A1 segments is hypoplastic (i.e., <1.5 mm), then an approach on the dominant A1 side is preferred to ensure early proximal control and optimal viewing of the aneurysmal neck and dome. Regardless of surgical approach, careful dissection of the surrounding structures, particularly the optic nerve, internal carotid artery (ICA), ipsi- and contralateral A1 segments, ipsi- and contralateral frontopolar and orbitofrontal arteries, and neighboring perforator vessels must be methodically carried out. The aneurysmal neck must be carefully defined, and cleavage planes should be dissected around the neck of the aneurysm after proximal and distal control has been attained. Neighboring perforator arteries, namely, the MSA and RAH, should be dissected proximally and distally and then carefully displaced to allow clip application without occlusion of these vessels. If clip application cannot be accomplished without occlusion of adherent or intimately associated perforator vessels, a fenestrated aneurysmal clip should be employed to incorporate these delicate vessels into the construct without disturbing their flow.

Tumors of the anterior skull base and suprasellar compartment are a diverse group that encompass pathologies such as meningioma, hemangiopericytoma, pituitary adenoma, craniopharyngioma, chordoma, esthesioneuroblastoma, sarcoma, and lymphoma, among many others. These tumors may involve the anterior skull base's contents and can displace or even encase critical neurovascular structures of this region. Accordingly, maximal safe or gross total resection can be difficult without sacrificing or disturbing flow of associated perforators. Some tumor types, such as pituitary adenomas, tend to encase nearby cerebral vasculature (e.g., ICAs) but in most cases can be separated relatively easily, whereas other tumors, like aggressive fibrous meningiomas, have a proclivity for invasion of nearby vessel adventitia—making the surgical separation of tumor from involved vessels difficult or impossible without sacrifice or leaving residual tumor behind. Preservation of involved perforators should be attempted at all costs and mandates the skull base neurosurgeon to understand the involved parent and branching perforator vessels by studying each patient's preoperative magnetic resonance imaging (MRI) and vascular imaging.

In the case of large clinoidal meningiomas, which tend to encase neighboring vessels and perforator branches, surgical treatment of these typically benign tumors can prove particularly difficult.[30,31] In our experience, a pterional transsylvian approach is favored, with careful dissection of the middle cerebral artery in distal-to-proximal fashion toward the ICA bifurcation. Encased perforators (e.g., LSA, MSA, and AChA) must be meticulously dissected and freed from the tumor using a combination of microdissection, bipolar electrocautery, and microscissors to facilitate their separation. The surgeon should carefully explore the entrance points of the perforator vessels into the tumor along with their exit points (when applicable) and dissect along the anatomical layer that separates the vessels from the tumor. Knowledge of the parent vessel course relative to the tumor and perforator entrance points is essential when dissecting these small, often friable perforators free, as intratumoral vasculature can further complicate their identification and dissection. When identification of these branches is difficult, dividing the tumor into several segments or carefully debulking can improve visualization and ease of identification of involved perforator vessels—aiding in their safe dissection and separation from the tumor. Carefully debulking a tumor that encases the perforators can help minimize the risk of progressive compression and disruption of normal perforator flow dynamics, leading to vessel thrombosis and stroke.

Understanding of the preoperative anatomy is essential for intraoperative decision-making, because inadvertent sacrifice of a perforator branch will likely lead to a significant postoperative neurological deficit. Leaving behind a small amount of tumor that can be treated postoperatively with adjuvant radiotherapy or chemotherapy is almost always preferable to an aggressive gross total resection with significant postoperative neurological deficit.

16.5.2 Open Skull Base Surgery for Pathology Near the Posterior Circulation

Posterior circulation aneurysms broadly encompass PComA aneurysms, basilar apex aneurysms, and those of major branches of the vertebral and basilar arteries (anterior inferior cerebellar artery and posterior inferior cerebellar artery). PComA aneurysms represent roughly 30% of all intracranial aneurysms.[32] These aneurysms have unique variability in their projection orientation. In large PComA aneurysms, the microvascular anatomy can be significantly distorted on preoperative DSA. Large PComA aneurysms can appear to arise from an absent or hypoplastic PComA, which results from direct aneurysmal compression. The neighboring AChA can also be displaced posteromedially and mistaken for an MSA, and the thalamoperforate artery (TPA) branches can be similarly pushed posteromedially by the aneurysm. PComA aneurysms can be approached via pterional, orbitozygomatic, or lateral supraorbital approaches and may require anterior clinoidectomy for expansion of the paraclinoid space (i.e., optic-carotid and carotid-oculomotor windows) to ensure adequate visualization and proximal control. Regardless of the approach, the same principles for safe, effective surgical clipping apply. The PComA

aneurysm dome may be adherent to the oculomotor nerve and is often not dissected free because of the risk of injury to the third nerve. A temporary clip can be placed across a perforator-free zone of the supraclinoid ICA to facilitate aneurysmal neck dissection. Opening of the cistern of the lamina terminalis enables better visualization of collateralization of the PComA with the AComA and anterior cerebral artery, nearby perforator vessels, and eventual placement of a permanent clip without perforator flow disturbance. A medial trajectory is then used to check the distal clip interface to ensure no perforators are caught in the clip. This is facilitated by mild lateral displacement of the ICA.

Basilar apex aneurysms comprise approximately 5 to 8% of all intracranial aneurysms and are associated with a high risk of rupture.[32] Although most basilar apex aneurysms are now treated endovascularly, these aneurysms are particularly prone to recanalization and regrowth after coiling, necessitating subsequent definitive open neurosurgical treatment.[33] These aneurysms are technically difficult to access because of their deep-seated location, extremely narrow surgical corridors, difficulty attaining sufficient proximal and distal exposure of the basilar artery, and close association with basilar apex perforator arteries. Interestingly, the basilar bifurcation complex has significantly less anatomic variability and complexity than the AComA complex.[34] Nevertheless, inadvertent occlusion of the basilar apex perforators carries significant risk of severe neurological impairment and death. Basilar apex aneurysms can be approached via subtemporal, pterional, transcavernous, and other extended skull base approaches. The region of the interpeduncular fossa is crowded by several different groups of perforators, namely, the TPA of the P1 segment, thalamogeniculate artery of the P2 segment, AChA, medial posterior choroidal artery, lateral posterior choroidal artery, and perforators deriving from the superior cerebellar artery. Like with all aneurysm surgery, direct visualization of the nearby perforators is essential during the clipping process. In the case of the transcavernous approach for basilar apex aneurysms, the posterior clinoid process may need to be removed to improve visualization of the contralateral P1 segment and its perforators, which can be inadvertently included in the clip construct—as they are often hidden behind the aneurysm. In the case of perforators adherent to the aneurysmal dome, placement of temporary clips alone or in combination with adenosine-induced cardiac pause (0.3–0.4 mg/kg body weight) to soften the aneurysmal dome prior to their dissection can be particularly helpful. The senior author often prefers a lateral subtemporal approach to basilar apex aneurysms, as described by Drake,[35] to better visualize the posterior P1 perforators during clip placement.

Preoperative understanding of the aneurysmal neck and fundus, its projection orientation, its relationship to the dorsum sellae, the angle of bifurcation and height of the basilar apex, and the angle between the P1 segments can help dictate the most appropriate neurosurgical approach for a patient with this type of aneurysm. An approach that maximizes visualization of the aneurysm neck and fundus, nearby neurovascular structures, and perforators is likely to decrease inadvertent perforator injury and thereby minimize postoperative morbidity and mortality.

Tumors involving the posterior circulation encompass a wide variety of neoplastic pathologies and include meningioma, schwannoma, glioma, giant cell tumor, chordoma, chondrosarcoma, epidermoid tumors, and metastases, among many others. Like tumors near the anterior circulation, these tumors can vary in their involvement of surrounding vasculature. Petroclival meningiomas are often large and can encase the nearby surrounding posterior circulation vasculature and perforator vessels and can also displace and adhere to the brainstem and its associated cranial nerves. They may also parasitize the brainstem perforating vasculature. These collective features make petroclival meningiomas technically challenging tumors to resect despite their typically benign pathology. Approaches to petroclival meningiomas are patient-specific; depend on tumor size, location, and extension; and span frontotemporal, orbitozygomatic, subtemporal-transzygomatic, presigmoid, retrosigmoid, anterior, posterior, and combined petrosal, retrolabyrinthine, translabyrinthine, transcochlear, far lateral, and extreme lateral approaches.[36] Because of the close anatomic relationships these lesions have to critical neurovascular structures, a systematic, multidisciplinary approach must be employed to improve long-term patient outcomes.[37] Nevertheless, the same surgical principles apply in the successful resection of these tumors. Preoperative understanding of the tumor's relationship to the posterior circulation, perforator branches, draining veins and dural venous sinuses, and cranial nerves is essential when planning a skull base approach for these tumors. The senior author favors developing a plane between the tumor capsule and adjacent vessels, when possible. Again, in the case of tumor encasement of the posterior circulation and perforators, identification of their entry and exit points aids in the careful microsurgical dissection and separation of these vessels from the tumor. In cases where the main cerebral vessels and perforators cannot be safely separated from the tumor, a near-total or subtotal resection of the tumor is favored to avoid major ischemic complications. This is especially true when the tumor shares blood supply with brainstem perforators. The skull base surgeon must incorporate a patient's preoperative functional status and quality of life, likelihood of progression-free survival, and possibility of durable disease control with adjuvant therapies into the surgical decision-making process. Leaving behind a small amount of tumor that can be treated with adjuvant radiotherapy is almost always preferable to attempting a curative, aggressive gross total resection with significant postoperative neurological deficit and subsequent poor quality of life.

16.6 Case Examples

16.6.1 Optic Tract Glioma Near the Posterior Clinoid

A 76-year-old man with a history of hypertension, type 2 diabetes, and prostate cancer (status post radical prostatectomy) presented initially to ophthalmology with 1 year of worsening vision and was found to have a right homonymous superior quadrantanopia. MRI of brain with and without contrast revealed a contrast-enhancing lesion of the left optic tract and posterior clinoid region (▶ Fig. 16.2a–c). He underwent a left frontotemporal approach for biopsy and gross total resection (**Video 16.1**). Pathology was consistent with pilocytic

astrocytoma of the optic tract. Upon completion of tumor resection, the patient was noted to have diminished motor-evoked potentials involving the right hand. At this point, a dilute solution of papaverine (3 mg/mL) was applied to the ICA, A1, M1, P1, superior cerebellar artery, PComA, and all visualized perforator vessels. Microvascular Doppler ultrasonography and ICG video angiography were then performed, which both demonstrated delayed flow of the left PComA, consistent with dissection. The patient's blood pressure was liberalized with a mean arterial pressure (MAP) goal of greater than 85 mm Hg, and an additional aliquot of papaverine solution (3 mg/mL) was irrigated onto the left PComA and nearby perforators. Repeat ICG video angiography was performed, which demonstrated left PComA vessel patency with similar slightly diminished filling. The patient's motor evoked potentials improved but did not return to baseline. Of note, the left AChA demonstrated normal flow on intraoperative microvascular Doppler ultrasonography and ICG video angiography. Despite additional intraoperative papaverine, documented perforator vessel patency on microvascular Doppler ultrasonography and ICG video angiography, and postoperative care with permissive hypertension, high-rate intravenous fluids (125 mL/hour), and aspirin (325 mg) on postoperative day 1, the patient sustained an infarction in a left AChA distribution with right upper and right lower extremity weakness postoperatively (▶ Fig. 16.2e). Postoperative MRI of brain with and without contrast demonstrated gross total resection (▶ Fig. 16.2d).

16.6.2 Basilar Apex Aneurysm Clipping

A 57-year-old woman with no significant past medical history presented to an outside hospital with left-sided Bell's palsy; she underwent a noncontrast CT of the head that revealed a hyperdensity in the area of the basilar apex that was concerning for aneurysm. She was transferred to our hospital where she received a CT angiogram of the head and neck, which demonstrated an unruptured, 1-cm, anterosuperiorly projecting basilar apex aneurysm (▶ Fig. 16.3a–c). A DSA was performed to evaluate the morphology of the aneurysm and cerebral vasculature, which revealed a neck width of 4.2-mm, anterosuperior projection, and multilobulated dome morphology (▶ Fig. 16.3d, e). Given the abovementioned features, the patient elected to undergo definitive surgical treatment with clipping of the aneurysm. She underwent a right-sided subtemporal approach for basilar apex aneurysm clipping with preoperative placement of a lumbar drain. Liberal egress of CSF via the lumbar drain was employed to improve brain relaxation. In addition, intermittent adenosine-induced cardiac pause along with burst suppression was used to permit safe dissection of the aneurysmal dome, ipsilateral posterior cerebral artery (PCA), superior cerebellar artery, contralateral PCA, and accompanying P1 perforators. A temporary clip was placed across the basilar artery followed by adenosine-induced cardiac pause. The aneurysmal neck was subsequently dissected free of perforators, and a single permanent clip was placed across the neck of the aneurysm. The temporary basilar clip was removed, and motor and somatosensory evoked potentials were unchanged. ICG video angiography showed that all major vessels and surrounding perforators remained patent with normal filling (▶ Fig. 16.3f); however, there was some residual aneurysmal neck filling noted. A temporary clip was placed

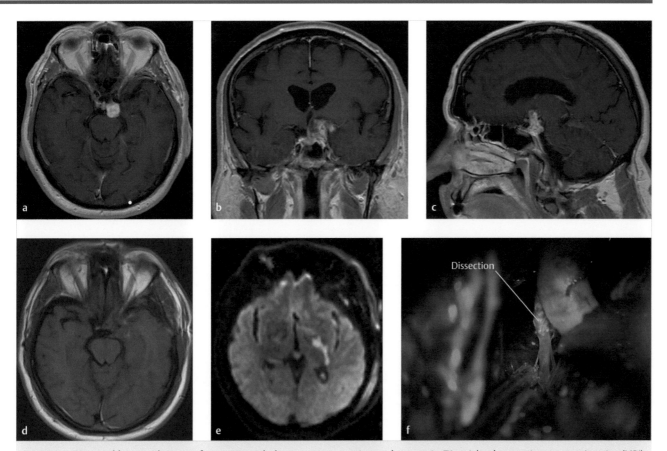

Fig. 16.2 A 76-year-old man with 1 year of worsening right homonymous superior quadrantanopia. T1-weighted magnetic resonance imaging (MRI) of the brain with contrast in **(a)** axial, **(b)** coronal, and **(c)** sagittal views demonstrates a 2.5-cm contrast-enhancing mixed solid and cystic mass encasing the left internal carotid artery (ICA) and abutting the left optic chiasm and tract and left hippocampus. The patient underwent a left frontotemporal craniotomy for resection of this tumor, which was found to be an optic tract glioma on final pathology. **(d)** Postoperative axial T1-weighted MRI of the brain with contrast demonstrated a gross total resection. **(e)** Postoperative axial diffusion-weighted MRI sequence demonstrates a capsular infarct resulting from left anterior choroidal artery vasospasm. **(f)** Intraoperative microscope view of arterial dissection and spasm of left posterior communicating artery (PComA) as it arises from the ipsilateral ICA.

on the basilar artery once more, adenosine cardiac pause was employed, and the clip was repositioned more obliquely to incorporate the entirety of the aneurysmal neck. The temporary clip was removed, and ICG video angiography demonstrated the aneurysmal neck was now completely occluded and all major vessels and surrounding perforators remained patent with normal filling. The perforators and parent vessels were irrigated with papaverine solution (3 mg/mL) and motor and somatosensory evoked potentials remained unchanged. Postoperatively, the patient was extubated and remained neurologically intact with the exception of mild right third and fourth cranial nerve palsies. Her postoperative convalescence was uncomplicated, and she was discharged home on postoperative day 4. Her cranial nerve deficits and diplopia had fully resolved at 1-month follow-up, and repeat CT angiogram of the head at that time demonstrated complete occlusion of the aneurysm (▶ Fig. 16.3g, h).

16.7 Management Algorithm

If vasospasm or arterial dissection of the perforating vessels is visualized or if there is loss of motor or somatosensory evoked potentials, the anesthesiologist is immediately notified and

MAP is increased above 85 mm Hg to induce hypertension (maintained for up to 5–7 days postoperatively, depending on degree of vasospasm). Manipulation and dissection are discontinued. Dilute papaverine (3 mg/mL) is used to bathe the vessels suspected to be in vasospasm. If the potentials normalize, dissection is judiciously continued to complete resection of the tumor or clipping of the aneurysm. If the potentials do not quickly return or only mildly improve, an ICG angiographic evaluation is performed to determine if there is gross disruption of perforator flow on which further therapy should be directed.

If the above maneuvers do not achieve an optimal outcome, an intraoperative or immediate postoperative angiogram (DSA) is performed to assess vascular anatomy and look for any disruption of important vascular perforators. Postoperative MRI is performed to determine whether any ischemia that would further direct therapy is evident.

16.8 Root Cause Analysis

Patient: A 76-year-old male with hypertension, type 2 diabetes, and left optic tract glioma whose resection was complicated by left PComA arterial dissection and infarction causing right upper and lower extremity weakness.

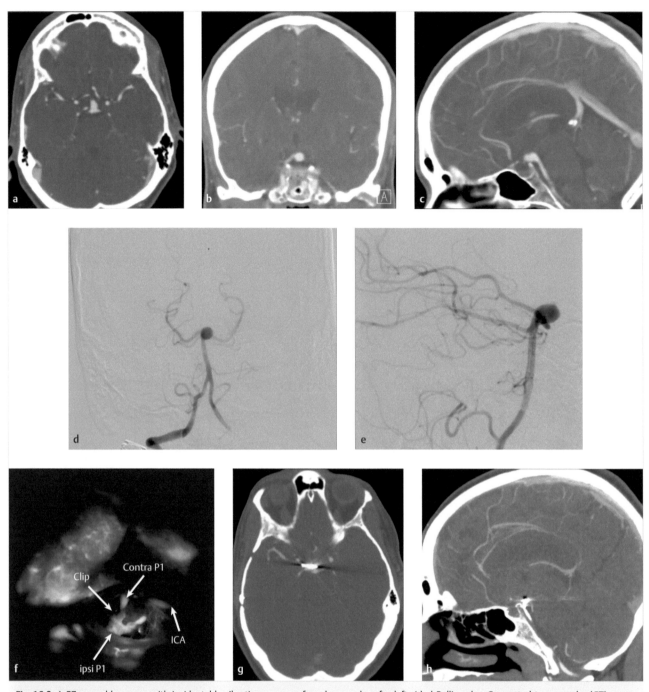

Fig. 16.3 A 57-year-old woman with incidental basilar tip aneurysm found on workup for left-sided Bell's palsy. Computed tomography (CT) angiogram of the head in **(a)** axial, **(b)** coronal, and **(c)** sagittal views demonstrates a 1-cm basilar tip aneurysm. **(d, e)** Digital subtraction angiography was performed preoperatively and demonstrates a 1-cm anterosuperiorly projecting basilar tip aneurysm without visible perforators emanating from the aneurysmal neck or dome. The patient underwent a right subtemporal craniotomy with clipping of the basilar tip aneurysm. **(f)** Right-sided subtemporal view of intraoperative indocyanine green (ICG) video angiography showing ipsilateral and contralateral P1 segments, basilar apex, and clip occluding the basilar tip aneurysm. Perforators coming from basilar apex were inspected and not included in clip construct. Postoperative CT angiogram of the head in **(g)** axial and **(h)** sagittal views demonstrates no residual contrast filling of the aneurysmal neck or dome.

Problem: Left PComA vasospasm and/or dissection causing infarction

Factors: Surgical manipulation of ICA and left PComA and AChA is the most likely cause of arterial dissection and vasospasm in this patient. Other potential factors that could contribute to vasospasm in this setting include intraoperative under-

resuscitation resulting in a hypovolemic state, mild hyponatremia (Na 133 intraoperatively), or unknown underlying vasculopathy related to patient's long-standing hypertension and/or type 2 diabetes. Additional tumor-related factors include tumor invasiveness and enveloping of the involved perforator vessel. Given the location of this tumor near the posterior clinoid region, attempted maximal safe or gross total resection mandates careful vessel manipulation and dissection of nearby perforators to successfully resect this lesion.

Preventative/therapeutic measures: Once arterial dissection and vasospasm were recognized on motor evoked potentials, appropriate counter measures with copious papaverine irrigation of perforator vessels, induced hypertension (MAP >85 mm Hg), visual inspection of the affected vessel (to ensure no compressive/mechanical obstruction of flow), and high-rate intravenous normal saline (125 mL/h) and aspirin 325 mg daily (on postoperative day 1) were implemented.

16.9 Conclusion

Sacrifice or flow disruption of delicate intracranial perforator arteries can lead to significant postoperative neurological deficits. The neurosurgeon must have a thorough understanding of normal microvascular perforator anatomy, its common variations, and how normal anatomy is altered by a patient's particular skull base pathology. This mandates significant preoperative planning on the part of the skull base surgeon. The most appropriate surgical approach should thoughtfully incorporate the location of a particular patient's pathology and preoperative vascular imaging. The use of the operating microscope and other intraoperative tools and technologies can decrease the risk of inadvertent perforator injury. A combination of intraoperative tools and technologies should be utilized to assess perforator flow dynamics. Nevertheless, these modalities remain imperfect and cannot substitute for careful dissection, adequate visualization and inspection, understanding of a patient's unique anatomy, and clinical judgment based on years of experience.

Acknowledgment

The author thank Kristin Kraus, M.Sc., for her assistance with preparation of this chapter.

References

[1] Marinković S, Milisavljević M, Kovacević M. Anatomical bases for surgical approach to the initial segment of the anterior cerebral artery. Microanatomy of Heubner's artery and perforating branches of the anterior cerebral artery. Surg Radiol Anat. 1986; 8(1):7–18

[2] Perlmutter D, Rhoton AL, Jr. Microsurgical anatomy of the anterior cerebral-anterior communicating-recurrent artery complex. J Neurosurg. 1976; 45(3): 259–272

[3] Rosner SS, Rhoton AL, Jr, Ono M, Barry M. Microsurgical anatomy of the anterior perforating arteries. J Neurosurg. 1984; 61(3):468–485

[4] Umansky F, Gomes FB, Dujovny M, et al. The perforating branches of the middle cerebral artery. A microanatomical study. J Neurosurg. 1985; 62(2): 261–268

[5] Marinković S, Gibo H, Brigante L, Nikodijević I, Petrović P. The surgical anatomy of the perforating branches of the anterior choroidal artery. Surg Neurol. 1999; 52(1):30–36

[6] Rhoton AL, Jr, Fujii K, Fradd B. Microsurgical anatomy of the anterior choroidal artery. Surg Neurol. 1979; 12(2):171–187

[7] Marinković SV, Milisavljević MM, Marinković ZD. The perforating branches of the internal carotid artery: the microsurgical anatomy of their extracerebral segments. Neurosurgery. 1990; 26(3):472–478, discussion 478–479

[8] Gibo H, Marinković S, Brigante L. The microsurgical anatomy of the premamillary artery. J Clin Neurosci. 2001; 8(3):256–260

[9] Saeki N, Rhoton AL, Jr. Microsurgical anatomy of the upper basilar artery and the posterior circle of Willis. J Neurosurg. 1977; 46(5):563–578

[10] Marinković S, Milisavljević M, Kovacević M. Interpeduncular perforating branches of the posterior cerebral artery. Microsurgical anatomy of their extracerebral and intracerebral segments. Surg Neurol. 1986; 26(4): 349–359

[11] Milisavljević MM, Marinković SV, Gibo H, Puskas LF. The thalamogeniculate perforators of the posterior cerebral artery: the microsurgical anatomy. Neurosurgery. 1991; 28(4):523–529, discussion 529–530

[12] Zeal AA, Rhoton AL, Jr. Microsurgical anatomy of the posterior cerebral artery. J Neurosurg. 1978; 48(4):534–559

[13] Fischer G, Oertel J, Perneczky A. Endoscopy in aneurysm surgery. Neurosurgery. 2012; 70(2) Suppl Operative:184–190, discussion 190–191

[14] Tantuwaya LS, Fukushima T, Schurman GW, Davis D. Intraoperative microvascular Doppler sonography in aneurysm surgery. Neurosurgery. 1997; 40(5):965–970, discussion 970–972

[15] Stendel R, Pietilä T, Al Hassan AA, Schilling A, Brock M. Intraoperative microvascular Doppler ultrasonography in cerebral aneurysm surgery. J Neurol Neurosurg Psychiatry. 2000; 68(1):29–35

[16] Baker DW. Pulsed ultrasonic Doppler blood-flow sensing. IEEE Trans Sonics Ultrason. 1970; 17:65

[17] Malinova V, von Eckardstein K, Rohde V, Mielke D. Neuronavigated microvascular Doppler sonography for intraoperative monitoring of blood flow velocity changes during aneurysm surgery—a feasible monitoring technique. Clin Neurol Neurosurg. 2015; 137:79–82

[18] Charbel FT, Hoffman WE, Misra M, Ostergren L. Ultrasonic perivascular flow probe: technique and application in neurosurgery. Neurol Res. 1998; 20(5): 439–442

[19] Lundell A, Bergqvist D, Mattsson E, Nilsson B. Volume blood flow measurements with a transit time flowmeter: an in vivo and in vitro variability and validation study. Clin Physiol. 1993; 13(5):547–557

[20] Suzuki K, Kodama N, Sasaki T, et al. Intraoperative monitoring of blood flow insufficiency in the anterior choroidal artery during aneurysm surgery. J Neurosurg. 2003; 98(3):507–514

[21] Sakuma J, Suzuki K, Sasaki T, et al. Monitoring and preventing blood flow insufficiency due to clip rotation after the treatment of internal carotid artery aneurysms. J Neurosurg. 2004; 100(5):960–962

[22] Horiuchi K, Suzuki K, Sasaki T, et al. Intraoperative monitoring of blood flow insufficiency during surgery of middle cerebral artery aneurysms. J Neurosurg. 2005; 103(2):275–283

[23] Choi HH, Ha EJ, Cho W-S, Kang H-S, Kim JE. Effectiveness and limitations of intraoperative monitoring with combined motor and somatosensory evoked potentials during surgical clipping of unruptured intracranial aneurysms. World Neurosurg. 2017; 108:738–747

[24] Ishizaki T, Endo O, Fujii K, et al. Usefulness and problems of intraoperative monitoring for unruptured aneurysm surgery with the motor evoked potential]. No Shinkei Geka. 2016; 44(4):283–293

[25] Tang G, Cawley CM, Dion JE, Barrow DL. Intraoperative angiography during aneurysm surgery: a prospective evaluation of efficacy. J Neurosurg. 2002; 96 (6):993–999

[26] Klopfenstein JD, Spetzler RF, Kim LJ, et al. Comparison of routine and selective use of intraoperative angiography during aneurysm surgery: a prospective assessment. J Neurosurg. 2004; 100(2):230–235

[27] Raabe A, Nakaji P, Beck J, et al. Prospective evaluation of surgical microscope-integrated intraoperative near-infrared indocyanine green videoangiography during aneurysm surgery. J Neurosurg. 2005; 103(6):982–989

[28] Kassell NF, Torner JC, Jane JA, Haley EC, Jr, Adams HP. The International Cooperative Study on the Timing of Aneurysm Surgery. Part 2: Surgical results. J Neurosurg. 1990; 73(1):37–47

[29] Hernesniemi J, Dashti R, Lehecka M, et al. Microneurosurgical management of anterior communicating artery aneurysms. Surg Neurol. 2008; 70(1):8–28, discussion 29

[30] Attia M, Umansky F, Paldor I, Dotan S, Shoshan Y, Spektor S. Giant anterior clinoidal meningiomas: surgical technique and outcomes. J Neurosurg. 2012; 117(4):654–665

[31] Bassiouni H, Asgari S, Sandalcioglu IE, Seifert V, Stolke D, Marquardt G. Anterior clinoidal meningiomas: functional outcome after microsurgical resection in a consecutive series of 106 patients. Clinical article. J Neurosurg. 2009; 111(5):1078–1090

[32] Wiebers DO, Whisnant JP, Huston J, III, et al. International Study of Unruptured Intracranial Aneurysms Investigators. Unruptured intracranial aneurysms: natural history, clinical outcome, and risks of surgical and endovascular treatment. Lancet. 2003; 362(9378):103–110

[33] Henkes H, Fischer S, Mariushi W, et al. Angiographic and clinical results in 316 coil-treated basilar artery bifurcation aneurysms. J Neurosurg. 2005; 103 (6):990–999

[34] Tulleken CAF, Luiten MLFB. The basilar artery bifurcation: microscopical anatomy. Acta Neurochir (Wien). 1987; 85(1–2):50–55

[35] Drake CG. The surgical treatment of aneurysms of the basilar artery. J Neurosurg. 1968; 29(4):436–446

[36] Xu F, Karampelas I, Megerian CA, Selman WR, Bambakidis NC. Petroclival meningiomas: an update on surgical approaches, decision making, and treatment results. Neurosurg Focus. 2013; 35(6):E11

[37] Natarajan SK, Sekhar LN, Schessel D, Morita A. Petroclival meningiomas: multimodality treatment and outcomes at long-term follow-up. Neurosurgery. 2007; 60(6):965–979, discussion 979–981

17 Endovascular Options to Treat Iatrogenic Vascular Injury and Tumor Involvement of the Skull Base

Jacob F. Baranoski, Colin J. Przybylowski, Bradley A. Gross, Felipe C. Albuquerque, and Andrew F. Ducruet

Summary

Internal carotid artery tumor encasement, concomitant aneurysms, and iatrogenic injury pose formidable surgical and clinical management challenges during skull base surgery. When encountering these scenarios, it is critical to understand the potential endovascular treatment and salvage options if an injury does occur. Better yet is understanding how preoperative endovascular techniques can help protect against intraoperative vascular injury and facilitate safe and efficacious tumor resection. This chapter describes the endovascular treatment options for acute and delayed vascular injury after skull base surgery, the utility and interpretation of balloon test occlusion (BTO), preoperative stenting for arterial protection during skull base tumor resection, and treatment strategies for concomitant internal carotid artery aneurysms and skull base tumors.

Keywords: Internal carotid artery (ICA), ICA aneurysms, ICA injury, preoperative stenting, skull base tumors

17.1 Key Learning Points

- Although rare, iatrogenic internal carotid artery (ICA) injury is a potentially fatal complication of skull base surgery.
- Preoperative evaluation of ICA anatomy, tumor involvement, and concomitant aneurysms is essential before skull base tumor resection surgery.
- After recognition and attempted repair of an iatrogenic ICA injury, all patients should undergo an immediate angiogram to assess the extent of injury and the efficacy of the attempted repair.
- Endovascular techniques can be used to treat the sequelae of iatrogenic ICA injury.
- Depending on the endovascular repair performed and the severity of the injury, short-term follow-up angiograms may be warranted. Regardless of the technique used, 6-month follow-up vascular imaging is prudent.
- Judicious use of preoperative endovascular techniques, including preoperative stenting, can help prevent ICA injury during skull base tumor surgery and can facilitate safe and efficacious tumor resection.
- Treatment of ICA aneurysms before surgical or medical management of skull base tumors may prevent iatrogenic injury or subarachnoid hemorrhage.

17.2 Introduction

Surgical treatment of vascular injuries along the skull base is challenging because of the proximity of other critical structures, the complex surgical corridor, limited access, and technical limitations of endoscopic and even open instruments. Extreme care must be taken to avoid iatrogenic injury during skull base dissection and tumor resection while working in this critical region.

If a vascular injury occurs during skull base surgery that cannot be repaired surgically at the time, it is critical to understand the potential endovascular salvage options. Further, judicious use of preoperative endovascular treatments to help protect against intraoperative vascular injury can be beneficial. In this chapter, we discuss the endovascular treatment options for acute and delayed vascular injury after skull base surgery, balloon test occlusion (BTO), preoperative stenting for arterial protection during skull base tumor resection, and treatment strategies for concomitant internal carotid artery (ICA) aneurysms and skull base tumors.

17.3 Endovascular Treatment for Iatrogenic Skull Base Vascular Injuries Sustained During Skull Base Surgery

Vascular injuries are rare but potentially fatal complications of both open microsurgical and endoscopic surgery for skull base tumors. Although ICA injury occurs in <2% of cases of pituitary adenomas,[1,2] treatment of these vascular injuries is markedly challenging. Historically, ICA injuries that could not be primarily repaired required vessel sacrifice with or without attempted high-flow bypass, a treatment strategy that contributes to the morbidity associated with the injuries.[2,3,4,5,6] Vascular injuries may be immediately apparent intraoperatively or can present in a delayed fashion, days to even years after the index surgery.[1,2,6,7,8,9]

In general, the ideal strategy for managing ICA injury during skull base surgery is prevention. This requires a combination of anatomical knowledge, experience, and adherence to established surgical principles. Primary repair of vascular injuries, particularly during endonasal approaches, is very challenging because of the long working corridor, limited surgical freedom, and limitations in available instrumentation. Recently, dedicated teaching efforts using both live courses and simulator models have been designed to help prepare surgeons to manage endonasal ICA injuries intraoperatively.[10,11,12,13] However, the combination of the challenging anatomy and technical limitations currently prevents definitive primary repair of ICA injuries in a majority of these cases.

Various endovascular options have been used to treat iatrogenic ICA injuries after endonasal and open microsurgical skull base surgery. These options differ for injuries that are immediately evident and require emergent treatment[2,3,4,6,8,14-20] and those that present in a delayed fashion after surgery,[2,5,7,9,21-27] radiosurgery,[26,28] or medical management.[29]

Acute injuries with active extravasation require immediate treatment. Traditionally, ICA hemorrhage control was accomplished via vessel sacrifice. However, this was often performed at the cost of ICA territory perfusion. This technique has also been used for injuries that present in a delayed fashion if the patient is determined to be tolerant of vessel occlusion after BTO.

As endovascular treatment technologies have evolved, so too have the treatment options and strategies for iatrogenic ICA injuries. In 2013, Gardner et al[3] reported on seven ICA injuries during endonasal cases that occurred over a 13-year period. They proposed an endovascular treatment algorithm that involved the use of covered stents or coil sacrifice of the ICA to treat pseudoaneurysms or lacerations with active hemorrhage, respectively. Additional studies have reported favorable outcomes treating acute injuries with covered stents to control bleeding and preserve vessel patency.[17,18,19,20] With the advent of flow-diverting devices, potential treatment options have expanded further and cases of iatrogenic ICA injuries have been successfully treated with these devices.[14,15] When using flow-diverting devices, covered stents, and stent-assisted coiling techniques, the need for antiplatelet therapy must be considered.

In 2016, Sylvester et al[2] reported on seven patients with an ICA injury after endonasal surgery who were treated with endovascular therapy, and these authors performed a comprehensive review of the literature. Combining their patients' data with the available published data, they identified 105 total patients with ICA injuries after endonasal surgery who received endovascular treatment. Of these, 46 patients were treated with ICA sacrifice, 28 with focal embolization of the lesion with or without stent assistance, and 31 with parent vessel reconstruction via a covered stent or flow-diverter device. They found that ICA sacrifice provided durable hemorrhage control but carried a relatively high rate of persistent neurological complication (22%). Lesion coil embolization with or without stent assistance was likewise successfully accomplished but carried a high rate of technical complication (31 and 22%, respectively) and resulted in new or persistent neurologic deficits. Endoluminal reconstruction via a covered stent or flow-diverting device was successfully used for select cases. Although the cases for which this technique was used were carefully selected for this therapy, endoluminal reconstruction produced favorable results with a relatively low complication rate. Based on these data, the authors propose a treatment algorithm that takes into account numerous factors including vascular anatomy, injury characteristics, response to BTO, and relative risk of dual antiplatelet therapy (DAPT). Combining the treatment strategies discussed above with our own institutional experience, we propose a similar treatment algorithm (▶ Fig. 17.1). If an iatrogenic injury occurs that cannot be readily repaired, the injury is packed off to limit bleeding. Regardless of whether the bleeding appears to be controlled by surgical packing, the patient is taken immediately to the angiography suite. The first critical decision-making branch point is to determine whether the patient is a candidate for DAPT. DAPT is required for any covered stent, stent-assisted coiling, or flow-diverter treatment. Of course, the use of DAPT puts patients at a higher risk for postoperative hematoma, and the use of these agents must be weighed against the benefits of the attempted endovascular repair. If the bleeding is controlled with packing and there is no angiographic evidence of active extravasation or large pseudoaneurysm, it may be reasonable to consider delaying treatment until DAPT can be initiated; however, proceeding with treatment urgently is favored, even with the risk of initiating DAPT earlier. Factors that may make patients poor candidates for DAPT are a large residual tumor volume that may predispose them to hematoma development from disrupted tumor vasculature or injuries resulting from trauma.[2,30]

If a patient has been determined to be not a candidate for DAPT, but emergent intervention is required, BTO evaluation is recommended next. Because patients with iatrogenic ICA injuries remain intubated and under general anesthesia, the BTO must be completed and interpreted without neurological examination. In these scenarios, the determination of whether the patient can tolerate occlusion must be made on the basis of radiographical and electrophysiological data (discussed below). If the patient can tolerate occlusion, vessel sacrifice can be performed endovascularly using coils with or without liquid embolysates or microvascular plugs. If the patient cannot tolerate occlusion and active extravasation is noted at the injury site and if DAPT is contraindicated for the patient, a high-flow extracranial to intracranial bypass is needed to supplement blood flow before the ICA is sacrificed. In this situation, if a pseudoaneurysm is identified, it can be treated with primary coiling, if possible, or with high-flow bypass followed by vessel sacrifice.

If a patient is deemed an acceptable candidate for DAPT, the endovascular treatment selected is on the basis of angiographic findings. All patients are heparinized during the procedure. Because these patients were not treated with DAPT before stent placement, we use intraoperative intravenous and intra-arterial administration of abciximab, followed postoperatively by aspirin and clopidogrel. Our group recently showed that this strategy was not associated with an increased risk of perioperative thromboembolic complications.[31] We typically continue DAPT for 6 months to allow time for endothelialization of the stent and then repeat angiography. If no in-stent thrombosis is noted, we then consider discontinuing clopidogrel and maintaining the patient on an aspirin regimen. With regard to treatment selection for the ICA injury, if active extravasation is noted, the injury is treated by placing a covered stent across the site of injury. Traditional covered stents, such as those used to treat extracranial carotid injuries and pseudoaneurysms, can be difficult to place in the intracranial circulation. However, smaller covered stents, such as the Jostent (Abbott Vascular Devices, Abbott Medical, Abbott Park, IL), can be delivered through catheters capable of navigating through the cranial ICA and can be used to treat iatrogenic ICA injuries and cavernous carotid fistulas.[20,32,33,34] If a pseudoaneurysm is noted, the endovascular treatment options include deployment of a covered stent, stent-assisted coiling, or deployment of a flow-diverter device. The specific treatment selected should be based on the patient's individual injury and the operator's discretion. In general, stent-assisted coiling or flow-diverter placement is favored, because of the technical nuances involved with the deployment of covered stents and because they are associated with an increased risk of thromboembolic complications. If these techniques are unsuccessful, BTO followed by ICA sacrifice is recommended either with or without high-flow bypass based on the results of the BTO, as discussed above. Depending on the type of endovascular repair performed and the severity of the injury, short-term follow-up angiograms may be warranted. These may be particularly necessary in the situations where a stent was placed across a pseudoaneurysm to ensure stabilization of the lesion. Regardless of technique used, 6-month follow-up vascular imaging is prudent.

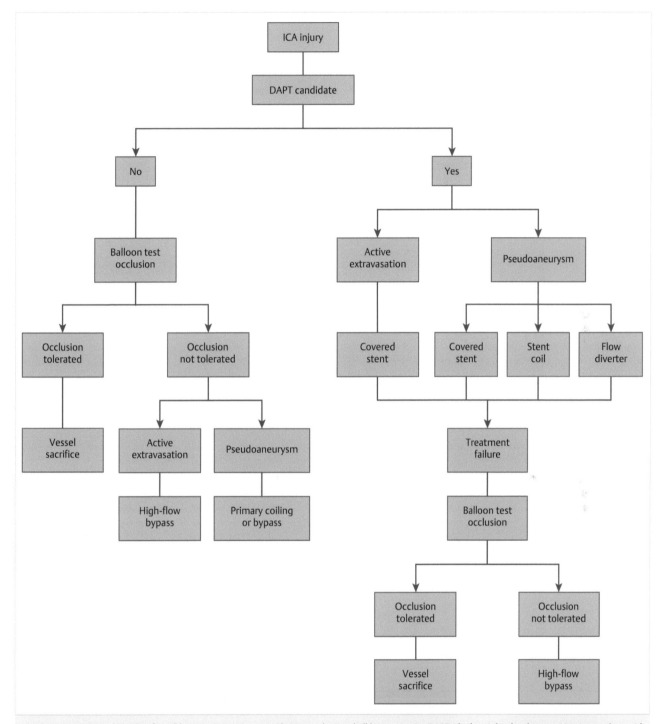

Fig. 17.1 Treatment algorithm for addressing iatrogenic vascular injury during skull base surgery. DAPT, dual antiplatelet therapy; ICA, internal carotid artery. (Used with permission from Barrow Neurological Institute, Phoenix, Arizona.)

As the technology and experience with flow-diverting devices continues to progress, endoluminal reconstruction techniques may continue to improve outcomes for these challenging cases. Additional techniques have also been reported. Cobb et al[35] reported an iatrogenic ICA injury that was repaired primarily after an endovascular balloon was inflated at the injury site during an intraoperative angiogram.[35]

Regardless of the endovascular treatment strategy selected, timely recognition of the event and effective communication between the teams involved are essential. If an iatrogenic injury occurs, the surgical team should immediately alert the anesthesia team, so that they can prepare for blood pressure augmentation and necessary fluid resuscitation and transfusions. If primary control or repair of the injury cannot be achieved immediately, the surgical team should inform the endovascular team, conveying important details, including the side, site, mechanism, and likely extent of the injury, and ask them to have an angiography suite prepared. In cases that have a higher risk for a carotid artery injury (such as surgery for tumors encasing the carotid, revision surgeries, etc.), it is of paramount importance to discuss this elevated risk with all the teams involved and to have a plan in place before beginning surgery. We recommend that an endovascular team be available whenever central skull base surgery is to be performed. Furthermore, it is recommended that high-risk procedures be performed exclusively at institutions with immediately available endovascular services, such as comprehensive stroke centers.

Skull base vascular injuries are not limited only to the ICA. Cases of posterior cerebral artery injury following endonasal and open surgery have also been reported.[36,37,38]

17.3.1 Case Example

One example is a case of a hemorrhagic posterior communicating artery (PComA) pseudoaneurysm after endoscopic endonasal surgery. A 41-year-old man was diagnosed with a midline intracranial dermoid cyst and underwent endoscopic endonasal resection (▶ Fig. 17.2a). No vascular injury was noted during surgery. On postoperative day 9, the patient experienced a sudden-onset severe headache and neurologic decline from a subarachnoid hemorrhage. An angiogram demonstrated a right

PComA pseudoaneurysm (▶ Fig. 17.2b). Vertebral artery injection demonstrated robust filling of bilateral posterior cerebral arteries (▶ Fig. 17.2c), and the pseudoaneurysm was treated with coil embolization with focal sacrifice of the distal PComA (▶ Fig. 17.2d). The patient did not experience any neurologic complication associated with this treatment.

Similar treatment strategies and techniques can be applied to skull base vascular injuries secondary to other etiologies, including trauma or sinus surgery.[14] Patients with an ICA injury and pseudoaneurysm development have also presented in a delayed fashion after radiosurgery for tumors, and these injuries necessitated endovascular therapy.[26,28,39]

17.4 Preoperative Evaluation, Endovascular Stenting or Vessel Sacrifice Prior to Resection of Skull Base Tumors

Skull base tumors that abut or encase the carotid artery represent a technically challenging surgical problem. Aside from tumor resection, the primary goal of surgery and often one of the most difficult aspects of management involves preservation of the ICA. As surgical skull base techniques continue to evolve, surgeons are able to attempt resection of tumors formerly considered inoperable. Nevertheless, attempted resection of tumors

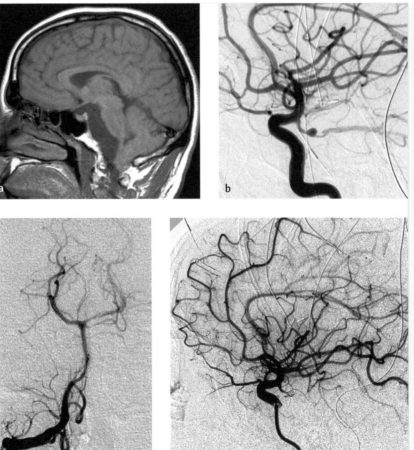

Fig. 17.2 **(a)** Sagittal magnetic resonance imaging (MRI) demonstrating a midline intracranial dermoid cyst. **(b)** Lateral projection angiogram of a right internal carotid artery (ICA) injection demonstrating a pseudoaneurysm of the right posterior communicating artery. **(c)** Townes projection angiogram of a right vertebral artery injection demonstrating robust filling of bilateral posterior cerebral arteries, suggesting that the right posterior communicating artery could be safely sacrificed. **(d)** Posttreatment lateral projection angiogram of a right ICA injection demonstrating successful treatment of the pseudoaneurysm and sacrifice of the distal posterior communicating artery. (Used with permission from Dr. Bradley Gross of the University of Pittsburgh.)

that encase the ICA is associated with a significant risk of morbidity stemming from carotid artery rupture, dissection, and stroke.[40] Though carotid artery reconstruction has been attempted in patients with these lesions, this treatment itself is technically difficult and carries a high rate of morbidity. Subtotal lesion resection is also an option; however, this predisposes the patient to a high likelihood of recurrence with these often-aggressive tumors. As we continue to push the boundary of skull base surgery, endovascular techniques have also evolved to aid in the treatment of these challenging lesions.

These endovascular techniques include preoperative permanent occlusion of the ICA, external carotid artery to ICA bypass followed by vessel sacrifice, and ICA reinforcement with carotid stents. All of these techniques carry associated risks and limitations and must be used cautiously and judiciously. Application of any of these techniques requires thorough preoperative evaluation, and technique selection must be tailored on the basis of patient-specific characteristics, including the degree of ICA involvement, overall patient prognosis and clinical presentation, and the anatomic integrity of collaterals and the circle of Willis. A BTO can also assist in the decision-making process by helping to determine whether a patient can tolerate vessel sacrifice without risking ischemic injury. To assist in planning salvage options if an ICA injury occurs, BTO is recommended for all patients with tumors where the risk of carotid artery injury is elevated (e.g., circumferential involvement, revisions, postradiation) and when preoperative endovascular manipulation of the ICA (either permanent occlusion or stenting) procedures are being planned or en bloc ICA resection considered.

To perform a BTO, the awake patient is taken to the angiography suite. After femoral access is obtained, the patient is systemically heparinized to a goal activated clotting time of 250 to 300 seconds. A balloon is then inflated in the ipsilateral cervical or petrous ICA. A dual-lumen, compliant microcatheter balloon is preferred as it allows the flow of heparinized saline distal to the balloon occlusion, which can help limit stagnation and subsequent thrombus formation. Complete occlusion of the ICA is confirmed with ipsilateral contrast injection demonstrating complete angiographic block. With the balloon inflated, a clinical neurological examination is performed every 2 to 5 minutes. The development of any neurologic deficit or a decreased level of consciousness indicates that the patient is intolerant of occlusion, and the balloon should be deflated immediately. Additional assessments include angiographic visualization of collateral flow via injection of the contralateral ICA or vertebral arteries or use of somatosensory evoked potential (SSEP) and electroencephalogram (EEG) recordings. The ICA must be completely occluded for at least 30 minutes with no development of neurologic dysfunction before the BTO is considered to have been successful. Adjunctive testing that includes a hypotensive challenge component of the BTO is also recommended, in which the patient's systolic blood pressure is decreased by 25 to 30% and neurologic testing is done for an additional 10 to 20 minutes. This technique increases the sensitivity of the BTO by further diminishing collateral reserves. Another technique uses single-photon emission computed tomography (SPECT) to extrapolate cerebral blood flow. To perform this technique, a baseline SPECT study of the patient is obtained before the BTO is performed. During the BTO, the patient is injected intravenously with a radioisotope. After the BTO is completed, repeat SPECT imaging is performed. The

assessment is considered to be unsuccessful if a >10% change occurs between the pre- and post-BTO SPECT imaging.

The aforementioned assessment of collaterals from the contralateral ICA and vertebral arteries is also valuable. With the balloon inflated in the ipsilateral ICA, if the distal ipsilateral ICA branch arteries and hemispheres fill adequately during contralateral ICA or vertebral artery injections via the circle of Willis, the patient is deemed to be able to tolerate occlusion. If the ipsilateral ICA branches and hemisphere do not adequately fill, the patient may not tolerate occlusion. If the BTO and supplemental testing are successful, they are deemed acceptably low risk for ischemic complication secondary to ICA occlusion and are considered for permanent ICA sacrifice. If patients fail any portion of the BTO, they should be considered at higher risk of permanent occlusion, and an alternative technique (e.g., stenting, bypass, subtotal resection) should be considered instead. As discussed above, in emergent situations following iatrogenic ICA injury, the determination of whether a patient passed the BTO and will be able to tolerate ICA sacrifice must be based solely on radiographical and electrophysiological data.

17.4.1 Case Example

A 47-year-old man with a history of aggressive retinoblastoma who had undergone previous surgical resection with bilateral enucleations followed by radiation developed a radiation-induced leiomyosarcoma involving the nasal septum and anterior skull base. This lesion was resected but recurred (▶ Fig. 17.3a). Given that the lesion circumferentially encased the right ICA, carotid artery sacrifice was considered prior to attempting re-resection (▶ Fig. 17.3b). Angiography revealed robust collaterals with widely patent posterior and anterior communicating arteries (▶ Fig. 17.3c, d). The patient tolerated a BTO of his right ICA based on clinical and nuclear medicine radiographic assessment. Given these results, we proceeded with endovascular sacrifice of the right ICA using a combination of coils and liquid embolysate (▶ Fig. 17.3e). This procedure resulted in complete occlusion of the right ICA (▶ Fig. 17.3f). Injection of the left ICA and vertebral arteries demonstrated robust opacification of the right middle cerebral artery and anterior cerebral artery territories (▶ Fig. 17.3g). The patient then successfully underwent gross total resection of his tumor without vascular complication.

A number of endovascular techniques can be used to sacrifice the ICA, including placement of coils with or without liquid embolysates, detachable balloons, or microvascular plugs. In general, we recommend performing all of these procedures in the angiography suite with the patient under general anesthesia, although some surgeons may opt to perform the vessel sacrifice with the patient awake immediately following the BTO. Transarterial access is achieved, and the patient is systemically heparinized. When coils, with or without liquid embolysates, are used—as in this case—a balloon is inflated in the ICA proximal to the site of the desired occlusion. If a single-lumen balloon catheter is used, a coil delivery catheter must be positioned distal to the balloon catheter before the balloon is inflated. The use of a dual-lumen balloon catheter can obviate the need for an additional catheter system. With the balloon inflated, coiling can be performed, and the balloon can then be deflated and removed. The advent and refinement of vascular plug devices

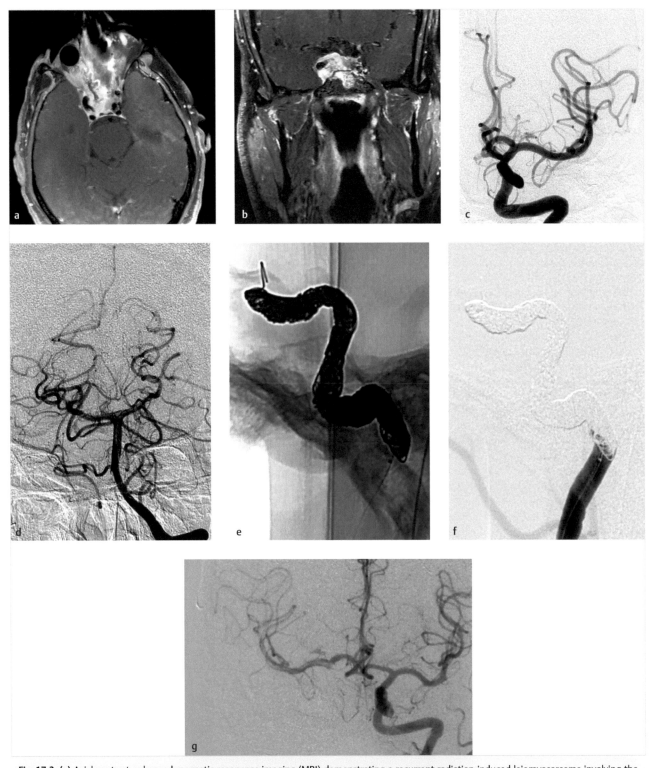

Fig. 17.3 **(a)** Axial contrast-enhanced magnetic resonance imaging (MRI) demonstrating a recurrent radiation-induced leiomyosarcoma involving the nasal septum and anterior skull base. **(b)** Coronal MRI demonstrating that this lesion has circumferentially encased the right internal carotid artery (ICA). **(c)** Townes projection angiogram of a left ICA injection demonstrating robust filling of right anterior circulation via a widely patent anterior communicating artery. **(d)** Townes projection angiogram of a left vertebral artery injection demonstrating robust filling of bilateral posterior cerebral arteries. **(e)** Lateral projection angiogram demonstrating the coil mass deployed into the right ICA resulting in complete occlusion of the vessel **(f)**. **(g)** Post-treatment Townes projection angiogram of a left ICA injection demonstrating robust filling of bilateral anterior and middle cerebral artery territories with the contralateral side filling via a widely patent anterior communicating artery. (Used with permission from Dr. Bradley Gross of the University of Pittsburgh.)

provide endovascular surgeons with additional options for achieving permanent ICA occlusion. The location of ICA sacrifice should take into account the origins of the ICA branches and the relative location of the tumor. In general, we tend to perform ICA occlusion in the distal petrous segment.

Sanna et al[41] reported their series of tympanojugular paragangliomas that were resected with preoperative endovascular ICA augmentation. Complex tympanojugular paragangliomas can infiltrate the ICA; this infiltration represents a significant risk of surgical morbidity and limits the ability to achieve a gross total resection. For patients with tympanojugular paragangliomas, the ICA is classically involved along the posterolateral surface of the vertical segment near the jugular bulb. Although carotid artery manipulation at this location can often be accomplished safely, tympanojugular paragangliomas that have invaded the ICA preclude manipulation of the ICA and can result in incomplete tumor resection or ICA injury. To address this, endovascular techniques have been used to protect the ICA and promote gross total resection of the tumor while minimizing the potential surgical morbidity.

In the study reported by Sanna and colleagues,[41] 20 patients with tympanojugular paragangliomas planned for gross total resection were evaluated for preoperative ICA intervention. Ten patients underwent a preoperative permanent balloon occlusion for carotid sacrifice after a BTO indicated they were tolerant of vessel occlusion. Two of these patients had an external carotid artery to ICA bypass before balloon occlusion. Out of these 10 patients, 8 patients underwent subsequent surgery that resulted in gross total resection in 7 cases and subtotal resection in 1 case. There were no endovascular or intraoperative complications in these 8 patients. Two patients died before surgical resection could be performed because of intracranial hypertension, which may or may not be directly related to the endovascular treatment.[41]

The other 10 patients who were deemed intolerant of vessel occlusion after evaluation by a BTO underwent preoperative ICA stenting using one of three types of self-expanding nitinol stents: Xpert Stent System (Abbott Laboratories Vascular Enterprises, Dublin, Ireland), Neuroform 3 (Boston Scientific, Fremont, CA), and LEO (Balt Extrusion, Montmorency, France). In this series, patients who underwent stenting were started on antiplatelet therapy 1 week before stent placement that consisted of either a combination of ticlopidine (250 mg twice daily) and aspirin (100 mg daily) or clopidogrel (75 mg daily) and aspirin (100 mg daily). Patients were continued on a dual antiplatelet regimen for a minimum of 30 days after stenting and were then transitioned to an aspirin-only regimen. The interval between stenting and surgery varied from 1 to 3 months. In this series, antiplatelet therapy was suspended 1 week before surgery and resumed 1 week afterward. During the interim, patients were maintained on a heparin regimen.[41]

For these 10 patients, the selected stents deployed spanned the petrous and cervical carotid artery. This was achieved without difficulty in eight of these patients. One patient developed vasospasm that was successfully treated with intra-arterial vasodilators without clinical consequence and another patient required permanent occlusion of the ICA after stent placement. No other thromboembolic or periprocedural complications were encountered during endovascular treatment or surgical resection. Of the nine patients who underwent

surgical resection after preoperative stent placement, eight patients were able to have a surgical plane established, which resulted in a gross total resection in six cases and near-total resection in two patients. In one patient with a recurrent tumor who underwent preoperative stenting, it was not possible to establish a cleavage plane between the recurrent tumor and the ICA, which resulted in a subtotal resection. On the basis of these results, these authors conclude that preoperative stenting can be advantageous in the surgical management of complex tympanojugular paragangliomas.[41]

Similarly, Markiewicz et al[40] describe a series of five patients with squamous cell carcinoma of the head and neck who underwent preoperative stenting of the ICA before surgical resection. In this study, patients underwent placement of a heparin-bonded Viabahn covered stent(s) (W.L. Gore and Associates, Inc., Flagstaff, AZ) spanning the portion of the ICA that was encased in tumor with an additional 1 cm of proximal and distal coverage. All patients were initiated on a dual-antiplatelet regimen of clopidogrel (75 mg daily) and aspirin (325 mg daily) that was continued for at least 6 months. After stent placement, all five patients underwent surgical resection. The interval from stent placement to surgery was 1 to 22 days. The short interval was due to the aggressive nature of the patients' tumors that required immediate surgical intervention upon presentation. In all five patients, a gross total resection was achieved, including resection of the carotid artery adventitia from the stent. No intraoperative complications were reported. One stent-related complication occurred in one patient that was caused by in-stent thrombosis, which resulted in decreased visual acuity. No spontaneous hemorrhage or pseudoaneurysm formation was noted in any patient at the site of carotid artery adventitia resection. Based on these results, these authors conclude that preoperative covered stent placement can facilitate safe and efficacious resection of tumors encasing the ICA with minimal associated morbidity.[40]

Carotid body tumors represent another technically challenging lesion due to their vascularity and proximity to the carotid artery. McDougall et al[42] reported on two patients on whom preoperative deployment of a covered stent was used during resection of carotid body tumors. Two patients with carotid body tumors were selected for preoperative covered stent deployment, the first because of bilateral tumors and the second because evaluation by BTO determined the patient was intolerant of vessel occlusion. The stents used were either a Wallgraft covered stent (Boston Scientific, Marlborough, MA) or a Fluency covered stent (Bard Peripheral Vascular Inc, Tempe, AZ). Both patients were maintained on dual antiplatelet regimen of clopidogrel and aspirin for 6 weeks after stent placement followed by an aspirin-only regimen that was then held 1 week prior to surgery. Patients were admitted 3 days preoperatively and started on an intravenous heparin drip that was then held 6 hours preoperatively. Aspirin was restarted postoperatively. Gross total resection of the tumor was able to be achieved with preserved patency of the ICA in both cases.[42]

Overall, preoperative stenting for tumors that abut or involve the carotid artery may provide significant benefit in the management of these difficult lesions. The primary goal of stenting should be carotid artery preservation with potential secondary benefits of tumor devascularization and assisting with achievement of a gross total resection. The stent may provide a physical and hemodynamic barrier that protects the artery, promotes laminar arterial flow, devascularizes the tumor, and allows for tactile feedback facilitating subadventitial dissection and complete tumor removal. This technique may allow surgeons to perform a more aggressive anatomical dissection of the artery while decreasing overall risk. This may be particularly useful in cases where the ICA sacrifice cannot be tolerated. However, it is important to note that carotid stenting, particularly using a covered stent, carries its own risk and potential morbidity. The risks of thromboembolic complications, vessel rupture or dissection, in-stent stenosis, and the lifelong requirement for antiplatelet medication must be considered. Therefore, careful consideration on a case-by-case basis and judicious use of these techniques is of paramount importance in making treatment decisions.

17.5 Treatment Considerations for Concomitant ICA Aneurysms and Skull Base Tumors

Although rare, the co-occurrence of an intracranial ICA aneurysm with a tumor of the anterior skull base poses a significant clinical challenge and influences treatment priorities, strategy, and outcomes. Prior studies have reported an incidence of ICA aneurysms in patients with pituitary tumors ranging from 0.5 to 7.4%.[43] The incidence of ICA aneurysm and anterior skull base tumor co-occurrence may be higher in patients with tumors that invade the cavernous sinus and with growth hormone–secreting lesions.[44] Because of the proximity of the ICA to the midline of the anterior skull base, these aneurysms may project into a sellar or suprasellar tumor. It is also critical to remember that ICA aneurysms can have intrasellar extension even without a concomitant skull base lesion and patients can present with symptoms of mass effect and endocrine dysfunction that mimic the presence of a pituitary tumor.[45] Successful management of these complex scenarios requires anatomical analysis of both lesions and a patient-personalized intervention strategy based on the individual's anatomy and clinical presentation. This co-occurrence can be particularly challenging in the setting of progressive neurologic decline due to the mass effect of the tumor or aneurysmal subarachnoid hemorrhage. Before proceeding with an intervention for either lesion, the following should be considered:

- The natural history and potential rupture risk of the aneurysm in question.
- The need for surgical resection of the skull base lesion based on serial growth assessment or progression of endocrinologic or neurologic symptoms.
- Proximity and involvement of the ICA and the aneurysm with the skull base tumor.

Many authors recommend preoperative endovascular management of the aneurysm prior to skull base surgery for tumor resection.[44,46,47] Raper et al[43] reported their results in treating 13 patients with an anterior skull base lesion and concomitant ICA aneurysm. These authors employed various treatment strategies determined on a patient-by-patient basis. Five patients underwent endovascular treatment before skull base sur-

gery, 1 patient's aneurysm was treated after skull base surgery, 2 patients underwent endovascular treatment for their aneurysm and conservative/medical management of their skull base lesion, 4 patients underwent surgery for their skull base lesion and conservative management of their aneurysm, and 1 patient was followed conservatively for both the tumor and aneurysm. On the basis of their experience, these authors state that preoperative evaluation of the ICAs with vigilance to the presence of aneurysms is critical before the patient undergoes skull base surgery. Optimal management is case-specific, but these authors report that preoperative coiling is well tolerated and does not necessitate a significant delay for surgical resection due to the need for dual-antiplatelet therapy associated with stenting procedures.[43] For cases in which a stent is necessary for aneurysm treatment, a minimum of 3 months of DAPT is necessary and should not be interrupted for an elective skull base surgery. As with iatrogenic ICA injury during skull base surgery, addressed above, aneurysm rupture during skull base surgery can be managed using direct surgical clipping, coiling, flow diversion, or ICA sacrifice. However, careful preoperative planning and clinical decision-making will often successfully obviate the likelihood of encountering this potentially devastating scenario.

Even if the skull base lesion is planned to be managed medically or conservatively, treatment for the concomitant aneurysm should still be considered. Khalsa et al[29] reported a case of subarachnoid hemorrhage due to a ruptured cavernous ICA aneurysm after medical treatment of a large prolactinoma. The patient ultimately required permanent occlusion of the ICA to control the rupture. Treatment of the aneurysm at the time of presentation may have prevented aneurysm rupture after medication-induced shrinkage of the prolactinoma. This was not the first report of subarachnoid hemorrhage due to a cavernous aneurysm rupture after medical treatment of a large prolactinoma,[48] and the risk warrants consideration in treatment planning. Indeed, Soni et al[49] report successfully treating a fusiform ICA aneurysm encased in a large prolactinoma via endovascular obliteration of the aneurysmal segment and concurrent medical management of the prolactinoma.

17.6 Conclusion

ICA tumor encasement, the presence of concomitant aneurysms, and iatrogenic injury pose formidable surgical and clinical management challenges during skull base tumor surgery. Although fortunately rare, iatrogenic ICA injury is a potentially fatal complication of skull base surgery. Endovascular techniques—including primary coiling, stent-assisted coiling, flow-diverting or covered stent deployment, and vessel sacrifice—can be used to treat the sequelae of ICA injury and limit the clinical consequences. Furthermore, preoperative utilization of endovascular techniques, including BTO, stenting, vessel occlusion, and concomitant aneurysm treatment, can help prevent ICA injury during skull base tumor surgery and can facilitate safe and efficacious tumor resection. Supplemented by the judicious use of preoperative endovascular techniques, preoperative evaluation of ICA anatomy, tumor involvement, and the presence of concomitant aneurysms is essential before any planned skull base surgery.

References

[1] Raymond J, Hardy J, Czepko R, Roy D. Arterial injuries in transsphenoidal surgery for pituitary adenoma; the role of angiography and endovascular treatment. AJNR Am J Neuroradiol. 1997; 18(4):655–665

[2] Sylvester PT, Moran CJ, Derdeyn CP, et al. Endovascular management of internal carotid artery injuries secondary to endonasal surgery: case series and review of the literature. J Neurosurg. 2016; 125(5):1256–1276

[3] Gardner PA, Tormenti MJ, Pant H, Fernandez-Miranda JC, Snyderman CH, Horowitz MB. Carotid artery injury during endoscopic endonasal skull base surgery: incidence and outcomes. Neurosurgery. 2013; 73(2) Suppl Operative:ons261–ons269, discussion ons269–ons270

[4] Rangel-Castilla L, McDougall CG, Spetzler RF, Nakaji P. Urgent cerebral revascularization bypass surgery for iatrogenic skull base internal carotid artery injury. Neurosurgery. 2014; 10 Suppl 4:640–647, discussion 647–648

[5] Wang L, Shi X, Liu F, Qian H. Bypass surgery to treat symptomatic fusiform dilation of the internal carotid artery following craniopharyngioma resection: report of 2 cases. Neurosurg Focus. 2016; 41(6):E17

[6] Lawton MT, Spetzler RF. Internal carotid artery sacrifice for radical resection of skull base tumors. Skull Base Surg. 1996; 6(2):119–123

[7] Elliott RE, Wisoff JH. Fusiform dilation of the carotid artery following radical resection of pediatric craniopharyngiomas: natural history and management. Neurosurg Focus. 2010; 28(4):E14

[8] Lee JH, Sade B, Park BJ. A surgical technique for the removal of clinoidal meningiomas. Neurosurgery. 2006; 59(1) Suppl 1:ONS108–ONS114, discussion ONS108–ONS114

[9] Liu SS, Zabramski JM, Spetzler RF. Fusiform aneurysm after surgery for craniopharyngioma. J Neurosurg. 1991; 75(4):670–672

[10] Shen J, Hur K, Zhang Z, et al. Objective validation of perfusion-based human cadaveric simulation training model for management of internal carotid artery injury in endoscopic endonasal sinus and skull base surgery. Oper Neurosurg (Hagerstown). 2018; 15(2):231–238

[11] Pacca P, Jhawar SS, Seclen DV, et al. "Live cadaver" model for internal carotid artery injury simulation in endoscopic endonasal skull base surgery. Oper Neurosurg (Hagerstown). 2017; 13(6):732–738

[12] Pham M, Kale A, Marquez Y, et al. A perfusion-based human cadaveric model for management of carotid artery injury during endoscopic endonasal skull base surgery. J Neurol Surg B Skull Base. 2014; 75(5):309–313

[13] Rowan NR, Turner MT, Valappil B, et al. Injury of the carotid artery during endoscopic endonasal surgery: surveys of skull base surgeons. J Neurol Surg B Skull Base. 2018; 79(3):302–308

[14] Ghorbani M, Shojaei H, Bavand K, Azar M. Surpass streamline flow-diverter embolization device for treatment of iatrogenic and traumatic internal carotid artery injuries. AJNR Am J Neuroradiol. 2018; 39(6):1107–1111

[15] Karadag A, Kinali B, Ugur O, Oran I, Middlebrooks EH, Senoglu M. A case of pseudoaneurysm of the internal carotid artery following endoscopic endonasal pituitary surgery: endovascular treatment with flow-diverting stent implantation. Acta Med (Hradec Kralove). 2017; 60(2):89–92

[16] Iancu D, Lum C, Ahmed ME, et al. Flow diversion in the treatment of carotid injury and carotid-cavernous fistula after transsphenoidal surgery. Interv Neuroradiol. 2015; 21(3):346–350

[17] Cinar C, Bozkaya H, Parildar M, Oran I. Endovascular management of vascular injury during transsphenoidal surgery. Interv Neuroradiol. 2013; 19(1):102–109

[18] Park YS, Jung JY, Ahn JY, Kim DJ, Kim SH. Emergency endovascular stent graft and coil placement for internal carotid artery injury during transsphenoidal surgery. Surg Neurol. 2009; 72(6):741–746

[19] Leung GK, Auyeung KM, Lui WM, Fan YW. Emergency placement of a self-expandable covered stent for carotid artery injury during trans-sphenoidal surgery. Br J Neurosurg. 2006; 20(1):55–57

[20] Kocer N, Kizilkilic O, Albayram S, Adaletli I, Kantarci F, Islak C. Treatment of iatrogenic internal carotid artery laceration and carotid cavernous fistula with endovascular stent-graft placement. AJNR Am J Neuroradiol. 2002; 23(3):442–446

[21] Reynolds MR, Heiferman DM, Boucher AB, Serrone JC, Barrow DL, Dion JE. Fusiform dilatation of the internal carotid artery following childhood craniopharyngioma resection treated by endovascular flow diversion—a case report and literature review. J Clin Neurosci. 2018; 54:143–145

[22] Bougaci N, Paquis P. Cerebral vasospasm after transsphenoidal surgery for pituitary adenoma: case report and review of the literature. Neurochirurgie. 2017; 63(1):25–27

[23] Eneling J, Karlsson PM, Rossitti S. Sphenopalatine arteriovenous fistula complicating transsphenoidal pituitary surgery: a rare cause of delayed epistaxis treatable by endovascular embolization. Surg Neurol Int. 2016; 7 Suppl 41:S1053–S1056

[24] Li Q, Wang C, Xu J, You C. Endovascular treatment for fusiform dilation of internal carotid artery following craniopharyngioma resection: a case illustration. J Child Neurol. 2015; 30(10):1354–1356

[25] Fu M, Patel T, Baehring JM, Bulsara KR. Cavernous carotid pseudoaneurysm following transsphenoidal surgery. Neuroimaging. 2013; 23(3):319–325

[26] Endo H, Fujimura M, Inoue T, et al. Simultaneous occurrence of subarachnoid hemorrhage and epistaxis due to ruptured petrous internal carotid artery aneurysm: association with transsphenoidal surgery and radiation therapy: case report. Neurol Med Chir (Tokyo). 2011; 51(3):226–229

[27] Tirakotai W, Sure U, Benes L, et al. Successful management of a symptomatic fusiform dilatation of the internal carotid artery following surgery of childhood craniopharyngioma. Childs Nerv Syst. 2002; 18(12):717–721

[28] Ito H, Onodera H, Sase T, et al. Percutaneous transluminal angioplasty in a patient with internal carotid artery stenosis following gamma knife radiosurgery for recurrent pituitary adenoma. Surg Neurol Int. 2015; 6 Suppl 7:S279–S283

[29] Khalsa SS, Hollon TC, Shastri R, Trobe JD, Gemmete JJ, Pandey AS. Spontaneous subarachnoid hemorrhage due to ruptured cavernous internal carotid artery aneurysm after medical prolactinoma treatment. J Neurointerv Surg. 2017; 9(3):e9

[30] Nerva JD, Mantovani A, Barber J, et al. Treatment outcomes of unruptured arteriovenous malformations with a subgroup analysis of ARUBA (A Randomized Trial of Unruptured Brain Arteriovenous Malformations)-eligible patients. Neurosurgery. 2015; 76(5):563–570, n570, quiz 570

[31] Levitt MR, Moon K, Albuquerque FC, Mulholland CB, Kalani MY, McDougall CG. Intraprocedural abciximab bolus versus pretreatment oral dual antiplatelet medication for endovascular stenting of unruptured intracranial aneurysms. J Neurointerv Surg. 2016; 8(9):909–912

[32] Briganti F, Tortora F, Marseglia M, Napoli M, Cirillo L. Covered stent implantation for the treatment of direct carotid-cavernous fistula and its mid-term follow-up. Interv Neuroradiol. 2009; 15(2):185–190

[33] Kalia JS, Niu T, Zaidat OO. The use of a covered stent graft for obliteration of high-flow carotid cavernous fistula presenting with life-threatening epistaxis. J Neurointerv Surg. 2009; 1(2):142–145

[34] Kim BM, Jeon P, Kim DJ, Kim DI, Suh SH, Park KY. Jostent covered stent placement for emergency reconstruction of a ruptured internal carotid artery during or after transsphenoidal surgery. J Neurosurg. 2015; 122(5):1223–1228

[35] Cobb MI, Nimjee S, Gonzalez LF, Jang DW, Zomorodi A. Direct repair of iatrogenic internal carotid artery injury during endoscopic endonasal approach surgery with temporary endovascular balloon-assisted occlusion: technical case report. Neurosurgery. 2015; 11 Suppl 3:E483–E486, discussion E486–E487

[36] Lee CH, Chen SM, Lui TN. Posterior cerebral artery pseudoaneurysm, a rare complication of pituitary tumor transsphenoidal surgery: case report and literature review. World Neurosurg. 2015; 84(5):1493.e1–1493.e3

[37] Chalil A, Staudt MD, Lownie SP. Iatrogenic pseudoaneurysms associated with cerebrospinal fluid diversion procedures. Surg Neurol Int. 2019; 10:31

[38] Ciceri EF, Klucznik RP, Grossman RG, Rose JE, Mawad ME. Aneurysms of the posterior cerebral artery: classification and endovascular treatment. AJNR Am J Neuroradiol. 2001; 22(1):27–34

[39] Mak CH, Cheng KM, Cheung YL, Chan CM. Endovascular treatment of ruptured internal carotid artery pseudoaneurysms after irradiation for nasopharyngeal carcinoma patients. Hong Kong Med J/Xianggang yi xue za zhi. 2013; 19(3):229–236

[40] Markiewicz MR, Pirgousis P, Bryant C, et al. Preoperative protective endovascular covered stent placement followed by surgery for management of the cervical common and internal carotid arteries with tumor encasement. J Neurol Surg B Skull Base. 2017; 78(1):52–58

[41] Sanna M, Piazza P, De Donato G, Menozzi R, Falcioni M. Combined endovascular-surgical management of the internal carotid artery in complex tympanojugular paragangliomas. Skull Base. 2009; 19(1):26–42

[42] McDougall CM, Liu R, Chow M. Covered carotid stents as an adjunct in the surgical treatment of carotid body tumors: a report of 2 cases and a review of the literature. Neurosurgery. 2012; 71(1) Suppl Operative:182–184, discussion 185

[43] Raper DM, Ding D, Evans E, et al. Clinical features, management considerations and outcomes in case series of patients with parasellar intracranial aneurysms undergoing anterior skull base surgery. World Neurosurg. 2017; 99:424–432

[44] Xia X, Ramanathan M, Orr BA, et al. Expanded endonasal endoscopic approach for resection of a growth hormone-secreting pituitary macroadenoma coexistent with a cavernous carotid artery aneurysm. J Clin Neurosci. 2012; 19 (10):1437–1441

[45] Hanak BW, Zada G, Nayar VV, et al. Cerebral aneurysms with intrasellar extension: a systematic review of clinical, anatomical, and treatment characteristics. J Neurosurg. 2012; 116(1):164–178

[46] Wang CS, Yeh TC, Wu TC, Yeh CH. Pituitary macroadenoma co-existent with supraclinoid internal carotid artery cerebral aneurysm: a case report and review of the literature. Cases J. 2009; 2:6459

[47] Yamada S, Yamada SM, Hirohata T, et al. Endoscopic extracapsular removal of pituitary adenoma: the importance of pretreatment of an adjacent unruptured internal carotid artery aneurysm. Case Rep Neurol Med. 2012; 2012:891847

[48] Akutsu N, Hosoda K, Ohta K, Tanaka H, Taniguchi M, Kohmura E. Subarachnoid hemorrhage due to rupture of an intracavernous carotid artery aneurysm coexisting with a prolactinoma under cabergoline treatment. J Neurol Surg Rep. 2014; 75(1):e73–e76

[49] Soni A, De Silva SR, Allen K, Byrne JV, Cudlip S, Wass JA. A case of macroprolactinoma encasing an internal carotid artery aneurysm, presenting as pituitary apoplexy. Pituitary. 2008; 11(3):307–311

18 Extracranial Anterior Cranial Base Surgery for Vascular Tumors

Carl H. Snyderman

Summary

Vascular tumors of the head and neck include both benign and malignant neoplasms. In the head and neck region, paragangliomas are the most common vascular tumors and are discussed in Chapter 19 given their involvement of the lateral cranial base. In the sinonasal region, the most common vascular tumor is the angiofibroma. Whereas paragangliomas prominently involve the temporal bone and lateral skull base, angiofibromas more commonly affect the sinonasal region and ventral skull base. Angiofibromas are the focus of this chapter and provide a good model for discussion of principles of management of all vascular tumors.[1] These include preoperative assessment of tumor vascularity, tumor staging based on vascularity, preoperative devascularization, surgical strategy including role of endoscopy, hemostatic surgical techniques, and prevention of complications. Other benign and malignant tumors that are associated with increased vascularity are also discussed.

Keywords: Endoscopic endonasal surgery, juvenile nasopharyngeal angiofibroma, embolization, ethmoidal arteries, sphenopalatine artery, sinonasal malignancy

18.1 Key Learning Points

- For vascular tumors such as angiofibroma, intraoperative bleeding is a major risk factor for complications and oncologic control.
- The University of Pittsburgh Medical Center staging system for angiofibroma incorporates tumor vascularity as a significant prognostic factor.[2]
- Angiography with embolization provides useful information regarding the vascular supply of a tumor and devascularization of the extracranial component of the vasculature.
- Large tumors can be divided into vascular territories to facilitate stepwise surgical removal.
- Intraoperative sacrifice of the ethmoidal arteries further devascularizes a tumor prior to dissection.
- Patient positioning, specialized hemostatic instruments, and warm saline irrigation are useful adjuncts in managing intraoperative hemorrhage.
- Staging of surgery is sometimes necessary with highly vascular tumors.
- Endoscopic and open approaches may be combined in a complementary fashion to optimize access and minimize morbidity.
- A team-based approach including a surgical team facilitates more effective management of highly vascular tumors.

18.2 Introduction

The sinonasal tissues naturally have a rich blood supply due to bilateral contributions of the external carotid artery (ECA) and internal carotid artery (ICA) with abundant anastomoses. Some tumor types are particularly characterized by increased vascularity and pose additional challenges. Vascular tumors of the sinonasal region may extend to the ventral skull base through direct tissue invasion or erosion and may be in close proximity to major vessels and nerves. Traditional surgical management required open approaches with wide exposure to provide necessary control of the blood supply. With advances in endovascular techniques and improved management strategies with surgical innovation, the majority of these tumors can be successfully managed using less invasive endoscopic techniques.

18.3 Vascular Challenge

Bleeding is the greatest challenge during surgery for sinonasal tumors, especially vascular tumors such as angiofibroma. Poor visualization due to bleeding obscures landmarks, increasing the odds of injury to the orbit, optic nerve, dura/brain, or a major vessel or cranial nerve. Poor visualization compromises oncologic resection, increasing the risk of positive resection margins and residual tumor. Excessive intraoperative blood loss may require transfusion of blood products and contribute to perioperative morbidity such as infection, and pulmonary and cardiac problems. There is also an increased risk of bleeding complications postoperatively due to inadequate replacement of coagulation factors. In some cases, surgery may need to be staged due to excessive blood loss.

The challenges of surgical treatment of vascular tumors are maintaining visualization during tumor dissection and minimizing intraoperative blood loss. Widespread adoption of endoscopic techniques introduces new challenges in dealing with tumor vascularity. A variety of hemostatic tools and techniques have greatly improved the ability to control intraoperative hemorrhage.

18.4 Injury Avoidance

Avoidance of bleeding complications starts with a thorough preoperative assessment. Clues to the vascularity of a tumor are often provided by the history and physical examination. A history of mild intermittent epistaxis is a common presentation for vascular sinonasal tumors such as angiofibromas or sinonasal malignancies. A history of other malignancies such as renal cell carcinoma, prostate cancer, or breast cancer raises the possibility of metastasis to the skull base. Associated nonspecific symptoms include nasal obstruction, headache, nasal discharge, loss of olfaction, epiphora, and eustachian tube dysfunction. Extension beyond the nasal cavity may result in orbital symptoms (diplopia, proptosis, and visual loss), facial hypesthesia (V_2), and trismus. Nasal endoscopy often reveals a hypervascular tumor with blood clots, but tumor may be hidden from view within the sinuses or submucosally.

A proper preoperative diagnosis is essential to avoid untoward consequences. A preoperative biopsy in an outpatient setting is not always possible due to inaccessibility of the tumor or is ill-advised due to risk of bleeding. In such cases, radiologic imaging can narrow the range of possibilities and may offer a near-definitive diagnosis. Computed tomography (CT) and magnetic resonance imaging (MRI) provide complementary information and are often obtained in concert. Brisk enhancement with contrasted CT and evidence of flow voids with MRI from large vascular channels are indicators of increased vascularity. Masses that are in proximity to a major vessel need to be considered carefully since they may represent an aneurysm or pseudoaneurysm; diagnostic biopsy is to be avoided in such situations. A CT angiogram (image guidance protocol) is often obtained in anticipation of surgery to provide precise localization of the ICA relative to the tumor.

Angiography has dual roles: confirmation of diagnosis and assessment of vascular architecture for preoperative planning. As discussed below, angiography is an important part of the staging process for angiofibromas. Angiography with embolization further provides an opportunity for devascularization of the extracranial vascular contributions to the tumor.

Neurophysiological monitoring should be employed in all cases where there is potential for vascular injury. Monitoring of cortical function with somatosensory evoked potentials provides an early warning system for global ischemia and can guide intraoperative decision-making in the event of ICA injury. Intraoperative navigation with a CT angiogram improves identification of the course of the ICA relative to the tumor. Intraoperative Doppler and indocyanine green fluoroscopy provide additional confirmation of the course of the ICA during tumor dissection.[3]

18.5 Related Pathologies

Benign vascular lesions include arteriovenous malformations, aneurysms, and pseudoaneurysms. True vascular tumors of the extracranial anterior cranial base region are rare and include both benign and malignant pathologies (▶ Table 18.1).

18.5.1 Fibro-osseous Tumors

Fibro-osseous tumors include osteoma, ossifying fibroma, and fibrous dysplasia.[4] Of these, ossifying fibroma and fibrous

Table 18.1 Vascular pathologies of the anterior cranial base

Benign	Malignant
Aneurysm/pseudoaneurysm	Adenocarcinoma
Aneurysmal bone cyst	Metastatic renal cell carcinoma
Angiofibroma	Mucosal melanoma
Arteriovenous malformation	Neuroendocrine carcinoma
Fibrous dysplasia	Olfactory neuroblastoma
Giant cell tumor	Plasmacytoma
Glomangiopericytoma	Sarcoma
Juvenile ossifying fibroma	Sinonasal undifferentiated carcinoma
Osteoblastoma	Squamous cell carcinoma
Solitary fibrous tumor	

dysplasia may be hypervascular. Juvenile ossifying fibroma (JOF) is seen in younger patients and is a locally aggressive tumor that can be quite extensive with skull base involvement and optic nerve compression (▶ Fig. 18.1). Recurrence is common in the absence of complete surgical excision.

With fibrous dysplasia, normal bone marrow and cortical bone are replaced by immature fibro-osseous tissue intermixed with woven bone (▶ Fig. 18.2). Fibrous dysplasia exists as monostotic or polyostotic forms. Patients may present with painless swelling and facial asymmetry, but it is often discovered incidentally when imaging is obtained for other reasons. Rarely, visual loss due to nerve compression occurs. Rapid growth may be observed during adolescence and may indicate cystic degeneration. Rarely, malignant transformation can occur. Surgery is performed for relief of compressive symptoms or cosmesis.

Aneurysmal bone cysts are nonneoplastic expansile bone lesions characterized by cystic cavities, usually filled with blood (▶ Fig. 18.3). They occur predominantly in children and may be associated with JOF, fibrous dysplasia, and giant cell tumors. Complete surgical excision is necessary to prevent further cystic expansion and destruction of bone.

In all of these fibro-osseous lesions, distortion of anatomy with loss of surgical landmarks in association with increased bleeding increases the risks of surgery.

18.5.2 Angiofibroma

Angiofibromas are benign highly vascular tumors arising from the basisphenoid region in proximity to the sphenopalatine foramen. They occur almost exclusively in adolescent males. Nasal obstruction and epistaxis are the most common presenting symptoms. Due to their location and nonspecific symptoms, tumors are often advanced at presentation. Tumors grow through existing foramina

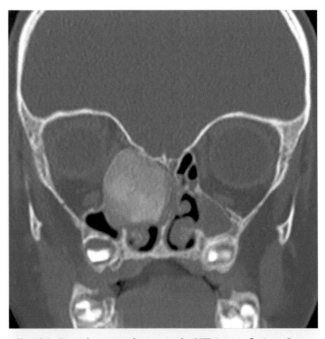

Fig. 18.1 Coronal computed tomography (CT) image of a juvenile ossifying fibroma of the right nasal cavity in a child.

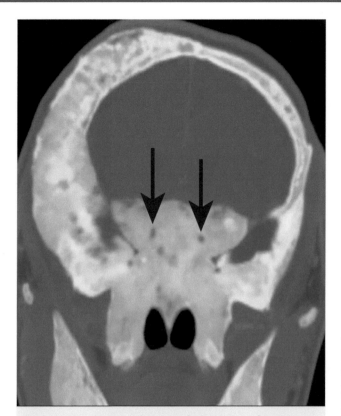

Fig. 18.2 Coronal computed tomography (CT) image of extensive fibrous dysplasia with compression of the optic canals (*arrows*).

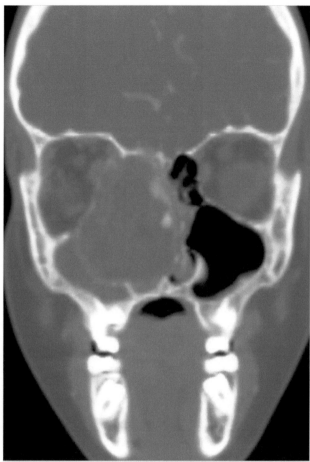

Fig. 18.3 Coronal computed tomography (CT) image of an aneurysmal bone cyst in the setting of juvenile ossifying fibroma.

and fissures to extend to the nasopharynx and paranasal sinuses, pterygopalatine space and infratemporal fossa, and the orbit and middle cranial fossa.

The vascularity of these tumors is derived from branches of both the external and internal carotid arteries. The predominant blood supply is typically from the internal maxillary artery. In large tumors, blood supply from the ICA is derived from the vidian artery in the pterygoid canal and other small branches from the cavernous ICA.

The preferred treatment for angiofibroma is complete surgical excision.[1,5,6] The greatest operative challenge with these tumors is hemorrhage due to residual vascularity. Intraoperative bleeding and proximity to the ICA increase the risk of vascular injury.

18.5.3 Glomangiopericytoma

Glomangiopericytoma is a highly vascular tumor of borderline or low malignant potential that can occur in the nasal cavity.[7] These indolent tumors should not be confused with solitary fibrous tumor, previously called hemangiopericytoma, which has greater malignant potential. Surgical excision is the treatment of choice.

18.5.4 Solitary Fibrous Tumor

Similar to glomangiopericytoma, solitary fibrous tumors are rare fibroblastic tumors that may be highly vascular.[7] Complete surgical excision is usually curative.

18.5.5 Sinonasal Malignancy

Malignancies of the sinonasal region include a wide variety of pathologies, including squamous cell carcinoma, adenocarcinoma, olfactory neuroblastoma, neuroendocrine carcinoma, sinonasal undifferentiated carcinoma, adenoid cystic carcinoma, melanoma, lymphoma, plasmacytoma, and sarcoma. Although not vascular tumors, there is risk of increased bleeding due to their invasive nature, friability, and proximity to major vessels. Intraoperative blood loss is understandably greater with advanced stage tumors.

18.5.6 Metastasis

Metastatic tumors to the nasal cavity and sinuses include tumors that metastasize to bone such as cancers of the prostate, thyroid, breast, and kidney.[8] In particular, metastatic renal cell carcinoma is notorious for its hypervascularity. Metastasis to the sinonasal cavity may be the first presentation. When surgery is considered, preoperative embolization may help minimize blood loss.

18.6 Case Examples

18.6.1 Angiofibroma

A 14-year-old boy presented with complaints of left nasal congestion and left hearing loss. Visual acuity was 20/40 OS and 20/20 OD. He had no complaints of diplopia, facial hypesthesia, or trismus. Physical examination including nasal endoscopy revealed an obstructive left nasal mass with displacement of the nasal septum to the contralateral side (▸ Fig. 18.4). CT and MRI revealed an obstructive tumor filling the left nasal cavity/nasopharynx, and sphenoid sinus with extension to the masticator space and middle cranial fossa (▸ Fig. 18.5). Based on the presentation, endoscopic appearance, and radiographic appearance, a presumptive diagnosis of angiofibroma was made.

Angiography demonstrated blood supply from the right ECA and ICA (cavernous segment) and the left ECA and ICA (cavernous and petrous segments). Following embolization of the ECA branches with Onyx, the tumor blush was reduced by approximately 50% (▸ Fig. 18.6). Based on residual vascularity, tumor extent, and route of spread, the tumor was staged UPMC stage V-L (▸ Table 18.2).

For surgical planning, the tumor was divided into vascular territories: nasal cavity, sphenoid sinus, masticator space, and middle fossa (▸ Fig. 18.7). The extracranial segments without ICA proximity were addressed first, followed by the portion of the tumor receiving feeders from the ICA. If bleeding was not excessive, the intracranial (middle cranial fossa) portion of the tumor would be resected; otherwise, the surgery would be staged.

An endoscopic right spheno-ethmoidectomy with resection of the posterior nasal septum was first performed to establish a nasal corridor lateral to the tumor and mobilize the sphenoid portion of the tumor. Vascular contributions from the right ICA (vidian artery) were controlled with bipolar electrocautery (▸ Fig. 18.8). At this stage, it is best to avoid transecting the tumor until it is fully mobilized around its periphery. The intranasal portion of the

tumor on the left side was mobilized as much as possible. This includes an ethmoidectomy superior to the tumor and a medial maxillectomy for full access to the maxillary component.

A left Caldwell-Luc approach (anterior maxillotomy) was performed next to provide access to the lateral extent of the tumor including the middle and infratemporal fossae. The medial maxillectomy was completed and the central compartment of tumor (nasal cavity and sphenoid sinus) was further mobilized from the skull base and sphenoid sinus and amputated with the Harmonic scalpel (Ethicon, Raritan, New Jersey, USA). The nasopharyngeal mucosa was incised with electrocautery to release the inferior attachment of the tumor. Large segments of tumor can be extracted through the oral cavity.

The infraorbital nerve was identified and dissected free from the superior surface of the tumor. Remodeled bone of the posterior maxilla was removed, and the periosteum and soft tissues of the pterygopalatine fossa were dissected in a medial to lateral direction to expose the surface of the tumor. If possible, the descending palatine branch of the maxillary nerve (second division of trigeminal nerve) is preserved; it is typically stretched over the surface of the tumor. The extracranial portion of the tumor in the masticator space was carefully mobilized from the pterygoid muscles. Lobules of tumor posterior to the hard palate can be delivered into the surgical field using a bimanual technique of pulling on the tumor endoscopically while pushing on the palatal mucosa posterior to the maxillary tuberosity intraorally. This portion of the tumor was then detached from the remaining segments using a Harmonic scalpel or bipolar electrocautery. Tumor was followed back to the

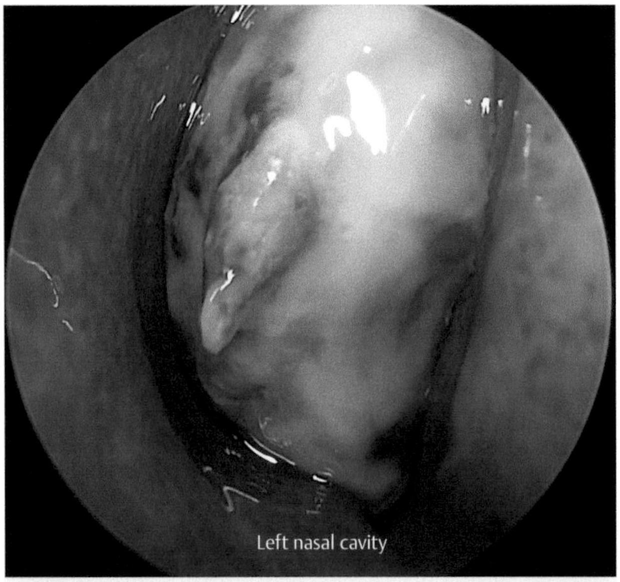

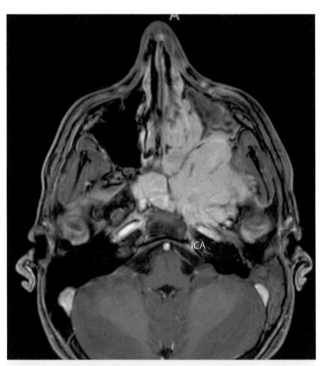

Fig. 18.5 Axial magnetic resonance imaging (MRI) demonstrates an extensive angiofibroma filling the left nasal cavity/nasopharynx, and sphenoid sinus with extension to the masticator space and middle cranial fossa. Note the proximity of the tumor to the petrous segment of the internal carotid artery.

Left nasal cavity

Fig. 18.4 Endoscopic view of angiofibroma obstructing the left nasal cavity.

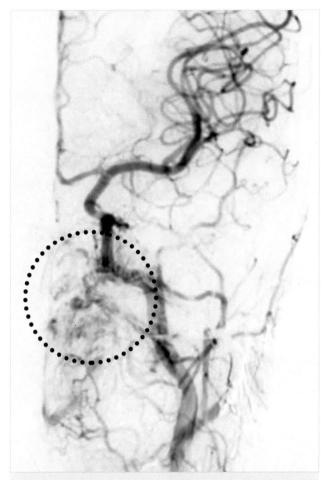

Fig. 18.6 Residual vascularity from the left internal carotid artery (ICA) (*dotted circle*) is seen following embolization of the external carotid artery (ECA) supply.

Table 18.2 UPMC staging system for angiofibroma

Stage I	Nasal cavity, medial PPF
Stage II	≥1 sinus, lateral PPF; no residual vascularity*
Stage III	Skull base erosion, orbit, ITF; no residual vascularity*
Stage IV	Skull base erosion, orbit, ITF; residual vascularity*
Stage V	Intracranial extension, residual vascularity*; M: medial extension; L: lateral extension

Abbreviations: ITF, infratemporal fossa; PPF: pterygopalatine fossa.
Note: *From internal carotid artery (ICA) after embolization of external carotid artery (ECA) supply.

18.6.2 Chondrosarcoma

A 65-year-old female presented with complete nasal obstruction of 7 months duration and recent periorbital swelling. Examination including nasal endoscopy revealed a large obstructive mass with displacement of the anterior nasal septum to the left side. Bilateral dacryocystitis with expansion of the nasal dorsum was present (▶ Fig. 18.10). Biopsy demonstrated cartilaginous tissue consistent with a chondrosarcoma. CT and MRI demonstrated a large expansile mass with displacement of the medial maxilla and orbits bilaterally with obstruction of the paranasal sinuses (▶ Fig. 18.11).

A bilateral endoscopic endonasal approach with medial maxillectomies, Draf 3 frontal sinusotomy, and sphenoidotomies was performed with piecemeal removal of the entire tumor. Hemostasis was achieved intraoperatively using reverse Trendelenburg position, Aquamantys (Medtronic, Dublin, Ireland) device in addition to other endoscopic bipolar electrocautery devices (KARL STORZ Endoscopy-America, Inc., El Segundo, CA; Sutter Medical Technologies USA, Atlanta, GA), application of Surgiflo, and warm saline irrigation. The lacrimal sac infections were drained and stented. Estimated blood loss was 1,500 cc and she received one unit of blood. Final pathology confirmed a low-grade chondrosarcoma.

18.7 Management Strategy

There are a variety of staging systems that have been proposed for the staging of angiofibromas.[2,10] The UPMC staging system is the only one that incorporates the vascularity of the tumor as a criterion (▶ Table 18.2). It has been shown to provide the strongest correlation with intraoperative blood loss and the risk of residual/recurrent disease for angiofibromas. Early-stage tumors (I and II) are readily managed using endoscopic techniques (▶ Fig. 18.12). Preoperative embolization is optional for these cases, depending on availability. Stage III tumors may be quite extensive but have no appreciable blood supply from the ICA and can be effectively devascularized with preoperative embolization of the ECA blood supply (▶ Fig. 18.13). These tumors are extracranial and there is little risk to the ICA. Stage IV and V tumors are extensive tumors with significant residual vascularity from the ICA following embolization of the ECA (▶ Fig. 18.14). Despite skull base erosion, there is typically a good plane of dissection. Stage V tumors are further characterized based on their route of intracranial extension: *medial* to the ICA (anterior cranial fossa, medial cavernous sinus compartments); *lateral* to the ICA (inferior orbital fissure, Meckel's cave, lateral cavernous sinus, middle cranial fossa). The route of extension dictates the surgical approach: a midline approach for

base of pterygoid and the vidian artery and other feeders from the ICA were cauterized. The base of pterygoid was drilled to remove all remnants of tumor invading the bony spaces. Adequate hemostasis is obtained after each vascular unit is resected with a combination of bipolar electrocautery, application of absorbable morselized gelatin sponge (Floseal [Baxter, Deerfield, IL], Surgiflo® [Johnson & Johnson, New Brunswick, NJ], Surgifoam [Johnson & Johnson, New Brunswick, NJ]), and warm saline irrigation.[9]

A decision was made to stage the surgery due to the amount of blood loss; tumor remained around the paraclival ICA and middle cranial fossa. The second-stage surgery was performed 5 days later, combining an endoscopic endonasal/transmaxillary approach with a left lateral orbitotomy to access extradural tumor of the middle cranial fossa. This provided a better window for extradural dissection and drilling of tumor-involved bone of the middle fossa floor, lateral to the orbital apex. Reconstruction consisted of coverage of the exposed dura with a fat graft.

Postoperatively, the patient had intact vision and extraocular motility. Hypesthesia of the left maxillary nerve was present as expected. Motor function of the mandibular nerve was intact, and the patient was discharged on postoperative day 2. Postoperative MRI confirmed complete removal of tumor (▶ Fig. 18.9).

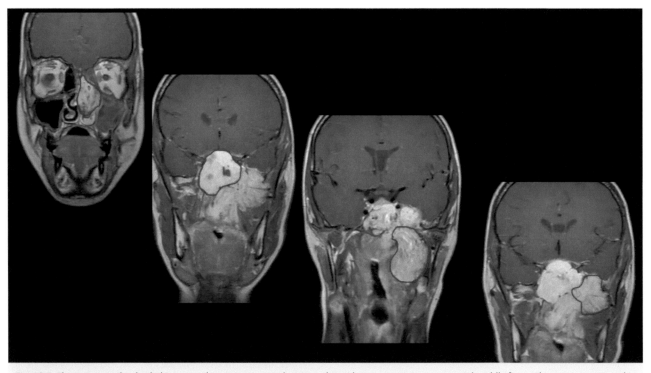

Fig. 18.7 The tumor can be divided into vascular territories: nasal cavity, sphenoid sinus, masticator space, and middle fossa. The tumor is removed in these vascular units to limit hemorrhage and optimize visualization of key anatomical areas.

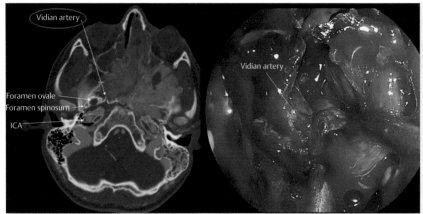

Fig. 18.8 Axial view of computed tomography (CT) angiogram and intraoperative endoscopic image showing tumor relationship to the major internal carotid artery (ICA) supply via the vidian artery. Early identification and cauterization of major feeders (vidian artery) from the ICA help devascularize the tumor.

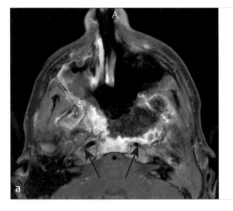

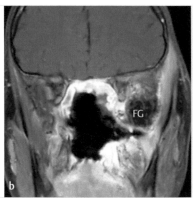

Fig. 18.9 Early postoperative magnetic resonance imaging (MRI) demonstrates complete removal of the tumor on axial (a) and coronal (b) views. *Arrows*, internal carotid arteries (ICAs); FG, fat graft.

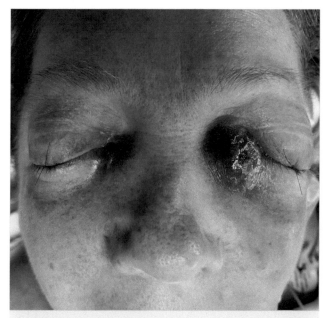

Fig. 18.10 Bilateral dacryocystitis with expansion of the nasal dorsum was present.

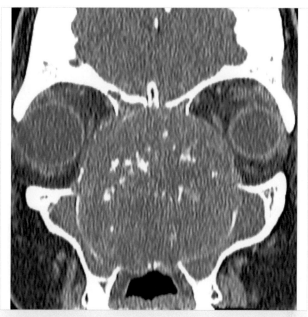

Fig. 18.11 Computed tomography (CT) demonstrating a large, expansile mass with displacement of the medial maxilla and orbits bilaterally with obstruction of the paranasal sinuses. Biopsy showed a chondrosarcoma (nasal septal origin) which underwent complete resection via endoscopic endonasal approach (EEA).

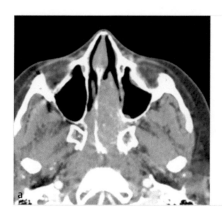 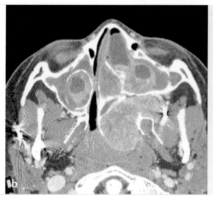

Fig. 18.12 UPMC stage I (a) and stage II (b) tumors have limited extension.

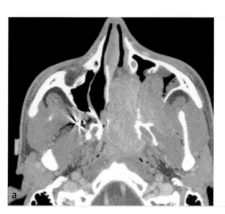 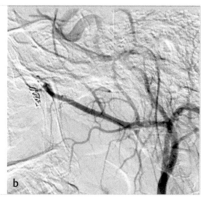

Fig. 18.13 UPMC stage III tumors are advanced (a) but lack residual vascularity from the internal carotid artery (ICA) following embolization of external carotid artery (ECA) supply (b).

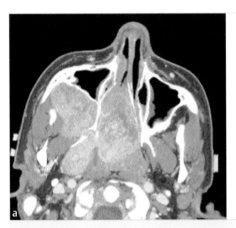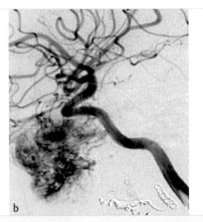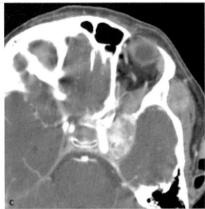

Fig. 18.14 UPMC stage IV (a) and stage V (b) tumors are advanced and have significant residual vascularity from the internal carotid artery (ICA) (c).

medial routes of extension and a midline approach in combination with a paramedian or lateral approach for lateral extension.

The goal of surgery is complete surgical excision in one surgical episode with the least morbidity for the patient. This is best accomplished with a surgical team with one surgeon providing endoscopic visualization, thus allowing a second surgeon to perform bimanual dissection. Bimanual dissection is necessary for visualization in the presence of hemorrhage and manipulation of tumor. Ideally, the surgical team consists of an otolaryngologist for sinus exposure and endoscopy and a neurosurgeon to manage neural and arterial dissection and potential complications. With an experienced endoscopic skull base team, even the most advanced stage tumors can be managed using less invasive endoscopic techniques. Larger tumors that extend laterally require a transmaxillary approach for introduction of endoscopic instruments. Rarely, a lateral infratemporal skull base approach with zygomatic osteotomy is necessary to dissect the lateral margin of the tumor. A lateral orbitotomy can be used to supplement an endoscopic approach for tumors that involve bone lateral to the orbital apex (**Video 18.1**).

Advanced stage tumors with residual vascularity may require staging of surgery to achieve a complete resection with acceptable blood loss. Tumors can be segmented based on their vascular supply: laterality and extracranial/intracranial. Generally, the extracranial components are addressed first. If blood loss is acceptable (<50% total blood volume), dissection of the skull base/intracranial components can proceed. Otherwise, it is advantageous to stage the surgery and avoid complications related to coagulopathy or transfusion reaction. A second-stage surgery can be performed when the patient is hemodynamically stable, typically within 1 to 2 weeks.

18.8 Potential Complications

The greatest risks of surgery are those related to excessive bleeding. Risks of excessive hemorrhage include poor visualization with injury to the orbit, optic nerve, ICA, divisions of the trigeminal nerve, or dura. Poor visualization during dissection of feeders from the ICA increases the risk of ICA injury. Excessive intraoperative bleeding with multiple transfusions may result in a coagulopathy if clotting factors are not adequately replaced. This can make it difficult to achieve hemostasis when dissecting the most critical areas of the tumor. Large volume transfusions increase the risk of a transfusion reaction and associated pulmonary complications.

In angiofibromas, injury to the descending palatine branch of the maxillary division of the trigeminal nerve is often not avoidable due to stretching of the nerve over the maxillary portion of the tumor. This results in ipsilateral palatal numbness. The vidian nerve must be sacrificed to remove all remnants of tumor in the pterygoid base, resulting in the loss of ipsilateral emotional tearing. This could result in a dry eye in susceptible individuals but is usually well tolerated in younger patients.

18.9 Management Algorithm

Intraoperative management of extracranial vascular tumors builds on preoperative devascularization of the tumor provided by embolization of the ECA blood supply. Intraoperatively, further devascularization prior to dissection of the tumor can be achieved with ligation of other contributing vessels. The anterior and posterior ethmoidal arteries are branches of the ophthalmic arteries and are not accessible for preoperative embolization without risk of vision loss. External ligation of the vessels can be performed using a small incision between the nasal dorsum and medial canthus. Alternatively, they can be cauterized or ligated endonasally at the junction of the orbital roof and ethmoid sinus. For sinonasal malignancies that involve the anterior cranial base, this provides early devascularization and significantly limits bleeding. Vascular tumors can also be directly injected with an embolization material such as Onyx intraoperatively (see Chapter 3). This should be done with great caution, however, since there is risk of intracranial embolization through collateral anastomoses and should be done under fluoroscopic control.

Bleeding from the surface of vascular tumors requires the use of bipolar electrocautery. Endoscopic bipolars are a necessity for endoscopic surgery. Augmentation of the endonasal approach with a transmaxillary approach provides additional room for standard bayonet bipolars which can be more effective. For transection of large firm tumors such as angiofibromas, the Harmonic scalpel (Ethicon, Johnson & Johnson, New Brunswick, NJ) and Coblator (Smith & Nephew, London, UK) have both been used successfully.[1] For softer tumors such as a sinonasal malignancy, a fixed-distance irrigating bipolar such as the Aquamantys (Medtronic) is useful for debulking of tumor tissue or broad stroke coagulation prior to resection of tumor margins. Venous bleeding can be controlled with direct application of hemostatic materials such as Floseal (Baxter) and Surgiflo® (Ethicon). This is applied with a Frazier-tip suction with closed side port (KLS Martin, Jacksonville, FL). It is essential that arterial bleeding be differentiated from venous bleeding to avoid inadvertent arterial embolization. Additional measures that reduce venous bleeding include elevation of the head of bed (15–20 degrees) and warm saline irrigation (40 °C).[11] Systemic agents such as tranexamic acid (TXA), an antifibrinolytic agent, can be given prior to the onset of blood loss to lower blood loss[11] and transfusion rates.

"Time is blood loss" in sinonasal surgery. The longer it takes to remove a tumor, the greater the blood loss. Surgical efficiency is markedly improved with team surgery, two surgeons working simultaneously, with one surgeon driving the endoscope while the other has two hands free for tumor dissection. This allows constant suctioning with better visualization while dissecting the tumor. In addition, wide exposure of all aspects of the tumor prior to dissection allows for maximal control and freedom of movement.

18.10 Root Cause Analysis

A root cause analysis (RCA) provides useful information regarding the myriad potential factors that may contribute to an outcome (▶ Fig. 18.15). Standard categories of an RCA include

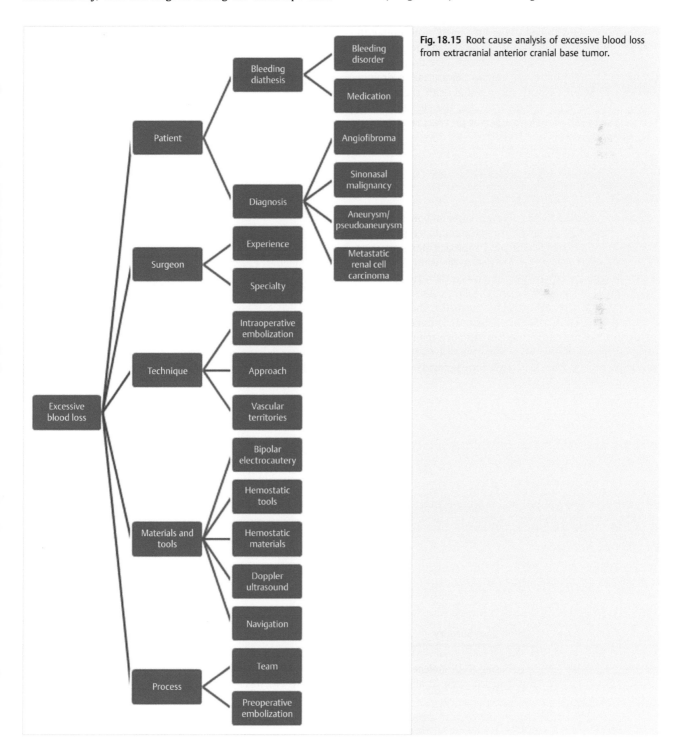

Fig. 18.15 Root cause analysis of excessive blood loss from extracranial anterior cranial base tumor.

patient, surgeon, technique, materials, and process. An RCA can be used for post-hoc analysis of a complication or undesirable outcome as part of a quality improvement program. A generic RCA can also be used prospectively as a checklist to identify potential risk factors and develop a prevention strategy.

18.11 Conclusion

With proper diagnosis and preparation, vascular tumors of the extracranial skull base can be managed effectively, often with endoscopic surgical techniques. Risk of hemorrhage can be anticipated based on the histology and staging of the tumor. Preoperative embolization, intraoperative devascularization in conjunction with hemostatic tools and materials, and team surgery all contribute to hemostasis.

References

[1] Snyderman CH, Pant H. Endoscopic management of vascular sinonasal tumors, including angiofibroma. Otolaryngol Clin North Am. 2016; 49(3):791–807

[2] Snyderman CH, Pant H, Carrau RL, Gardner P. A new endoscopic staging system for angiofibromas. Arch Otolaryngol Head Neck Surg. 2010; 136(6):588–594

[3] Geltzeiler M, Igami Nakassa AC, Setty P, et al. Evaluation of intranasal flap perfusion by intraoperative ICG fluorescence angiography. J Neurol Surg B Skull Base. 2017; 78 S1:S62

[4] Wilson M, Snyderman C. Fibro-osseous lesions of the skull base in the pediatric population. J Neurol Surg B Skull Base. 2018; 79(1):31–36

[5] López F, Triantafyllou A, Snyderman CH, et al. Nasal juvenile angiofibroma: current perspectives with emphasis on management. Head Neck. 2017; 39 (5):1033–1045

[6] Wang EW, Zanation AM, Gardner PA, et al. ICAR: endoscopic skull-base surgery. Int Forum Allergy Rhinol. 2019; 9 S3:S145–S365

[7] Thompson LDR, Flucke U, Wenig BM. Sinonasal glomangiopericytoma. In: El-Naggar AK, Chan JKC, Grandis JR, Takata T, Slootweg PJ, eds. WHO Classification of Head and Neck Tumours. 4th ed. Lyon, France: International Agency for Research on Cancer; 2017:44–45

[8] López F, Devaney KO, Hanna EY, Rinaldo A, F, erlito A. Metastases to nasal cavity and paranasal sinuses. Head Neck. 2016; 38(12):1847–1854

[9] Gan EC, Alsaleh S, Manji J, Habib AR, Amanian A, Javer AR. Hemostatic effect of hot saline irrigation during functional endoscopic sinus surgery: a randomized controlled trial. Int Forum Allergy Rhinol. 2014; 4(11): 877–884

[10] Rowan NR, Zwagerman NT, Heft-Neal ME, Gardner PA, Snyderman CH. Juvenile nasal angiofibromas: a comparison of modern staging systems in an endoscopic era. J Neurol Surg B Skull Base. 2017; 78(1):63–67

[11] Mebel D, Akagami R, Flexman AM. Use of tranexamic acid is associated with reduced blood product transfusion in complex skull base neurosurgical procedures: a retrospective cohort study. Anesth Analg. 2016; 122(2):503–508

19 Extracranial Lateral Cranial Base Vascular Tumor Surgery

Sampath Chandra Prasad Rao and Ananth Chintapalli

Summary

The chapter deals with the pathophysiology, anatomy, diagnostic workup, and intraoperative management of the extracranial vascular lesions of the lateral skull base. It focuses on the preoperative assessment of these tumors particularly involving the petrous internal carotid artery and makes an effort in providing valuable inputs to the reader in this regard.

Keywords: Vascular lesions of the head and neck, extracranial skull base vascular tumors, paragangliomas of the skull base

19.1 Key Learning Points

- Vascular lesions of the skull base, both benign and malignant need a thorough preoperative evaluation and meticulous workup.
- Paragangliomas are the most common extracranial skull base vascular tumors.
- Preoperative and intraoperative management of the petrous internal carotid artery is crucial in surgical excision of these tumors.
- A methodical classification of these tumors based on their extent and their relation to the adjacent anatomical structures is quintessential for surgical intervention of these tumors.

19.2 Introduction

Vascular tumors of the lateral skull base practically are divided into benign and malignant vascular tumors. Benign tumors include the more common paragangliomas and less common hemangiomas occurring in and around the temporal bone. The malignant group of vascular tumors in these areas are further grouped according to their malignant potential. Kaposi's sarcoma and hemangioendothelioma are of intermediate malignant potential, while angiosarcoma and hemangiopericytoma are more malignant variants. The paragangliomas (of the head and neck), the most common of vascular tumors involving the lateral skull base area, shall be discussed in greater detail than the other lesions mentioned above, which will be touched upon in brief.

19.3 Paragangliomas of the Head and Neck

Paragangliomas are predominantly nonsecreting tumors arising within the head and neck from aggregates of paraganglionic tissue, which are derivatives of the neural crest. The largest aggregation of this tissue in the head and neck is concentrated in the carotid body on the medial aspect of the carotid bifurcation. The remaining is within the confines of the temporal bone, approximately more than half of which is distributed in the adventitia of the jugular bulb, around the Jacobson's nerve, within the inferior tympanic canaliculus and over the promontory. The rest of this tissue is spread along the course of the Arnold's nerve and around the mastoid segment of the facial nerve on some occasions.

Clinically, head and neck paragangliomas are broadly classified as temporal bone paragangliomas and cervico-carotid paragangliomas. The former includes the tympanomastoid and the tympanojugular proper paragangliomas, the most common tumors of the middle ear and temporal bone, respectively. The cervico-carotid paragangliomas encompass carotid body paragangliomas and vagal paragangliomas. Paragangliomas of the head and neck make up about 3% of all paragangliomas occurring in the body with carotid body tumors accounting for 60% and their vagal counterpart less than 5% of them.[1,2,3,4,5,6,7] Paragangliomas have been reported to be both sporadic and familial and a germline defect in the succinate dehydrogenase complex has been implicated in a considerable proportion of these tumors.[8,9,10] Multicentricity has been reported to occur in about 5 to 20% of sporadic cases and as high as 80% in familial cases, with the most common being bilateral carotid body tumors followed by carotid and vagal paraganglioma.[8]

Despite being very slow growing tumors, skull base paragangliomas are aggressive with propensity to invade adjacent critical neurovascular structures and their slow growth rate often makes these tumors virtually impossible to detect early in their course. However, tympanomastoid paragangliomas present at an early stage with hearing impairment and/or pulsatile tinnitus. Tympanojugular paragangliomas, on the other hand, are not detected until they attain considerable size and quite often follow the path of least resistance into the middle ear cleft and other compartments of the temporal bone through the air cell tracts to involve the mastoid and petrous bone and not uncommonly, the cervico-petrous internal carotid artery (ICA), internal jugular vein (IJV), and in later stages, extend intracranially. Intracranial invasion of the paraganglioma occurs through the medial wall of the jugular foramen and in time along the inferior petrosal sinus. The involvement of the lower cranial nerves usually occurs at a very late stage after the tumor invades the medial wall of the jugular foramen, which acts as a barrier between the two and it is not very uncommon to come across cases with extensive tumors without lower cranial nerve palsy.[2,4,11,12,13,14] Characteristic bone erosion from ischemic necrosis is often extensive and underestimated. The cancellous portions of the temporal bone are extensively infiltrated, but the dense lamellar bone of the labyrinth is more likely to be spared.

This chapter focusses on temporal bone paragangliomas (tympanomastoid and tympanojugular proper paragangliomas) in greater detail from a surgical perspective and the carotid body tumor and vagal paraganglioma to a brief extent.

Classification: Tympanojugular paragangliomas, understood as tympanojugular proper and tympanomastoid categories, have been subjected to classification systems by several authors for better characterization of these tumors. Nonetheless, most of these classifications lacked a comprehensive understanding of these tumors from the surgical management standpoint. Glasscock and Jackson's classification[15] is based on the extent of the tumor alone. The De La Cruz classification system[16] makes a broad attempt to devise surgical approaches but lacks the description of finer details of tumor extension. The Ugo Fisch classification[17] categorizes the tumor according to its extension and location based on the computed tomography (CT) examination. Modification of Fisch classification by Sanna et al[18] provides further insight on temporal bone paragangliomas and allows precise surgical planning. Authors of this chapter adopt the modified Fisch classification system for all practical purposes.

Class A tumors are those which arise from the tympanic plexus over the promontory and are limited to the tympanic cavity without any extension into the hypotympanum. Modified Fisch classification further classifies these tumors into A1 and A2 based on their extent within the tympanic cavity. Class A1 tumors are small, well-defined tumors within the confinements of the mesotympanum, with all the tumor margins visible on otoscopy. Class A2 tumors are those which are confined to the tympanomastoid compartment of the temporal bone, completely involving the mesotympanum and the ossicles, and show a certain degree of extension beyond the tympanic annulus. The margins of A2 tumors are not entirely visible on otoscopy. Class A2 tumors may extend anteriorly into the eustachian tube or into the posterior mesotympanum and should always be thoroughly examined by imaging preoperatively considering the fact that their margins are obscured on otoscopy so as to differentiate them from tympanojugular proper tumors.

Class B tympanojugular paragangliomas limit themselves to the tympanomastoid compartment of the temporal bone, and do not breach the bony dome of the jugular bulb. They are categorized further by modified Fisch classification system into three types: Class B1 tumors are those which encroach the hypotympanum; Class B2 tumors involve the hypotympanum and the mastoid compartment of the temporal bone; Class B3 tympanomastoid paraganglioma is any tumor which involves the tympanomastoid compartment with erosion of the carotid canal. The more extensive B2 and B3 tumors show considerable encroachment into the external auditory canal and give a clinical picture of a polyp arising from the middle ear and taking a biopsy is never advised.

Class C tympanojugular paragangliomas are extensive tumors with involvement of the cervico-petrous ICA. This class of tumors arises from the paraganglionic tissue concentrated over the jugular bulb or within the inferior tympanic or mastoid canaliculi. Because of their location, this class of tumors poses a unique challenge in their management. Class C1 tumors destroy the anatomical integrity of the jugular bulb with limited involvement of the vertical portion of the carotid canal and rarely infiltrates the ICA. Class C2 tumors show a greater degree of destruction by invading the vertical portion of the carotid canal. Class C3 tumors invade the horizontal portion of the cervico-petrous carotid, and C4 paragangliomas reach up to the anterior foramen lacerum. All the class C tympanojugular paragangliomas, more so particularly C2 through C4, have the propensity of encasing the cervico-petrous carotid, a crucial aspect in surgical planning. Class C tumors also show varied degree of intracranial extension. The tympanojugular proper subset of paragangliomas spread to various adjacent compartments: intradural when the spread of the tumor is more medial; into the petrous compartment and the infratemporal fossa regions of the skull base when the tumor spread is anterior; into the upper cervical compartments along the course of the lower cranial nerves when they spread inferiorly; posteriorly along the sigmoid sinus and toward the occipital condyle and the vertebral artery when they spread posteroinferiorly. Class C tumors show varied degree of intracranial extension and are described accordingly along with Class D as described in the (▶ Table 19.1).

Table 19.1 Modified Fisch classification system for temporal bone paragangliomas

Class	Description
A	Tumors limited to the middle ear cleft without invasion of the hypotympanum
	• A1 Tumor completely visible on otoscopic examination
	• A2 Tumor margins not seen on otoscopy
B	Limited to the hypotympanum, mesotympanum and mastoid without erosion of the jugular bulb
	• B1 Confined to the middle ear cleft with extension into the hypotympanum
	• B2 Involving the middle ear cleft with extension to the hypotympanum and the mastoid
	• B3 Tumors confined to the tympanomastoid compartment with erosion of the carotid canal
C	Tympanojugular paraganglioma subclassification by the degree of carotid canal erosion
	• C1 Tumors destroying the jugular foramen and bulb with limited involvement of vertical portion of the carotid canal
	• C2 Tumors invading the vertical portion of the carotid canal
	• C3 Tumors invading the horizontal portion of the carotid canal
	• C4 Tumors reaching the anterior foramen lacerum
D	Defines only the intracranial tumor extension and should be reported as an addendum to the stage C. De, extradural; Di, intradural
	• De1 Tumors up to 2cm dural displacement
	• De2 Tumors with more than 2cm dural displacement
	• Di1 Tumors with up to 2cm intradural extension
	• Di2 Tumors with more than 2cm intradural extension
	• Di3 Tumors with inoperable intracranial intradural extension

19.4 Tympanomastoid Paragangliomas

The tympanomastoid paragangliomas, which correspond to the Fisch type A and type B classification, are tumors arising within the tympanomastoid compartment; they are relatively less common when compared to their tympanojugular proper counterparts. These tumors present typically with conductive hearing loss due to disruption of the middle ear conductive mechanism and are accompanied by pulsatile tinnitus. Clinically, the otoscopic findings are a red retrotympanic mass which blanches on pneumatic otoscopy (Brown's sign) at times, with perceivable pulsations.[19,20,21,22] Tympanomastoid paragangliomas are less aggressive than their counterparts arising within the jugular foramen. Seldomly, they present as a mass in the external auditory canal mimicking a polyp arising from the middle ear. Their extensions are often into the eustachian tube and though not common, direct involvement of the carotid can occur when the tumor extension is inferior toward the jugular bulb.

The tympanojugular proper paragangliomas, the class C tumors, present much later in their course, with the tumor having extended into the middle ear cleft after eroding the floor of the hypotympanum. Such clinical presentation in very advanced stages is attributed to their site of origin. They most commonly present with hearing impairment which is conductive type due to impingement of the tumor on the middle ear ossicles and with pulsatile tinnitus.[6,23,24,25,26,27,28,29,30,31,32] Though not very common, sensorineural type of hearing loss and vestibular symptoms depend on the extension of the tumor into the inner ear, internal auditory meatus, and the cerebellopontine angle. Lower cranial neuropathies develop very late in the course of the disease, as the extremely slow growth rate of the tumor allows progressive compensation, but when manifested denote the involvement of the medial wall of the jugular foramen, which essentially acts as an anatomical barrier between the tumor and these nerves. Glossopharyngeal and vagal palsies are more common followed by those of spinal accessory and the hypoglossal nerves and it is prudent to consider jugular foramen pathology when encountered with a compound lower cranial nerve palsy.[33,34,35,36] The facial nerve is by far the most common cranial nerve to be involved in extensive tympanojugular paragangliomas.

19.4.1 Preoperative Assessment

A comprehensive preoperative radiological assessment complemented with a well-planned surgery plays the most crucial role in effective management of these tumors. This includes high-resolution CT (HRCT) with reconstructions in the axial and coronal planes. In suspected cases with extension into the hypotympanum and in revision cases, T1- and T2-weighted images along with T1-weighted gadolinium-enhanced sequences with axial, coronal, and sagittal plane reconstruction are desired. Magnetic resonance angiography (MRA) and MR venography are additionally required to assess involvement of major vessels.[37] A thorough preoperative radiological evaluation not only gives insight of the extension and the size of the tumor, but also elucidates the intricacies of temporal bone invasion.

Class A tumors, as described earlier, arise from the tympanic plexus over the promontory and are limited to the tympanic cavity without any extension into the hypotympanum. Modified Fisch classification further classifies these tumors into A1 and A2 based on their extent within the tympanic cavity. Class A1 tumors are small, well-defined tumors confined to the mesotympanum, with all its margins visible on otoscopy. Class A2 tumors are those which are confined to the tympanomastoid compartment of the temporal bone, completely involving the mesotympanum, the ossicles, and show a certain degree of extension beyond the tympanic annulus; thus, the margins of the tumor not entirely visible on otoscopy. Class A2 tumors may extend anteriorly into the eustachian tube or into the posterior mesotympanum. These tumors should always be thoroughly examined by imaging preoperatively considering the fact that their margins are obscured on otoscopy so as to differentiate them from glomus jugulare tumors. Class A tumors on HRCT typically appear as small masses over the promontory without significant extension into the hypotympanum.

Class B tumors are those set of tumors which limit themselves to the confines of tympanomastoid compartment of temporal bone, but essentially do not breach the bony dome of the jugular bulb. They are categorized further by modified Fisch classification system into three types: Class B1 tumors are those which encroach upon the hypotympanum. Class B2 tumors involve the hypotympanum and the mastoid compartment of the temporal bone. Class B3 is any tumor involving the

tympanomastoid compartment with erosion of the carotid canal. The more extensive B2 and B3 tumors show considerable extension into the external auditory canal and give a clinical picture of a polyp arising from the middle ear and any attempt of biopsy is not advised.[38] HRCT confirms the findings of the tumor extension and no other imaging is mandatory once the integrity of the bone over the jugular bulb is confirmed. Nevertheless, it is essential to assess the extension of the tumor within the confinements of the temporal bone. Magnetic resonance imaging (MRI) differentiates the tumor from the middle ear effusions.

The degree of bone extension is crucial, particularly around the vital structures like the facial nerve, and oval and round windows. The degree of involvement is sometimes difficult to assess on HRCT; in a poorly pneumatized temporal bone with disease extending into its petrous apex, these areas of the skull base are often filled with marrow. MRI in such cases offers information regarding the bone marrow spaces in these areas and is very helpful in differentiating tumor from middle ear and mastoid effusions. Angiography is required for revision surgeries and extensive cases of class B tumors, B3 in particular which erode the carotid canal. In cases with suspected involvement of the sigmoid sinus, MR venogram offers vital information.

19.4.2 Surgical Approach

The management of the temporal bone paragangliomas continues to be a challenge despite several radiological and surgical advancements. Although paragangliomas are histologically benign, they are locally aggressive with extensive invasion of the bone and the soft tissue. With an initial innocuous growth pattern, their early diagnosis is often missed. The literature has rather little to offer regarding the fundamental aspects of these tumors such as their classification and protocols for surgical approaches. Thus, it really does not come as a surprise that the treatment of skull base paragangliomas in particular is yet to be standardized and there is still ambiguity on whether surgery, radiation, or simply observation is the best approach.

Nevertheless, surgical excision of the tumor offers a better treatment modality than radiotherapy. It is now well accepted that radiotherapy is not recommended at least for the cure of paragangliomas limited to the tympanomastoid compartment (classes A and B) but only in cases of recurrence and as a second option to the patient.[19,39] The selection of the optimal surgical approach mainly depends on the location, extension of the tumor, and the neurovascular structures involved by the tumor. The primary goals of surgery for class A and B tumors are complete disease clearance and hearing preservation. It was rather impractical in the past to achieve this twin objective and it was either a radical surgery for complete disease clearance or radiotherapy to preserve hearing, but with the latest advances in imaging and surgical equipment, it is now practically possible to preserve serviceable hearing while completely clearing the disease. It is now apparent, with substantial clinical evidence, that all tumors from classes A1 to B2 show good audiometric improvements in air conduction, the air-bone gap, and bone conduction postoperatively when a proper surgical technique is employed, the results which cannot be mimicked by radiotherapy.[40] Class B3 tumors, considering their extensiveness, require a more radical approach. This chapter unveils our perspective in managing these tumors from a surgical point of view.

19.4.3 Class A Tumors

Class A1 Tumors

For class A1 tumors which are very limited, with clear margins, and confined to the promontory, the approach is ideally transmeatal as for a stapes surgery. An aural speculum of optimal size is inserted into the external auditory canal and a tympanomeatal flap is raised as crafted for a stapes surgery. Canalplasty is done if deemed necessary. The tumor removal is essentially by coagulating its surface with bipolar electrocautery followed by blunt dissection using Surgicel (Johnson & Johnson, New Brunswick, NJ). The dissection ideally begins from the anterior margin of the tumor, away from more critical structures like the incudostapedial joint and round window area. It is recommended to flush the surgical field over the promontory periodically with cool saline to avoid thermal insult to the cochlea. The main feeding vessel of the tumor, the inferior tympanic artery from within the inferior tympanic canaliculus, is cauterized and the remaining tumor is dissected. The middle ear space is packed with Gelfoam (Pfizer, New York, NY) or with an adequately sized silastic sheet to prevent adhesions between the raw middle ear surface and the tympanic membrane.

Class A2 Tumors

For class A2 tumors, whose margins extend beyond the tympanic annulus, it is vital to preoperatively assess the inferior extent of the tumor in the hypotympanum radiologically and to be certain about the integrity of the dome of the jugular bulb, thereby ruling out the possibility of a tympanojugular paraganglioma. Of course, it is important to assess the integrity of other key middle ear structures like the facial nerve canal, petrous carotid canal, the ossicular chain, and the round window region. The approach for class A2 tumors is a retroauricular transmeatal approach (▶ Fig. 19.1). Optimal field visualization mandates a wide canalplasty along with widening of the tympanic annulus. This is facilitated by elevating the tympanomeatal flap along with the tympanic membrane in a glove finger fashion. The ossicular chain is invariably involved in class A2 tumors; if it is not disrupted, salvaging the middle ear hearing mechanism becomes a priority. Extreme care is taken to dissect the tumor around the ossicles. Addressing the superior extent of the tumor warrants caution to watch for a dehiscence in the facial nerve canal. Class A2 tumors bleed considerably; hence, the dissection ideally begins from the anterior margins of the tumor as described for class A1 tumor. Cauterizing the main feeding vessel, the inferior tympanic artery at its canaliculus, reduces the bleeding from the remaining tumor which eases the dissection at the more critical regions. The superior limit of those tumors which extend into the epitympanum can be accessed with a transmeatal epitympanotomy. Efforts are directed to maintain the integrity of the ossicular chain but should it be disrupted owing to the disease, ossiculoplasty is done either as a part of the same procedure or in a staged manner.

19.4.4 Class B Tumors

Class B paragangliomas are extensive but are limited to the confines of the temporal bone. Approach to class B1 and B2 tumors is quite similar. They both require a retroauricular transcortical approach. These procedures are ideally individualized for each case based on the extent of the disease.

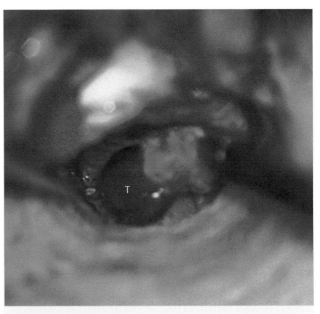

Fig. 19.1 Intraoperative image of class A2 tumor (marked as T) managed transmeatally.

Class B1 Tumors

Class B1 tumors are those which involve the hypotympanum, the facial recess and the tympanic sinus. The initial steps are similar to those of any retroauricular approach. It is recommended to create large posteroinferiorly based and small anteriorly based soft tissue flaps over the mastoid region. The tympanomeatal flap is either elevated in a glove finger fashion or just as done for a routine middle ear surgery if the anterior extent of the disease in the tympanic cavity is limited. But it is not uncommon that some of these tumors show an outward growth into the external auditory canal involving the meatal skin, in which case, the tympanomeatal flap needs to be crafted accordingly. Canalplasty to the extent possible optimizes the transmeatal surgical field. Canal wall up mastoidectomy is performed. The amount of bleeding can be significant in these cases owing to the high vascularity of the tumor and impeded drainage of the mastoid air cells system due to the disease. For class B1 tumors, an extended posterior tympanotomy is performed to access the facial recess area and the hypotympanum. Combined transmeatal and transcortical access provides optimal control over the tumor aiding in its total resection. A transcortical epitympanotomy is performed as needed to clear the disease from the epitympanum. The middle ear conduction mechanism in these cases is compromised more often than not and the reconstruction of the ossicular chain is either done as part of the procedure or in a staged manner.

Class B2 Tumors

The initial surgical strategy for class B2 tumors is no different from the one which is employed for class B1 tumors. For class B2 tumors, which have significant extension into the mastoid cavity, it is ideal to expose all margins before the tumor resection begins. Class B2 tumors are any paraganglioma confined to the tympanomastoid compartment of the temporal bone without breach of the petrous carotid canal. The elements which dictate the later course of the surgery for this class of the tumors are the breach in the tegmen with intracranial extension

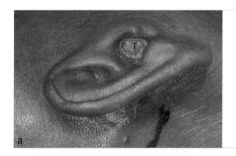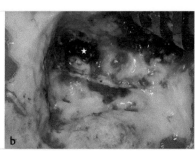

Fig. 19.2 **(a)** Class B3 tumor (T) extending into the external auditory canal. **(b)** Subtotal petrosectomy and complete tumor removal of class B3 paraganglioma. Note the exposed petrous carotid (*solid white star*) and the well-preserved facial nerve (*black asterisk*).

of the tumor, erosion of the sigmoid sinus plate with its possible involvement, and intraoperative finding of involvement of the jugular bulb. The extended posterior tympanotomy along with transmeatal access gives good control of the tumors in the mastoid and hypotympanum. The tumor which is further inferior in the hypotympanum and the deep tympanic sinus are accessed by a subfacial tympanotomy. Drilling out the presigmoid and postsigmoid bone over the posterior fossa dura facilitates the collapse of the posterior fossa dura along with the sigmoid sinus, thus giving extra working space to accommodate the instrumentation to drill the bone medial to the mastoid segment of the facial nerve and above the jugular bulb. Extreme care has to be taken while drilling the bone around this area to avoid injury to the facial nerve and the jugular bulb. A thin layer of bone is always left out around the mastoid segment of the facial nerve, particularly on its medial side. Learning the involvement of the jugular bulb intraoperatively is always a challenging scenario. The resection around this area proceeds with caution. Finding the plane between the tumor and the jugular bulb holds the key. It is wise to abandon the procedure if the plane is not achievable and prepare for a more comprehensive infratemporal fossa approach later.

Class B3 Tumors

Class B3 tumors are differentiated from other tympanomastoid paragangliomas by their involvement of the carotid canal with or without involving the carotid artery. These tumors are extensive involving the external auditory meatus (▶ Fig. 19.2a), mastoid cavity, facial recess, sinus tympani, eustachian tube, and hypotympanum. Tumors with such extensiveness derive their blood supply from a lot of feeding vessels and the possibility of torrential bleed intraoperatively from the tumor as well as the possibility of bleeding from the internal carotid and the jugular bulb are to be anticipated. The prospect of postoperative serviceable hearing in these cases is encouraging with intact preoperative bone conduction and every effort has to be made to preserve it.[41] Hence, an ideal approach would be a subtotal petrosectomy (▶ Fig. 19.2b) aiming for a near-total disease clearance and a blind sac closure of the middle ear cleft. It does not require special mention that such large tumors often involve the facial nerve in which case, the nerve is transected for tumor access and a nerve grafting is done later. In cases where the facial nerve can be preserved despite the magnitude of the tumor, the nerve is anteriorly rerouted.

The initial steps of retroauricular soft tissue dissection, elevation of soft tissue flaps, and canal wall down mastoidectomy remain the same as executed for class B2 tumors. After transecting the meatal skin leaving a healthy margin from the tumor, the canal is closed in a blind sac fashion, which we usually prefer to execute at the beginning of the procedure. To achieve optimal exposure of the carotid for tumor resection and

for gaining good control of the vessel in case of an injury, the tympanic bone is to be completely removed. Drilling the inferior portion of the tympanic bone exposes the vertical portion of the petrous carotid and removing the anterior wall of the tympanic bone gives unimpeded access to the horizontal segment of the carotid. After complete tumor resection, the rest of the procedure includes obliteration of the eustachian tube with pieces of periosteum and bone wax, obliteration of the cavity with the abdominal fat harvest, and closure of the wound in layers.

19.5 Tympanojugular Paragangliomas

Paragangliomas arising from the jugular foramen are more aggressive, in the sense that these tumors are often diagnosed very late in their course of evolution. Their slow growing nature often accommodates neural compensation of the lower cranial nerves, thereby going unnoticed. With the propensity of tumor spreading to various adjacent anatomical compartments, as described earlier, their surgical management depends on proper preoperative assessment of their extent, involvement of surrounding neurovascular architecture, and devising a surgical approach accordingly.

19.5.1 Preoperative Assessment

Tympanojugular paragangliomas (classes C3 and C4) invariably involve the ICA and the management of these tumors begins with a thorough preoperative radiological assessment of their size, their relation to the ICA and the surrounding other important vessels, and the extent of involvement of these vessels.

Indications for preoperative intervention for managing the ICA are based on tumor extension, related angiographic findings, and related patient characteristics:

- The competency of the collateral circulation in maintaining the perfusion of the areas that would be affected by manipulation or sacrifice of the involved vessel. The investigations available to achieve this aim include four-vessel angiography with manual cross-compression test for functional evaluation of the circle of Willis, xenon-enhanced CT of cerebral blood flow, single photon emission computed tomography, and carotid stump pressure management.
- The degree and extent to which the tumor has involved the ICA. The investigations available for this purpose include CT, MRI, MRA and digital subtraction angiography.
- Circumferential encasement of the distal cervical and petrous segment of the internal carotid (vertical and horizontal) by more than 180 degrees as evident on CT and MRI in the axial planes.

- Evidence of stenosis and irregularities of the arterial lumen on angiography of the distal cervical and the petrous carotid on angiography.
- Extensive feeders to the tumor from the internal carotid as evident on angiography.
- Classes C3 and C4 tympanojugular paragangliomas, vagal paragangliomas, and carotid body tumors.
- Previous radiotherapy or manipulation of the internal carotid in a previous surgery.

The modalities available for managing the ICA preoperatively in these scenarios include permanent balloon occlusion (PBO), cervical-to-petrous ICA saphenous vein bypass grafting, and intravascular reinforcement with stenting.

The intraoperative management of the ICA is by: (a) decompression with or without partial mobilization of the artery, (b) subperiosteal dissection, (c) subadventitial dissection, (d) subadventitial dissection with stent coverage, and (e) arterial resection (after preoperative PBO).

19.5.2 Permanent Balloon Occlusion (PBO)

Pretherapeutic knowledge of carotid artery dependence is essential in patients undergoing ICA sacrifice as vascular bypass or alternative interventional approaches may be necessary in those unable to tolerate ICA sacrifice. PBO involves a preprocedure balloon occlusion test (BOT), an angiographic test to assess ischemic tolerance after permanent occlusion of the ICA by assessing if there is a good cross-filling from at least one of the two communicating systems and also to study the circle of Willis.

Angiography is performed in two phases:

- To ascertain the patency of the anterior communicating system, the contralateral ICA is injected and the diseased carotid is manually compressed (Mata's test). Rapid and complete filling of the anterior and middle cerebral arteries indicate a patent anterior communicating system.
- Assessment of the posterior communicating system involves injecting the dominant vertebral artery while the ipsilateral common carotid artery is compressed (Allcock's test). Rapid and complete filling of the middle cerebral artery on the compressed side indicates a competent posterior communicating system.

BOT and PBO are performed under local anesthesia with mild sedation and systemic heparinization with anesthesiologist monitoring. Three balloons are usually placed, first one at the cavernous segment just proximal to the origin of the ophthalmic artery, the second in the petrous segment of the vessel at the level of the carotid canal, and the third in the cervical segment of the internal carotid just distal to the bifurcation of the common carotid. The angiographic studies during the Matas and Allcock maneuvers are evaluated for visualization of the anterior cerebral artery and middle cerebral artery on the tested side. The angiographic anatomy of the circle of Willis is studied according to the presence or absence of an anterior communication between the two ICAs via anterior communicating artery and the posterior communication of the tested ICA with the basilar artery system via posterior communicating artery. The neurological evaluation and electroencephalography (EEG) monitoring are carried out to detect ischemia during the procedure. Any signs suggesting intolerance to the procedure, which is quite apparent immediately after the occlusion,

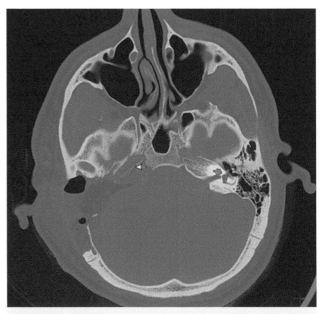

Fig. 19.3 Postoperative computed tomography (CT) image showing the stented intrapetrous internal carotid artery.

warrants deflation of the balloon and abandoning the procedure followed by planning for an alternative procedure.[42] After a successful PBO, the tumor resection is planned 3 to 4 weeks later.

19.5.3 Intraluminal Stenting of the Internal Carotid Artery

The intra-luminal reinforcement of the cervico-petrous carotid (▶ Fig. 19.3) is done when the tumor extent is significant and significant manipulation of the vessel intraoperatively is anticipated.[43,44,45,46] The number of stents required is based on the length of the vessel segment to be stented and the technical features of the stent. Occasionally two or even three stents are used. Ideally about 10 mm of tumor-free portion of the vessel is advised to be stented both proximal and distal to the limit of the tumor to avoid the possibility of accidental injury of ICA at the vessel–tumor interface and facilitate a radical tumor excision. The nature of the stent used for reinforcement is based on diameter (ideally 4 or 5 mm), length, flexibility (during endovascular deployment and positioning especially at the posterior loop of the ICA), and resilience of the stent to withstand manipulation during the surgery.[47,48] Occasionally, stenting is not technically possible when the ICA is significantly tortuous, in which case an alternative procedure is employed. A variety of intraluminal self-expanding nitinol stents are available which include Xpert Stent System (Abbott Laboratories Vascular Enterprises, Dublin, Ireland) and Astron (Biotronik SE, Berlin, Germany).

19.5.4 Facial and Hearing Rehabilitation

Facial and hearing rehabilitation is an integral part of the management of tympanojugular paragangliomas. In facial paralysis of less than 1-year duration, efforts are made to salvage the nerve intraoperatively. However, should the nerve be resected due to tumor infiltration, a sural nerve cable grafting is performed in such cases in the same sitting. Facial nerve palsy of greater than 1-year duration is ideally rehabilitated by reanimation procedures which include ipsilateral eyelid implant and facial–hypoglossal or facial–trigeminal nerve anastomosis. Hearing rehabilitation is best done by using a bone anchored hearing implant (BAHI). We routinely perform a simultaneous ipsilateral BAHI procedure along with facial nerve rehabilitation procedures as a part of the surgical treatment.

19.5.5 Surgical Approach

Class C tympanojugular paragangliomas, as described earlier, essentially arise from the jugular foramen area and hence are considered as tympanojugular proper paragangliomas. These tumors present very late in their course of evolution with significant extensions into the surrounding anatomical compartments of the skull base: medially to become intracranial or intradural, anteriorly into the infratemporal fossa and to the petrous compartment of the temporal bone, posteriorly into the sigmoid sinus, posteroinferiorly to involve the occipital condyle and the vertebral artery, and inferiorly into the upper cervical spaces. Class C tumors often present with varied degree of intracranial involvement with or without intradural involvement. The fundamental surgical principle of management of class C tumors is gaining access to the jugular foramen portion of the skull base. Despite the latest advances in preoperative imaging and in surgical equipment, these procedures are fraught with complications and anticipating them and managing these complications postoperatively are an integral part of the treatment of these difficult lesions.

Adequate exposure of the jugular foramen while minimizing associated morbidity with adequate proximal and distal exposure of the major vessels are the basic principles to be followed while operating in this region. The major impediments in achieving these objectives are management of the facial neve and salvaging the middle ear. Transposition with rerouting of the facial nerve gives uncompromised access to the petrous segment of the internal carotid, which invariably shows a certain degree of tumor encasement in all class C tumors.

Given the vascular nature of the tumor, its presentation in a very advanced stage, and its propensity to involve complicated anatomical domains in the vicinity of its origin, a wide and uncompromising exposure of the tumor is required, which optimally can be achieved by the infratemporal fossa approach type A (ITFA-A) allowing a safe and yet radical surgery. Although the ITFA-A is associated with a certain degree of morbidity, namely, conductive hearing loss, facial nerve dysfunction, and short-term masticatory difficulties, it nevertheless provides uncompromised access to the infralabyrinthine compartment, the jugular foramen and jugular bulb area, the cervico-petrous segment of the ICA, the upper cervical carotid artery, and poststyloid parapharyngeal spaces. Primarily designed for large extradural lesions of these areas, the ITFA-A can be utilized in combination with other skull base approaches.[49,50,51]

Several arguments against ITFA-A for these tumors do exist. Hypotympanic access to the jugular foramen area by partial petrosectomy and infralabyrinthectomy without facial nerve rerouting for limited C1 tumors is achievable, but only at the expense of limited carotid exposure and compromised control of the proximal and distal jugulosigmoid system.

Infratemporal Fossa Approach Type A

The ITFA-A has been a workhorse in surgical management of tympanojugular paragangliomas since it was described by Fisch and Pillsbury in 1979.[52] This is an extralabyrinthine approach passing below the otic capsule and is mainly designed for extensive extradural lesions involving the jugular foramen area, infralabyrinthine, and apical compartments of the petrous bone with anterior rerouting of the facial nerve as its key feature. Primarily designed as a cranio-temporo-cervical approach, gaining a wide access to the jugular bulb, jugular foramen, and the petrous apex of the temporal bone along with the mandibular fossa and posterior portion of the infratemporal fossa is the prime objective of ITFA-A.

A wide postaural cranio-temporo-cervical incision is applied that extends down to the neck. An anteriorly based subcutaneous flap is crafted followed by an inferiorly based musculoperiosteal flap. The inferiorly based musculoperiosteal flap is elevated in continuum with the sternocleidomastoid muscle up to splenius capitis. A posterior meatotomy is done and the external auditory meatal skin is transected. The meatal skin cuff is dissected and elevated from the surrounding tissue and delivered externally with the help of tissue hooks and sutured with an absorbable suture material. The conchal cartilage (within the pinna) and the tragal cartilage are released from their surrounding soft tissue and are sutured together creating a scaffold for blind sac closure to avoid iatrogenic fistula. The posterior belly of the digastric muscle is divided at its origin; the occipital artery encountered underneath the digastric is ligated. The glossopharyngeal nerve is identified traversing the ICA anteriorly. The vagus is identified coursing between the IJV and the ICA and the hypoglossal is seen crossing the ICA anteriorly toward the tongue. The spinal accessory nerve is identified lateral to the IJV (in majority of cases) and passing anterolateral to the transverse process of C1 vertebra. The condylar emissary vein which lies in close proximity to the CN XI is cauterized when needed. The great vessels are marked with vessel loops. The dissection so far exposes the lateral surface of the temporal bone from the root of zygoma anteriorly to the occipito-mastoid synchondrosis posteriorly along with its squamous and tympanic parts.

After cortical mastoidectomy, the canal wall down mastoidectomy is then performed; the tip of the mastoid is removed taking care to leave behind a cuff of soft tissue around the facial nerve at the stylomastoid foramen area. The tympanic bone is drilled and removed in toto. A neo bony canal is created at the root of the zygoma; the facial nerve is decompressed from the geniculate ganglion up to the stylomastoid foramen releasing the nerve from the fallopian canal. The dissection of the facial nerve (in its extra-tympanic segment) is carried within the parotid, thereby creating a soft tissue tunnel, which reduces the stretch injury of the nerve after its rerouting. The nerve is then positioned in the neo canal and secured with tissue glue. Now that the tympanic bone is excised and the facial nerve rerouted anteriorly, the jugular foramen is freely accessed after completion of subtotal petrosectomy. The sigmoid sinus is skeletonized and decompressed leaving behind a ledge of bone at its superior aspect under which Surgicel is packed, thereby compressing it extraluminally. Further compression is achieved by intraluminal packing of the sinus with Surgicel, completely ceasing the venous backflow from the transverse and the sigmoid sinuses.

After clipping the IJV in the neck with multiple Ligaclips (Johnson & Johnson, New Brunswick, NJ), the ligated portion of the IJV is then reflected superiorly. The lower cranial nerves are preserved by sparing the medial wall of the bulb and the upper portion of the IJV. Addressing the intradural extension of the tumors requires a thorough preoperative evaluation and needs to be done only after identifying and separating the anterior inferior cerebellar and anterior-inferior and posterior-inferior cerebellar arteries. The intradural component of the tumor is dealt with either in continuum with the extradural tumor resection or executed in a staged manner.

Clinical Case 1

Following (▸ Fig. 19.4, ▸ Fig. 19.5, ▸ Fig. 19.6, ▸ Fig. 19.7, ▸ Fig. 19.8, ▸ Fig. 19.9, and ▸ Fig. 19.10) are intraoperative pictures of a class C1 tympanojugular paraganglioma in a 56-year-old male who underwent ITFA-A with complete tumor removal.

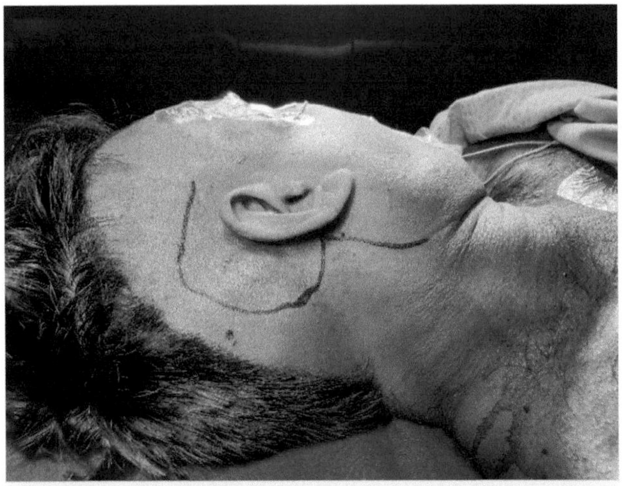

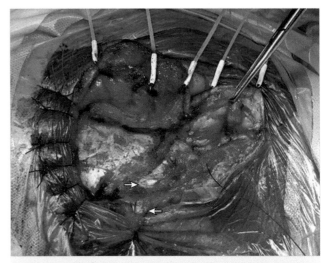

Fig. 19.5 Flaps reflected exposing the squamous and mastoid portions of the temporal bone. *Right arrow*, splenius capitis muscle; *left arrow*, posteriorly based musculoperiosteal flap in continuum with sternocleidomastoid muscle.

Fig. 19.4 Incision marking of a wide cranio-temporo-cervical incision.

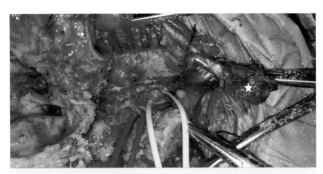

Fig. 19.6 Mastoidectomy and cervical exposure completed with gaining control over the great vessels. Note the posterior belly of the digastric muscle reflected inferiorly (*solid white star*).

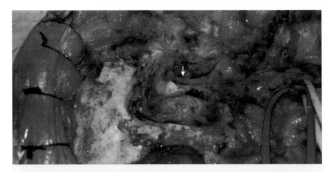

Fig. 19.7 The facial nerve (*solid white down arrow*) is decompressed all through its course from the geniculate ganglion to the extratemporal segment and carefully mobilized out of its bony canal.

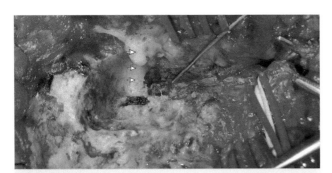

Fig. 19.8 The mobilized facial nerve is anteriorly transposed into the neo canal created and is secured with fibrin glue (*solid white arrows*).

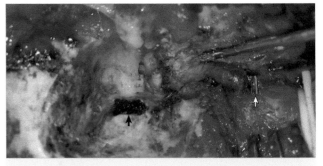

Fig. 19.9 The sigmoid sinus is obliterated by extraluminal packing with Surgicel (*solid black upward arrow*). The upper cervical portion of the internal jugular vein is ligated with multiple Ligaclips (*solid white upward arrow*).

Clinical Case 2

Following are the pictures (▶ Fig. 19.11, ▶ Fig. 19.12, ▶ Fig. 19.13, ▶ Fig. 19.14, ▶ Fig. 19.15, and ▶ Fig. 19.16) of a case of a tumor involving the mastoid and extratemporal segments of the facial nerve in a 62-year-old male with a preoperative House-Brackman grade V facial nerve palsy, managed with ITFA-A procedure, with resection of the facial nerve along with the tumor, followed by facial–trigeminal nerve anastomosis and bone-anchored hearing aid (BAHA) implantation.

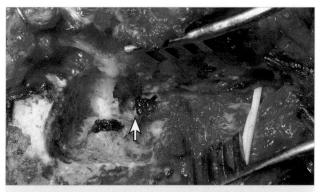

Fig. 19.10 The surgical field at the end of the procedure with the complete tumor having been removed; the jugular bulb area (*solid white arrow*) completely exposed.

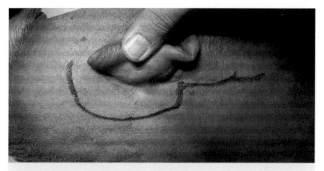

Fig. 19.11 The classical cranio-temporo-cervical incision marking.

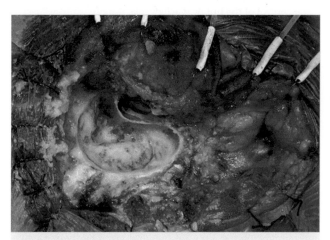

Fig. 19.12 Mastoid exploration and initial cervical exposure.

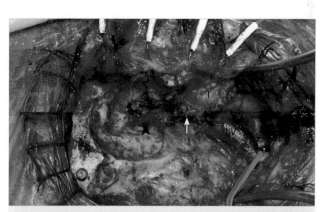

Fig. 19.13 The mastoid cavity after canal wall down and neck exposure. Note the tumor extending into the parotid gland (labelled T) involving the stylomastoid foramen area (*solid white upward arrow*) and the facial nerve (*solid black arrowhead*). IJV, internal jugular vein.

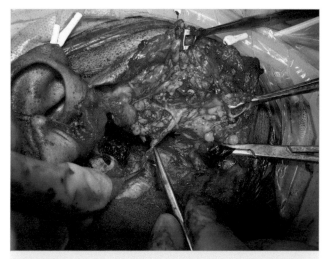

Fig. 19.14 The tumor along with the facial nerve resected with healthy proximal and distal nerve stumps. *Solid black arrow*, distal facial nerve stump.

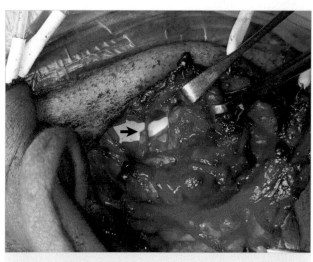

Fig. 19.15 After the facial–trigeminal nerve anastomosis (*solid black arrow*), the anastomosis is secured with fibrin glue over a bed that is created.

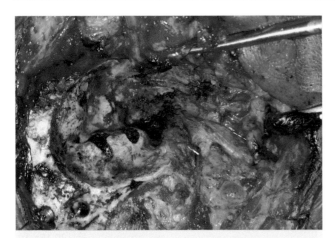
Fig. 19.16 The surgical field at the end of the procedure.

19.6 Carotid Body Tumors

Carotid body tumors are the commonest of the head and neck paragangliomas making up to 60% of them, arising from the dense aggregate of paraganglionic tissue at the bifurcation of the common carotid artery. Embryologically, these tumors are third branchial arch mesodermal and ectodermal derivatives of neural crest and play a vital role in oxygen homeostasis by sympathetic stimulation of the cardiovascular system during acute hypoxic conditions. A highly vascular gland measuring about 6 mm × 6 mm × 2 mm in size, it derives its blood supply from vasa vasorum, branches of vertebral artery, and from branches of the external carotid artery and is innervated by the glossopharyngeal nerve. As mentioned earlier, they occur as both sporadic and familial entities. Chronic hypoxemia either sustained or intermittent is a stimulus for hypertrophy and hyperplasia of the carotid body.

The carotid body tumor presents as a painless, pulsatile lateral neck mass exhibiting the characteristic restricted mobility in the cephalocaudal direction (Fontaine sign).[53,54] Neurological deficits with CN X and XII palsies can be seen in large tumors with manifestations of dysphagia, odynophagia, and hoarseness of voice. These tumors are occasionally secretory with endocrine products of the tumor being released into the systemic circulation causing fluctuations in blood pressure and other sympathetic manifestations. The differential diagnosis includes cervical lymphadenopathy, carotid artery aneurysm, and branchial cleft cyst.

Though these tumors are relatively very rare compared to other masses in the lateral neck, a high index of suspicion is required to exclude carotid body tumors. Fine needle aspiration cytology is hazardous and is avoided in suspicious cases. CT with contrast demonstrates the relationship of the tumor to adjacent structures and allows assessment of the extent of bone involvement in cases with skull base invasion. MRI with contrast usually reveals the characteristic "salt and pepper" appearance resulting from the flow voids of numerous vessels of the tumor which confirms the diagnosis. MRI also demonstrates the relationship of the tumor to adjacent soft tissue structures in the neck, details of vascular encasement, and infiltration of the ICA seen due to a poorly differentiated tumor–artery interface, and loss of enhancement of the precarotid

venous plexus which is otherwise normally seen. Digital subtraction angiography provides valuable information regarding the vascular structures around the tumor and other vital inputs such as the main feeding vessels of the tumor and the collateral circulation via the circle of Willis. Shamblin classification,[55] a widely applied grading system based on imaging, classifies the tumor according to its relation to the carotid vessel walls. Shamblin type I tumors are usually small tumors of less than 4 cm in size, rarely widen the carotid bifurcation, and the carotids are never encased. Type II tumors are adherent to and partially encase the carotids. Type III tumors are large tumors greater than 5 cm in size often widening the carotid bifurcation and encasing the vessels. The likelihood of cranial nerve involvement by the tumor depends on the degree of circumferential contact of the vessel by the tumor which is predictable on preoperative MRI. Evaluation of collateral cerebral circulation preoperatively by BOT of the ICA and manual compression in Shamblin type II and type III tumors provides critical information for tolerance of ICA clamping or sacrifice if necessary.

Surgical excision is the modality of treatment for these tumors with a transcervical approach adopted for tumors confined within the neck, with limited superior extension and where the distal control of the tumor is achievable. A more extensive retroauricular–transmastoid–transcervical approach (modified Fisch infratemporal fossa approach) with removal of the tip of the mastoid to gain control over the intrapetrous segment of the internal carotid is required for tumors with skull base involvement. Presurgical embolization is generally not performed since it makes the dissection planes more difficult and may increase the risk of carotid injury or sacrifice.

19.7 Vagal Paragangliomas

Vagal paragangliomas are rare neuroendocrine tumors comprising about 5% of all head and neck paragangliomas.[5,56,57,58,59] Though described to have the precursors of both epinephrine and norepinephrine, they are rarely secreted by them. Glomus vagale and glomus intravagale are commonly used terms in the literature but vagal paragangliomas denotes them more aptly.

Vagal paragangliomas arise from one of two ganglia present along the course of the nerve; the inferior ganglion or "nodose ganglion" presents high up in the neck immediately posterior to the ICA and is the one most commonly involved. Paragangliomas arising from the nodose ganglion present as a silent neck swelling which at times may have an oropharyngeal component with a medially displaced tonsil, pulsatile tinnitus, and deafness. Jugular foramen syndrome and Horner's syndrome have been described to occur with vagal paragangliomas. Those paragangliomas arising from the superior vagal ganglion within the jugular foramen present as a dumbbell-shaped tumor with an intracranial and cervical component.[59]

A three-stage staging system has been described by Netterville et al[57] and Browne et al:[60]

- Stage I tumor: Confined to the cervical region.
- Stage II tumor: Extending to the jugular foramen and the skull base with anterior displacement or/and encasement of the ICA.
- Stage III tumor: Extending into the jugular foramen often with intracranial extension.

HRCT and MRI both without and with contrast are essential for assessing the extent of these tumors and their relation with adjacent structures and in staging the tumors. Carotid body tumors arising from the carotid bifurcation splay the internal and external carotid vessels and may compress the vagus nerve.[61,62] Angiography confirms the diagnosis, assesses the extent of ICA involvement, and examines the collateral cerebral circulation via circle of Willis and venous drainage of the brain.

A transcervical approach is suitable for vagal paragangliomas confined to the neck within the parapharyngeal space, not invading the skull base and without significant ICA involvement. For stage II tumors with minimal skull base involvement, a transmastoid approach is added to the transcervical approach without sacrificing the external auditory canal. This gives access to the sigmoid sinus and the jugular bulb area. For extensive stage III tumors with intracranial extension, ITFA-A is required as this provides an uninterrupted exposure of the neck, jugular fossa, and sigmoid sinus.

19.8 Hemangiomas of the Temporal Bone

Temporal bone hemangiomas are extremely rare vascular tumors requiring a high degree of clinical suspicion to be diagnosed early in the course of their evolution.[63] Arising from areas with increased density of vascular anastomosis, they are histopathologically classified into capillary, venous, arteriovenous, and cavernous types.[64,65] The majority of them are found to originate at the perigeniculate ganglion region, with the capillary variant being more common and from the region of Scarpa's ganglion at the internal auditory canal, in which cases the cavernous variety is more common.[66,67] Other documented sites of their origin are the mastoid segment of the facial nerve, petrous part of the temporal bone, and jugular bulb.

Clinical signs of temporal bone hemangiomas typically depend on their site of origin. Hemangiomas arising from the perigeniculate region present early with progressive and significant facial palsy out of proportion to the size of the tumor, which is believed to be a consequence of the "vascular steal" phenomenon. Tumors of this region also tend to spread to the middle cranial fossa along the greater superficial petrosal nerve or into the middle ear cavity causing disruption of the ossicular chain and impaired hearing. Hemangiomas of the internal auditory canal show features of impaired hearing of retrocochlear type with or without facial weakness. Vertigo and tinnitus are relatively less common features in these tumors.

Preoperative radiological assessment is essential for evaluating a case of suspected temporal bone hemangioma and needs to be differentiated, if possible, from other more common tumors of these areas. The differential diagnosis includes facial neuromas, vestibular schwannomas, meningiomas, and metastatic deposits. The differentiation of hemangiomas from neuromas can be particularly difficult unless a classical "ossifying" or "salt and pepper" appearance of hemangiomas is present on HRCT.

The management of these tumors to a large extent depends on their site of origin and extent with aims of complete removal of the tumor with every attempt to preserve or restore facial nerve function and hearing. In contrast to earlier practice of subtotal resection of those tumors which are grossly adherent to the facial nerve with good preoperative function, contemporary long-term studies have proved the outcomes depend highly on early intervention and are better with complete tumor resection and primary facial nerve reconstruction. The hearing outcomes on the other hand solely depend on the tumor site with poorer results for tumors in the internal auditory canal.

19.9 Malignant Vascular Tumors

Extremely rare, malignant tumors of vascular origin within the temporal bone include the intermediate malignant variants, namely, Kaposi's sarcoma and the hemangioendothelioma, and the more malignant variants, namely, angiosarcoma and hemangiopericytoma.

19.9.1 Kaposi's Sarcoma

Kaposi's sarcoma usually occurs in the elderly as multiple bilateral cutaneous lesions of the lower extremities and their involvement in the head and neck region has been observed to be very low, with few cases involving the temporal bone being reported in the literature. Kaposi's sarcoma is a vascular tumor originating from the vascular and lymphatic endothelium, and characterized by multifocal angiogenic process.[68] Associated with viral infections, HIV in particular, the management of this tumor lacks a standard therapeutic guideline and depends on the tumor subtype, its stage, and the immune status of the patient.

19.9.2 Hemangioendothelioma

Forming thin-walled blood vessels and sheets of neoplastic cells, the hemangioendotheliomas are neoplastic proliferates of the endothelial cells of the blood vessels. They occur with variable malignant behavior depending on the degree of atypia. Hemangioendotheliomas are divided into three groups, grade I through III, with grade I having the least atypia and grade III showing the most anaplastic features.[69] Surgical resection offers the best modality of treatment for hemangioendothelioma while radiation is reserved for inoperable cases.

19.9.3 Angiosarcoma

Angiosarcoma of the bone usually occurs in the limbs and less likely in pelvis, ribs, and vertebra. The temporal bone is a very unusual site for angiosarcoma to occur with very few cases reported. These are unicentric lesions usually occurring in the third decade and manifest as a mass in the temporal bone region with hearing loss, tinnitus, and otalgia.[70] Their malignant behavior depends on the degree of vascularization and usually appear on CT as a well-demarcated lytic, hypervascularized hemorrhagic mass. Despite complete surgical excision of the tumor being the most effective treatment of temporal bone angiosarcoma, excision of these tumors with adequate margins is often difficult to achieve due to their involvement of the meninges and the brain.

19.9.4 Hemangiopericytoma

Hemangiopericytoma is proliferation of the pericytes, which are round or spindle-shaped contractile cells. It is an extremely rare tumor with the majority of the cases reported occurring in the head and neck being seen in the nasopharynx, nasal cavity, paranasal sinuses, mandible, maxilla, and orbit. Surgical treatment is the treatment of choice and radiotherapy may be helpful in cases where the excision has been incomplete.[71]

References

[1] Lee JH, Barich F, Karnell LH, et al. American College of Surgeons Commission on Cancer, American Cancer Society. National Cancer Data Base report on malignant paragangliomas of the head and neck. Cancer. 2002; 94(3):730–737

[2] Badenhop RF, Jansen JC, Fagan PA, et al. The prevalence of SDHB, SDHC, and SDHD mutations in patients with head and neck paraganglioma and association of mutations with clinical features. J Med Genet. 2004; 41(7):e99

[3] Baysal BE. Hereditary paraganglioma targets diverse paraganglia. J Med Genet. 2002; 39(9):617–622

[4] Sniezek JC, Netterville JL, Sabri AN. Vagal paragangliomas. Otolaryngol Clin North Am. 2001; 34(5):925–939, vi

[5] Zanoletti E, Mazzoni A. Vagal paraganglioma. Skull base. 2006; 16(3):161–167

[6] Pellitteri PK, Rinaldo A, Myssiorek D, et al. Paragangliomas of the head and neck. Oral Oncol. 2004; 40(6):563–575

[7] van der Mey AG, Jansen JC, van Baalen JM. Management of carotid body tumors. Otolaryngol Clin North Am. 2001; 34(5):907–924, vi

[8] Boedeker CC, Ridder GJ, Schipper J. Paragangliomas of the head and neck: diagnosis and treatment. Fam Cancer. 2005; 4(1):55–59

[9] Pawlu C, Bausch B, Neumann HP. Mutations of the SDHB and SDHD genes. Fam Cancer. 2005; 4(1):49–54

[10] Velasco A, Palomar-Asenjo V, Gañan L, et al. Mutation analysis of the SDHD gene in four kindreds with familial paraganglioma: description of one novel germline mutation. Diagn Mol Pathol. 2005; 14(2):109–114

[11] Schwaber MK, Glasscock ME, Nissen AJ, Jackson CG, Smith PG. Diagnosis and management of catecholamine secreting glomus tumors. Laryngoscope. 1984; 94(8):1008–1015

[12] Bradshaw JW, Jansen JC. Management of vagal paraganglioma: is operative resection really the best option? Surgery. 2005; 137(2):225–228

[13] Jansen JC, van den Berg R, Kuiper A, van der Mey AG, Zwinderman AH, Cornelisse CJ. Estimation of growth rate in patients with head and neck paragangliomas influences the treatment proposal. Cancer. 2000; 88(12):2811–2816

[14] Al-Mefty O, Teixeira A. Complex tumors of the glomus jugulare: criteria, treatment, and outcome. J Neurosurg. 2002; 97(6):1356–1366

[15] Jackson CG, Glasscock ME, III, Harris PF. Glomus tumors. Diagnosis, classification, and management of large lesions. Arch Otolaryngol. 1982; 108 (7):401–410

[16] Brackmann DE, Arriaga MA. Surgery for glomus tumors. In: Brackmann DE, Shelton C, Arriaga MA, eds. Otologic Surgery. Philadelphia, PA: W.B. Saunders; 1994

[17] Fisch U, Mattox D. Paragangliomas of the temporal bone. Microsurgery of the skull base. Stuttgart, New York: Georg Thieme Verlag; 1988:148–281

[18] Sanna M, Fois P, Pasanisi E, Russo A, Bacciu A. Middle ear and mastoid glomus tumors (glomus tympanicum): an algorithm for the surgical management. Auris Nasus Larynx. 2010; 37(6):661–668

[19] Moe KS, Li D, Linder TE, Schmid S, Fisch U. An update on the surgical treatment of temporal bone paraganglioma. Skull Base Surg. 1999; 9(3):185–194

[20] Sanna M, Shin SH, Piazza P, et al. Infratemporal fossa approach type a with transcondylar-transtubercular extension for Fisch type C2 to C4 tympanojugular paragangliomas. Head Neck. 2014; 36(11):1581–1588

[21] Sanna M, Flanagan S. The combined transmastoid retro- and infralabyrinthine transjugular transcondylar transtubercular high cervical approach for resection of glomus jugulare tumors. Neurosurgery. 2007; 61(6):E1340

[22] Jackson CG. Glomus tympanicum and glomus jugulare tumors. Otolaryngol Clin North Am. 2001; 34(5):941–970, vii

[23] Sanna M, Jain Y, De Donato G, Rohit, Lauda L, Taibah A. Management of jugular paragangliomas: the Gruppo Otologico experience. Otol Neurotol. 2004; 25(5):797–804

[24] Miman MC, Aktas D, Oncel S, Ozturan O, Kalcioglu MT. Glomus jugulare. Otolaryngol Head Neck Surg. 2002; 127(6):585–586

[25] Foote RL, Pollock BE, Gorman DA, et al. Glomus jugulare tumor: tumor control and complications after stereotactic radiosurgery. Head Neck. 2002; 24(4):332–338, discussion 338–339

[26] Robertson JH, Gardner G, Cocke EW, Jr. Glomus jugulare tumors. Clin Neurosurg. 1994; 41:39–61

[27] Brown JS. Glomus jugulare tumors revisited: a ten-year statistical follow-up of 231 cases. Laryngoscope. 1985; 95(3):284–288

[28] Jackson CG, Kaylie DM, Coppit G, Gardner EK. Glomus jugulare tumors with intracranial extension. Neurosurg Focus. 2004; 17(2):E7

[29] Michael LM, II, Robertson JH. Glomus jugulare tumors: historical overview of the management of this disease. Neurosurg Focus. 2004; 17(2):E1

[30] Watkins LD, Mendoza N, Cheesman AD, Symon L. Glomus jugulare tumours: a review of 61 cases. Acta Neurochir (Wien). 1994; 130(1–4):66–70

[31] Somasundar P, Krouse R, Hostetter R, Vaughan R, Covey T. Paragangliomas:a decade of clinical experience. J Surg Oncol. 2000; 74(4):286–290

[32] Prasad SC, Mimoune HA, Khardaly M, Piazza P, Russo A, Sanna M. Strategies and long-term outcomes in the surgical management of tympanojugular paragangliomas. Head Neck. 2016; 38(6):871–885

[33] Pareschi R, Righini S, Destito D, Raucci AF, Colombo S. Surgery of glomus jugulare tumors. Skull Base. 2003; 13(3):149–157

[34] Leonetti JP, Anderson DE, Marzo SJ, Origitano TC, Vandevender D, Quinonez R. Facial paralysis associated with glomus jugulare tumors. Otol Neurotol. 2007; 28(1):104–106

[35] Lustig LR, Jackler RK. The variable relationship between the lower cranial nerves and jugular foramen tumors: implications for neural preservation. Am J Otol. 1996; 17(4):658–668

[36] Jackson CG, McGrew BM, Forest JA, Netterville JL, Hampf CF, Glasscock ME, III. Lateral skull base surgery for glomus tumors: long-term control. Otol Neurotol. 2001; 22(3):377–382

[37] van den Berg R, Verbist BM, Mertens BJ, van der Mey AG, van Buchem MA. Head and neck paragangliomas: improved tumor detection using contrast-enhanced 3D time-of-flight MR angiography as compared with fat-suppressed MR imaging techniques. AJNR Am J Neuroradiol. 2004; 25(5):863–870

[38] Rohit, Jain Y, Caruso A, Russo A, Sanna M. Glomus tympanicum tumour: an alternative surgical technique. J Laryngol Otol. 2003; 117(6):462–466

[39] Krych AJ, Foote RL, Brown PD, Garces YI, Link MJ. Long-term results of irradiation for paraganglioma. Int J Radiat Oncol Biol Phys. 2006; 65(4):1063–1066

[40] Patnaik U, Prasad SC, Medina M, et al. Long-term surgical and hearing outcomes in the management of tympanomastoid paragangliomas. Am J Otolaryngol. 2015; 36(3):382–389

[41] Medina M, Prasad SC, Patnaik U, et al. The effects of tympanomastoid paragangliomas on hearing and the audiological outcomes after surgery over a long-term follow-up. Audiol Neurotol. 2014; 19(5):342–350

[42] Sanna M, Piazza P, Ditrapani G, Agarwal M. Management of the internal carotid artery in tumors of the lateral skull base: preoperative permanent balloon occlusion without reconstruction. Otol Neurotol. 2004; 25(6):998–1005

[43] Sanna M, Flanagan S. Surgical management of lesions of the internal carotid artery using a modified Fisch Type A infratemporal approach. Otol Neurotol. 2007; 28(7):994

[44] Sanna M, Khrais T, Menozi R, Piaza P. Surgical removal of jugular paragangliomas after stenting of the intratemporal internal carotid artery: a preliminary report. Laryngoscope. 2006; 116(5):742–746

[45] Sanna M, Piazza P, De Donato G, Menozzi R, Falcioni M. Combined endovascular-surgical management of the internal carotid artery in complex tympanojugular paragangliomas. Skull Base. 2009; 19(1):26–42

[46] Sanna M, Shin SH, De Donato G, et al. Management of complex tympanojugular paragangliomas including endovascular intervention. Laryngoscope. 2011; 121 (7):1372–1382

[47] Bacciu A, Prasad SC, Sist N, Rossi G, Piazza P, Sanna M. Management of the cervico-petrous internal carotid artery in class C tympanojugular paragangliomas. Head Neck. 2016; 38(6):899–905

[48] Prasad SC, Piazza P, Russo A, Taibah A, Galletti F, Sanna M. Management of internal carotid artery in skull base paraganglioma surgery. In: Wanna GB, Carlson ML, Netterville JL, eds. Contemporary Management of Jugular Paraganglioma. Cham: Springer; 2018:157–174

[49] Patel SJ, Sekhar LN, Cass SP, Hirsch BE. Combined approaches for resection of extensive glomus jugulare tumors. A review of 12 cases. J Neurosurg. 1994; 80(6):1026–1038

[50] Witiak DG, Pensak ML. Limitations to mobilizing the intrapetrous carotid artery. Ann Otol Rhinol Laryngol. 2002; 111(4):343–348

[51] Prasad SC, Paties CT, Schiavi F, et al. Tympanojugular paragangliomas: surgical management and clinicopathological features. In: Mariani-Costantini R, ed. Paraganglioma: A Multidisciplinary Approach [Internet]. Codon Publications; July 2, 2019

[52] Fisch U, Pillsbury HC. Infratemporal fossa approach to lesions in the temporal bone and base of the skull. Arch Otolaryngol. 1979; 105(2):99–107

[53] Williams MD, Phillips MJ, Nelson WR, Rainer WG. Carotid body tumor. Arch Surg. 1992; 127(8):963–967, discussion 967–968

[54] Baysal BE, Myers EN. Etiopathogenesis and clinical presentation of carotid body tumors. Microsc Res Tech. 2002; 59(3):256–261

[55] Shamblin WR, ReMine WH, Sheps SG, Harrison EG, Jr. Carotid body tumor (chemodectoma). Clinicopathologic analysis of ninety cases. Am J Surg. 1971; 122(6):732–739

[56] Lawson W. Glomus bodies and tumors. N Y State J Med. 1980; 80(10):1567–1575

[57] Netterville JL, Jackson CG, Miller FR, Wanamaker JR, Glasscock ME. Vagal paraganglioma: a review of 46 patients treated during a 20-year period. Arch Otolaryngol Head Neck Surg. 1998; 124(10):1133–1140

[58] Persky MS, Hu KS, Berenstein A. Paragangliomas of the head and neck. In: Harrison LB, Sessions RB, Hong WK, eds. Head and Neck Cancer: A Multidisciplinary Approach. Philadelphia: Lippincott Williams & Wilkins; 2004:678–713

[59] Eriksen C, Girdhar-Gopal H, Lowry LD. Vagal paragangliomas: a report of nine cases. Am J Otolaryngol. 1991; 12(5):278–287

[60] Browne JD, Fisch U, Valavanis A. Surgical therapy of glomus vagale tumors. Skull Base Surg. 1993; 3(4):182–192

[61] Noujaim SE, Pattekar MA, Cacciarelli A, Sanders WP, Wang AM. Paraganglioma of the temporal bone: role of magnetic resonance imaging versus computed tomography. Top Magn Reson Imaging. 2000; 11(2):108–122

[62] Borba LA, Al-Mefty O. Intravagal paragangliomas: report of four cases. Neurosurgery. 1996; 38(3):569–575, discussion 575

[63] Heckl S, Aschoff A, Kunze S. Cavernomas of the skull: review of the literature 1975–2000. Neurosurg Rev. 2002; 25(1–2):56–62, discussion 66–67

[64] Gottfried ON, Gluf WM, Schmidt MH. Cavernous hemangioma of the skull presenting with subdural hematoma. Case report. Neurosurg Focus. 2004; 17 (4):ECP1

[65] Reis BL, Carvalho GT, Sousa AA, Freitas WB, Brandão RA. Primary hemangioma of the skull. Arq Neuropsiquiatr. 2008; 66 3A:569–571

[66] Fierek O, Laskawi R, Kunze E. Large intraosseous hemangioma of the temporal bone in a child. Ann Otol Rhinol Laryngol. 2004; 113(5):394–398

[67] Liu JK, Burger PC, Harnsberger HR, Couldwell WT. Primary intraosseous skull base cavernous hemangioma: case report. Skull Base. 2003; 13(4):219–228

[68] Michaels L, Soucek S, Liang J. The ear in the acquired immunodeficiency syndrome: I. Temporal bone histopathologic study. Am J Otol. 1994; 15(4): 515–522

[69] Ibarra RA, Kesava P, Hallet KK, Bogaev C. Hemangioendothelioma of the temporal bone with radiologic findings resembling hemangioma. AJNR Am J Neuroradiol. 2001; 22(4):755–758

[70] Scholsem M, Raket D, Flandroy P, Sciot R, Deprez M. Primary temporal bone angiosarcoma: a case report. J Neurooncol. 2005; 75(2):121–125

[71] Magliulo G, Terranova G, Cordeschi S. Hemangiopericytoma and temporal bone. An Otorrinolaringol Ibero Am. 1999; 26(1):67–74

20 Venous Considerations in Skull Base Surgery

Chandranath Sen and Carolina Benjamin

Summary

Given the varied configurations of the venous system in both the normal and pathologic states, it is crucial to take venous anatomy into consideration when performing complex skull base surgery. In order to have a thorough understanding of the venous drainage for a particular case, dedicated imaging such as computed tomography venogram (CTV), magnetic resonance venogram (MRV), or diagnostic angiography is necessary. The best strategy remains avoidance of injury. Unlike arteries, veins are delicate and more easily susceptible to injury and therefore special attention has to be paid to this avoidance. This can be achieved by recognizing the relevant anatomy preoperatively and choosing the most direct and safest approach accordingly. However, in the case of sinus injury or involvement by the tumor, skull base surgeons must be prepared to repair and reconstruct major venous structures. Finally, surgeons must also be able to recognize and manage iatrogenic venous sinus thromboses in the postoperative setting.

Keywords: Venous complications, venous sinus thrombosis, venous thrombosis, venous sinus injury, venous sinus repair

20.1 Key Learning Points

- Skull base approaches often traverse important venous structures such as temporal lobe draining veins, the petrosal vein, the torcula, the sigmoid sinuses, and the jugular bulbs.
- Although the venous system can be assessed using magnetic resonance venogram (MRV) or computed tomography venogram (CTV), the only dynamic modality for understanding the venous outflow is an actual catheter-based angiogram. The optimal surgical approach can be planned while mitigating the risk of venous injury.
- Intraoperative techniques that can be used to maximize exposure of the tumor while preserving veins and sinuses include:
  - Arachnoid dissection to release the veins from the surface of the brain and the dural base.
  - When accessing the clivus, it may be advantageous to work on both sides of the sigmoid sinus.
  - Strategic placement of subtemporal retractors (e.g., placing a retractor underneath the posterior leaflet of a divided tentorium to elevate it with the temporal lobe can be used to prevent occlusion or avulsion of temporal lobe veins in a presigmoid transpetrosal approach).
- Venous sinuses or veins can be accidentally lacerated. Immediate repair and reconstruction have to be considered on an individual basis given that by the time brain edema or hemorrhage sets in, it is too late.
- If division of a dominant sigmoid or transverse sinus is contemplated, measurement of the intrasinus pressure on both sides of a temporary clip at the proposed site of ligation is helpful to predict the safety of such ligation.

- Patch grafts and venous interposition grafts are options to be considered in repairing sinus injuries.
- Postoperative sinus thrombosis after skull base surgery is rarely symptomatic and does not require intervention. However, occasionally patient may develop elevated intracranial pressure and may need a shunt or therapeutic anticoagulation.

20.2 Introduction

Venous sinuses and cerebral draining veins may be involved by tumors or may be encountered during the approach to most skull base tumors. Inadvertent injury to these structures can result in serious problems such as bleeding, air embolism, venous infarct, and intraparenchymal hemorrhage leading to intracranial hypertension requiring intervention. All of these can produce neurological deficits that range from asymptomatic to severe (▶ Fig. 20.1 and ▶ Fig. 20.2). In addition, excessive manipulation of these venous structures can result in thrombosis. Brain retraction coupled with sacrifice of some cortical veins can further complicate the situation, such as under the temporal lobe and in the sylvian fissure. Avoidance of venous injury is the best strategy. However, the surgeon needs to be aware of the options available for recognizing and dealing with these problems, should they arise.

20.3 Venous Anatomy

Although the venous drainage at the skull base follows a general pattern, normal variations can exist.

20.3.1 Temporal Lobe Draining Veins

Cortical veins from the basal temporal lobe drain into the lateral tentorial sinus which then joins the transverse sinus. Cortical veins from the lateral temporal lobe can drain directly into the transverse sinus or can also drain into tentorial venous lakes for a short course prior to draining into the transverse sinus (▶ Fig. 20.3). The anastomotic vein of Labbe typically drains to the transverse sinus directly but can occasionally drain into the lateral tentorial sinus.[1,2,3] Many skull base approaches require manipulation of or transection of the tentorium, which can lead to significant bleeding. Excessive coagulation of the tentorium can lead to compromise of the venous drainage of the temporal lobe leading to temporal lobe venous infarct as mentioned above.

20.3.2 The Petrosal Vein

The petrosal vein is composed of multiple tributaries that come together and drain into the superior petrosal sinus. The petrosal vein drains the lateral aspect of the cerebellum and the brainstem into the superior petrosal sinus which joins the transverse sinus to form the sigmoid sinus.[4,5,6,7] Although complication secondary to sacrifice of the superior petrosal vein is thought to

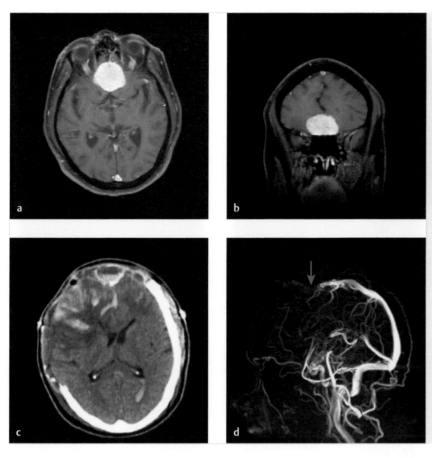

Fig. 20.1 (a) Axial and (b) coronal preoperative magnetic resonance imaging (MRI) of a patient with an olfactory groove meningioma. The superior sagittal sinus was ligated and transected distally for a subfrontal approach for the resection of this tumor. (c) Axial noncontrast computed tomography (CT) demonstrating the postoperative venous infarct with hemorrhagic conversion that was symptomatic and required a decompressive hemicraniectomy. It was discovered that the patient had Factor V Leiden mutation and therefore was hypercoagulable. (d) Postoperative magnetic resonance venogram (MRV) revealing the propagation of the superior sagittal sinus thrombosis (*arrow*) after sinus ligation.

be rare, there are reports of an incidence of up to 30%. The reported complications can range from mild cerebellar edema, peduncular hallucinosis, hearing loss, and cranial nerve palsies to more serious complications such as cerebellar venous infarct (with possible hemorrhagic conversion), midbrain or pontine infarct, acute hydrocephalus, or death.[2,8,9,10,11,12,13,14] Given that some of these complications can be very serious and even fatal, sacrifice of this vein should be avoided as much as possible.[15]

20.3.3 Torcula

The sinuses converge at the torcula in various configurations, which is best characterized on conventional angiogram or CTV. Anatomic studies show that the most common configuration is that the superior sagittal sinus (SSS) drains predominantly to the right transverse sinus (TS). The second most common configuration is that the SSS duplicates into right and left channels but still drains to a single transverse sinus. Another configuration seen is that the SSS drains to a true confluence of sinuses and then splits into bilateral transverse sinuses. The least commonly seen configuration is when the SSS drains predominantly to the left transverse sinus.[3,6,16,17,18,19] The drainage pattern of the SSS at the torcula becomes important in the preoperative planning of skull base approaches.

20.3.4 Sigmoid Sinuses and Jugular Bulb

The venous structures surrounding the vertebral artery in the suboccipital region form a complex network that is highly interconnected and has been likened to the cavernous sinus, hence the term the "suboccipital cavernous sinus." This venous plexus connects to the jugular bulb via the anterior, posterior, and lateral condylar emissary veins.[2,3,6] This relationship of the sigmoid sinus and jugular bulb with condylar emissary vein becomes important in cases of sigmoid or jugular bulb occlusion. In these cases, the condylar emissary acts as the alternate pathway for venous drainage and therefore care must be taken to preserve this vein during skull base approaches.

20.4 Avoidance of Injury

20.4.1 Understanding the Relevant Anatomy

The surgeon must have a thorough understanding of the relationship between the tumor and venous structures. There are several ways of assessing the venous system including MRV, CTV, and digital subtraction angiography (DSA). The only dynamic modality for understanding the venous outflow is an actual catheter-based angiogram or venogram. Interventionalists are becoming increasingly adept and comfortable with exploring the venous anatomy, which typically involves retrograde access from the ipsilateral internal jugular vein. We suspect this will become increasingly common as new techniques to assess venous flow or pressure, in combination with the ability to place venous stents, becomes mainstream.

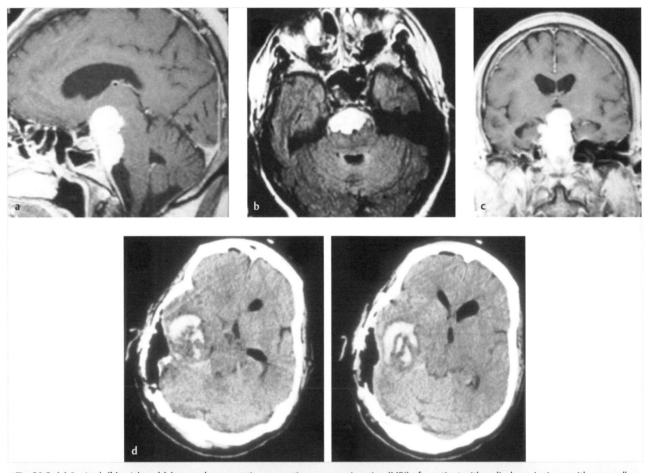

Fig. 20.2 (a) Sagittal, (b) axial, and (c) coronal preoperative magnetic resonance imaging (MRI) of a patient with a clival meningioma with suprasellar extension who underwent a transtemporal approach for resection. (d) Axial computed tomography (CT) images revealing a symptomatic hemorrhagic temporal lobe venous infarct which developed postoperatively.

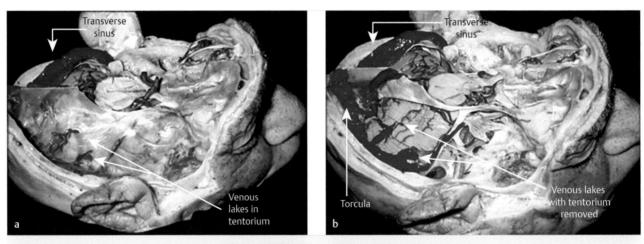

Fig. 20.3 Anatomic dissection illustrating the venous drainage of the temporal lobe (a) with and (b) without the tentorium in place. Lateral and basal temporal draining veins tend to drain into venous lakes in the tentorium; seen here prior to draining into the transverse sinus. Coagulation of these lakes intraoperatively for skull base approaches can lead to venous compromise.

Example 1: A 40-year-old female presented with facial numbness from a clival meningioma. As part of her workup, she also had an MRV performed (▶ Fig. 20.4a, b). The images suggested narrowing of a portion of the right transverse sinus (*blue arrow*). A preoperative cerebral arteriogram (▶ Fig. 20.4c, d) confirmed the area of stenosis on MRV (*blue arrow*). The temporal lobe

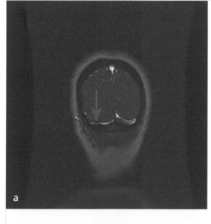
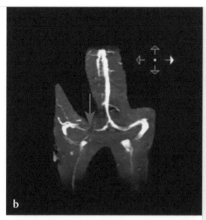
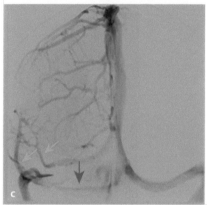
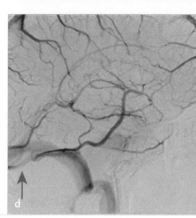

Fig. 20.4 (a) Coronal and (b) three-dimensional reconstruction of the preoperative magnetic resonance venogram (MRV) for a patient undergoing combined supratentorial and infratentorial approach for resection of a clival meningioma. These images revealed a suggested stenosis (*blue arrows*) which prompted a formal cerebral angiogram for further elucidation of the venous outflow. (c) Anteroposterior (AP) and (d) lateral views of the cerebral angiogram demonstrate that rather than a mere stenosis, there is an actual occlusion and discontinuity (*blue arrows*) in the transverse sinus which is not clear on the MRV. Furthermore, it reveals two major temporal lobe draining veins (*green arrows*) that converge at the sigmoid sinus and drain into the jugular bulb. It was, therefore, critical to avoid injury to the sigmoid sinus which can be compromised during this approach.

drainage (via two major veins, *green arrows*) was coming into the transverse-sigmoid junction that ultimately drained into the jugular bulb. Therefore, during the performance of a presigmoid supra- and infratentorial approach, it was imperative to avoid injury to the sinus which was the predominant pathway for draining the temporal lobe.

Example 2: A 37-year-old female suffered from palsy of the right hypoglossal nerve with atrophy of the right half of the tongue. Further workup with a cerebral arteriogram showed that the right jugular bulb and internal jugular veins were the dominant venous drainage (▶ Fig. 20.5). Direct surgery for removing the tumor could jeopardize the large jugular bulb. Also, given that she had a complete hypoglossal palsy, surgery was not considered and she was treated with stereotactic radiosurgery.

20.4.2 Using Alternate Approaches

Detailed study of the venous anatomy can reveal variations that may require a change in the planned approach. This becomes particularly important in cases involving an occluded sinus when collateral venous channels have to be carefully preserved.

Example case: A 63-year-old male had a dumbbell schwannoma arising from the left tenth cranial nerve (▶ Fig. 20.6a–c). A preoperative angiogram showed the left transverse and sigmoid sinus were the dominant venous outflow but the jugular bulb was occluded by the tumor. The venous drainage was via the condylar emissary vein (▶ Fig. 20.6d). A transtemporal approach was initially planned for a one-stage removal of the

intracranial and extracranial portions of the tumor. However, on reviewing the angiogram this approach would carry a high risk of injuring the condylar emissary vein with possibly serious consequences. It was therefore decided to perform the resection in two separate stages. A preauricular infratemporal approach was carried out in the first stage to allow resection of the extracranial and foraminal portion of the tumor. At a second stage, a retrosigmoid craniectomy was performed to remove the remaining posterior fossa portion of the tumor (▶ Fig. 20.6e). In this way, the venous drainage was safely avoided and preserved.

20.4.3 Dissection and Preservation of Veins

Cortical veins draining into a dural sinus travel in an oblique path from the cortex to the sinus. As they come from the brain surface, they have a subarachnoid course. This surrounding arachnoid can be carefully dissected to release the vein and provide room to mobilize the brain and open up a pathway for dissection. Similarly, veins can be freed up from the dura through careful microdissection until the point of entry into the venous sinus. Combining these two maneuvers can allow the surgeon to work around the veins while simultaneously preserving them.

In a presigmoid transpetrosal approach, careful and deliberate placement of a retractor after cutting the tentorium can also assist in preventing stretch injuries to temporal lobe veins. In this approach, the tentorium is divided into an anterior leaflet

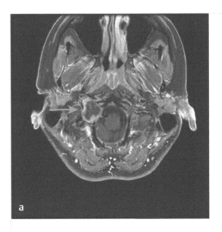
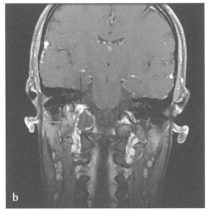
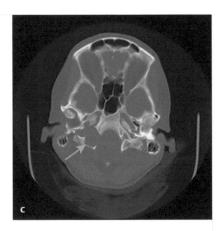
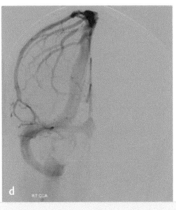
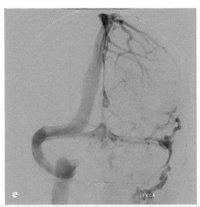

Fig. 20.5 (a) Axial magnetic resonance imaging (MRI), (b) coronal MRI, and (c) axial noncontrast computed tomography (CT) revealing an expansile lesion in the right hypoglossal canal (*green arrow*) with extension to the upper cervical region. Note the jugular bulb immediately superior to the tumor (*blue arrow*) which would have been at risk with surgery. Anteroposterior (AP) views of a cerebral angiogram of the (d) right carotid and (e) left carotid injections illustrating that the right-sided transverse and sigmoid sinus and the right internal jugular veins were dominant and the left-sided venous system was small. Given that this patient already had a fixed deficit (complete hypoglossal nerve palsy) which was unlikely to improve, surgery was not recommended and she was referred for stereotactic radiosurgery.

and a posterior leaflet after visualization and protection of the fourth cranial nerve. A retractor can be placed underneath the posterior leaflet such that the temporal lobe draining veins (that can drain into tentorial venous lakes prior to draining into the transverse sinus) are elevated with the posterior tentorial leaflet and the temporal lobe. The elevation of the veins with the temporal lobe together prevents stretch injury or avulsion of the veins.

20.4.4 Working on Both Sides of the Sinus

The clivus is flanked by the petrous temporal bones. Depending on the depth of the clivus, using the combined presigmoid retrolabyrinthine and subtemporal approach alone may pose a limitation for the surgeon to visualize the ventral surface of the clivus and the base of the tumor, especially the ipsilateral junction of the petrous bone and the clivus. A useful strategy is to use the presigmoid corridor to visualize and debulk the tumor and separate the brainstem and tumor interface (▶ Fig. 20.7a, b). Then the surgeon can open the retrosigmoid dura and access the ventral aspect of the clivus from a different angle (▶ Fig. 20.7c, d). This retrosigmoid dissection is

useful to access the lower pole of the tumor that may be extending below the caudal cranial nerves.

20.4.5 Planned Transection of the Sinus for Access to the Tumor and Reconstruction

Access to the pineal region can be done via a supracerebellar infratentorial approach, an occipital transtentorial approach, or a combined supra- and infratentorial trans-sinus approach. The choice of the approach is dictated by the location of the tumor, the relation with the deep venous system, and also the preference of the surgeon. Generally, the supra- and infratentorial trans-sinus approach works well for large tumors especially meningiomas arising from the tentorial incisura that may extend above and below the tentorium.

Example case: A 50-year-old male with neurofibromatosis type II had several prior operations for multiple intracranial meningiomas. A meningioma in the pineal region was found to be enlarging and surgical resection was planned (▶ Fig. 20.8). A cerebral arteriogram was done to study the arterial and venous anatomy. Due to prior operations and multiple meningiomas,

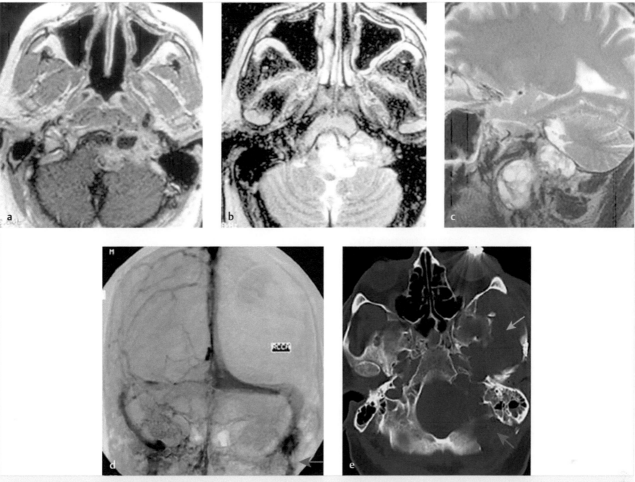

Fig. 20.6 (a) Axial postcontrast, **(b)** axial T2, and **(c)** sagittal T2 preoperative magnetic resonance imaging (MRI) of patient with an intracranial and extracranial dumbbell schwannoma arising from the tenth cranial nerve. **(d)** Preoperative angiogram was performed revealing that the left transverse and sigmoid sinuses were the dominant outflow but due to an occlusion of the jugular bulb, the drainage was being diverted through a condylar emissary vein (*arrow*). **(e)** Noncontrast head computed tomography (CT) demonstrating the surgical approach to this tumor. Given the risk of injury to the condylar emissary vein in a transtemporal approach, the surgical plan was changed to a two-stage resection, that is, a preauricular infratemporal approach first (*green arrow*) followed by a retrosigmoid approach (*blue arrow*).

his venous system was markedly abnormal. The superior sagittal sinus was draining through collateral cortical veins. The left transverse sinus was smaller than the right. Because of the size and extension of the tumor, the decision was made to use the combined supra- and infratentorial approach from the left side by dividing the transverse sinus.

In order to determine whether the transverse sinus could be safely transected, the intrasinus pressure was measured before and after application of a temporary clip. A 25-gauge needle was inserted into the sinus and connected to a transducer revealing a resting sinus pressure of 16 mmHg. A temporary clip was then used to occlude the sinus and the intrasinus pressure was measured proximally and distally. The pressure remained about the same with good waveforms and respiratory variations. Since there was no change in the intra-sinus pressure after placing the temporary clip, it was divided about midway between the torcula and the sigmoid-transverse junction (▶ Fig. 20.9a). The sinus bleeding was controlled by inserting #3 Fogarty catheters at each cut end and inflating the balloons.

It was important to intermittently release the balloons to let the sinus back bleed in order to confirm that it was not thrombosed (▶ Fig. 20.9b). The tumor was excised leaving a small piece, which was subsequently treated with gamma knife radiosurgery. After excision of the tumor the sinus was reconstructed so as to restore its continuity.

A small interposition saphenous vein graft was used to bridge the gap that occurred because of shrinkage of the two ends. The greater saphenous vein was harvested from the right lower leg anterior and superior to the right medial malleolus. The tributaries of the vein were ligated with hemoclips. Alternately, the tributaries can be suture ligated or coagulated and divided. A segment of the vein without valves was isolated, removed, and placed in heparinized irrigation. The cut ends of the saphenous vein graft were sutured ligated with 4–0 neurolon sutures. Heparinized irrigation was also used to flush the vein graft to clear the lumen of any blood clots. The proximal anastomosis was performed using 7–0 Prolene interrupted sutures. A small portion of this was left open to allow the sinus to back bleed. The distal anastomosis was also completed using 7–0 Prolene interrupted sutures. The distal end was also left open to allow for back

bleeding. There was some mismatch in the size of the vein and the sinus and this was compensated using fish-mouthing of the

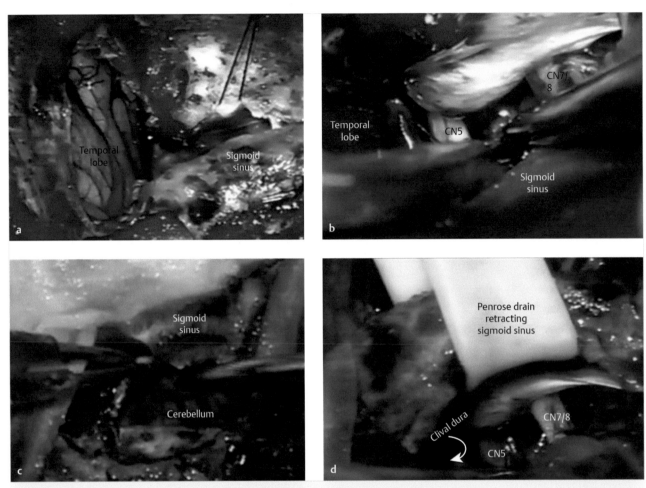

Fig. 20.7 (a) Intraoperative image of a combined transpetrosal approach to access deep clival pathology. (b) Intraoperative image where the surgeon is debulking the tumor in the presigmoid corridor first in order to separate the tumor from the brainstem. (c) Intraoperative image showing the retrosigmoid dura being opened. (d) Intraoperative image illustrating the technique of using a penrose drain to retract the sigmoid sinus anteriorly and therefore get improved access to the ventral aspect and the depths of the clivus.

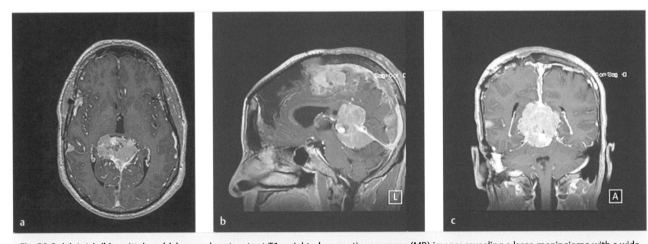

Fig. 20.8 (a) Axial, (b) sagittal, and (c) coronal postcontrast T1-weighted magnetic resonance (MR) images revealing a large meningioma with a wide attachment arising from the tentorial incisura causing severe compression of the brainstem, cerebellum, and occipital lobes in a patient with a history of neurofibromatosis type II.

vein at both ends. After releasing the Fogarty balloons and confirming good back bleeding from both sides, the anastomosis was closed. Heparinized saline irrigation was used throughout the process (▶ Fig. 20.9c, d). The patient was started on Aspirin postoperatively but systemic anticoagulation was not used. An angiogram 1-year postoperatively revealed that left transverse sinus remained open with the saphenous vein interposition graft, albeit less opacified than the right (▶ Fig. 20.10).

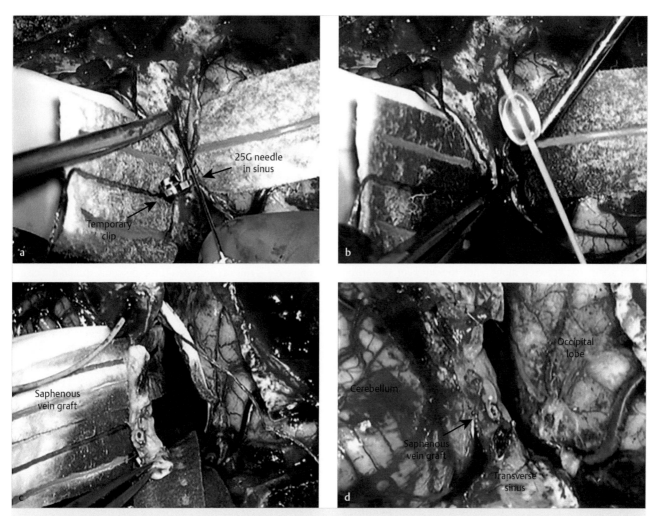

Fig. 20.9 Intraoperative images from a left-sided supra/infratentorial trans-sinus approach for resection of a falcotentorial meningioma. The transverse sinus was transected at the beginning of the case to access the tumor and reconstructed at the end. (a) Intraoperative image showing 25-gauge needle attached to a transducer measuring the intrasinus pressure before and after temporary clipping of the sinus. (b) Intraoperative image after the sinus was cut and a Fogarty balloon was inserted at either cut end of the sinus. (c, d) Once the tumor was resected, the sinus was then reconstructed by harvesting a saphenous vein graft and suturing it in using 7–0 Prolene sutures.

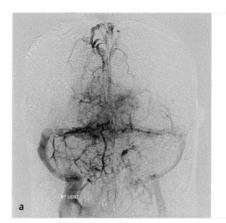
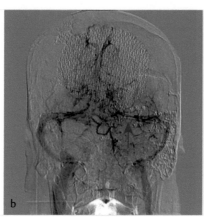

Fig. 20.10 (a) Preoperative and (b) postoperative angiogram at 1 year revealing that the left transverse sinus remained patent with the interposition saphenous vein graft (arrow). Note that on both images, the superior sagittal sinus is occluded. This patient had a history of neurofibromatosis type II and had multiple tumors, one of which was invading and occluding the superior sagittal sinus. This occlusion was not associated with this particular tumor or surgery.

20.4.6 Planned Sacrifice of the Transverse Sinus for Tumor Removal

A 60-year-old woman underwent a previous operation for removal of a right temporal meningioma. She had a second operation for a recurrence and fractionated radiation immediately after surgery. She then had progressive growth of the residual meningioma and had gamma knife radiosurgery. Despite this, the tumor progressed with associated extensive brain edema and postradiation changes. The tumor was centered in the transverse and sigmoid junction and the adjacent tentorium (▸ Fig. 20.11a, b). The preoperative angiogram showed that the sinus was occluded and there was a large temporal lobe draining vein entering the transverse sinus immediately posterior to the occluded transverse sinus (▸ Fig. 20.11c). At the time of surgery, the transverse sinus was opened longitudinally and followed posteriorly. The portion of the transverse sinus where the temporal lobe vein was entering was clearly involved by tumor. A Simpson Grade I resection was planned since there were no other options available for this patient. A temporary clip was placed on the temporal lobe draining vein and divided at the entry into the sinus. The involved portion of the transverse sinus was resected along with the adjacent tentorium. Once the tumor was removed and normal sinus bleeding was encountered, a #3 Fogarty catheter was inserted into the stump of the transverse sinus and the balloon was inflated to control the venous bleeding. After resection of the entire tumor, it was not possible to implant the temporal vein into the transverse sinus since the gap was too much. The decision was made to use a saphenous vein interposition graft.

The lower leg was prepped and a 5-cm segment of the greater saphenous vein anterior and superior to the medial malleolus was harvested. The tributaries of the vein were coagulated and divided. Both ends of the isolated vein were tied off with 4–0 neurolon sutures and a valve-less segment was removed. It was soaked in heparinized saline solution and irrigated thoroughly to ensure there weren't any clots inside the lumen. In order to compensate for the mismatch in the size of the greater saphenous vein and the sinus, the vein was fish mouthed. It was then sutured in an end-to-end manner to the cut end of

the transverse sinus using 8–0 Ethilon running sutures as well as interrupted sutures. Prior to placing the last two interrupted sutures, the Fogarty catheter was removed to allow the sinus to back bleed. Again, heparinized saline irrigation was used throughout this process to prevent formation of blood clots. The temporal vein was then sutured into the side of the saphenous vein. A small incision was made in the side wall of the saphenous vein graft to create an oval opening. The anastomosis was performed using 9–0 Ethilon interrupted and running sutures. The temporary clip was then removed from the temporal vein and good venous flow was noted. The stump of the saphenous vein was closed off with a hemaclip (▸ Fig. 20.12a–d). The patient was maintained on Aspirin only after the surgery without systemic anticoagulation. A postoperative MRV revealed patency of the saphenous vein graft and of the temporal lobe draining vein (▸ Fig. 20.13).

20.4.7 Iatrogenic Thrombosis of the Sinus

If a sinus is fully unroofed and subjected to prolonged retraction or manipulation, it is likely to thrombose either partially or completely. If this occurs, open thrombectomy should not be attempted. Once a venous channel clots, it is not possible to open it up because the clot gets stuck to the endothelium. Attempts to surgically remove formed clot will further traumatize the endothelium and is likely to cause clot propagation.

In a prospective study done at our institution, the incidence of sinus thrombosis after skull base and parasagittal surgery is up to 30%, a number much higher than previously cited in the literature. All patients in the cohort remained asymptomatic. There were no patient-related (age, gender, body mass index [BMI], tumor type) or surgery-related (length of surgery, fluid balance, mannitol use, surgical approach, or extent of resection) risk factors that were found to be statistically significant.[20] In some instances, such as a dominant sigmoid sinus or the superior sagittal sinus, it may become symptomatic with venous hypertension, papilledema, or hydrocephalus. Patients with hypercoagulable states may be prone to this. In such cases, early anticoagulation may have to be initiated despite the risks of

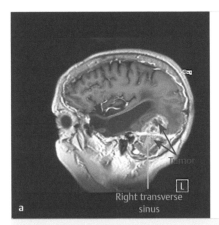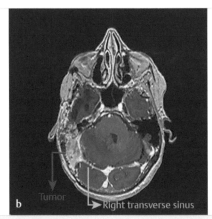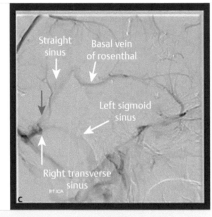

Fig. 20.11 (a) Sagittal and **(b)** axial T1 postcontrast preoperative magnetic resonance imaging (MRI) illustrating a recurrent right temporal meningioma centered in the transverse and sigmoid junction and extending to and involving the tentorium. **(c)** Preoperative angiogram highlights an occluded transverse sinus with a large temporal lobe vein (*arrow*) entering the medial transverse sinus proximal to the occlusion.

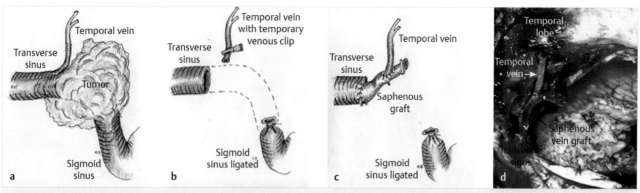

Fig. 20.12 Illustration showing the surgical plan for resection of the tumor as well as the portion of the sinus invaded by the tumor with reconstruction of the venous system to maintain the large temporal draining vein patent in order to avoid venous compromise and possible infarct. **(a)** Figure demonstrating the invasion of the transverse sigmoid junction by this tumor. **(b)** A temporary venous clip was placed on the temporal draining vein. The tumor was then removed en bloc with the portion of the sinus that it had invaded as well as the tentorium. The sigmoid sinus was ligated. **(c)** Since the temporal vein no longer reached the cut edge of the transverse sinus, a saphenous vein graft was harvested and sutured end to end to the transverse sinus and side to end to the temporal vein. The other end of the saphenous vein graft was then closed with a hemaclip. **(d)** Intraoperative image revealing the reconstructed venous configuration.

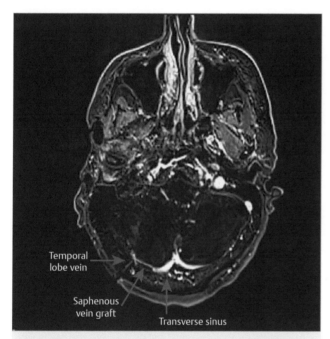

Fig. 20.13 Postoperative magnetic resonance venogram (MRV) revealing that the saphenous vein graft, temporal draining vein, and the transverse sinus which remained patent.

hemorrhage to prevent clot propagation. If this is the case, agents that are more easily reversed such as a heparin drip (without a bolus dose and close monitoring of the Anti Xa and partial thromboplastin time levels) should be utilized over agents such as Lovenox or Anti Xa inhibitors that cannot be fully reversed in case of hemorrhage. Close neurologic monitoring in an intensive care unit (ICU) setting is important when initiating anticoagulation in the immediate postoperative setting.

Example 1: A 29-year-old woman presented with a hemorrhage from a cavernoma in the middle cerebellar peduncle. Surgical resection was undertaken through a presigmoid retrolabyrinthine approach. There was prolonged retraction of the sigmoid sinus during the surgery. She was discharged home and had to be readmitted a week later for severe headaches. MRI venogram showed complete thrombosis of the sigmoid and transverse sinus on the surgical side (▶ Fig. 20.14a). She underwent hematological workup which revealed protein S deficiency. Given her hypercoagulable state as well as severe headaches with papilledema, she was treated with therapeutic anticoagulation with warfarin for 6 months. Follow-up imaging showed recanalization of the sinus (▶ Fig. 20.14b).

Example 2: A 55-year-old man presented with gait ataxia and diplopia. MRI shows a large posterior fossa epidermoid with brainstem compression. Surgical resection was performed through a combined supra- and infratentorial presigmoid retro-labyrinthine approach. Although a complete tumor resection was achieved, he developed symptomatic hydrocephalus with enlargement of the entire ventricular system (▶ Fig. 20.15a, b). A ventriculoperitoneal shunt was placed. Angiography revealed occlusion of the transverse and sigmoid sinuses on the side of the surgery (▶ Fig. 20.15c). Given his symptoms (that may have been compounded by progressive hydrocephalus) and the extent of thrombosis, he was anticoagulated in the postoperative setting with heparin and subsequently coumadin. An MRV at 6 months showed that the sinus did not recanalize but he was neurologically improved so the anticoagulation was stopped.

Example 3: A 63-year-old woman had a symptomatic, right-sided posterior fossa meningioma compressing and partially occluding the right transverse-sigmoid sinus junction (▶ Fig. 20.16a–c). MRV showed that the left-sided sigmoid and transverse sinus were atretic (▶ Fig. 20.16d). She also had hydrocephalus. The tumor was removed via a retrosigmoid approach. Immediately after surgery, she complained of headaches and an external ventricular drain was inserted which showed normal intracranial pressures. MRV showed complete occlusion of the right sigmoid sinus which was her predominant venous drainage prior to the surgery (▶ Fig. 20.16e). She remained intact and the venogram showed that she was now draining the superior sagittal sinus through bilateral cerebral

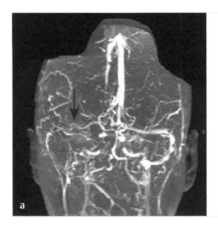
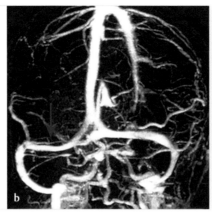

Fig. 20.14 (a) Postoperative magnetic resonance venogram (MRV) status of a patient post presigmoid retrolabyrinthine approach for a middle cerebellar peduncle cavernoma that shows complete thrombosis of the transverse and sigmoid sinus on the same side of the surgery (*arrow*). (b) Follow-up MRV after 6 months of anticoagulation revealed recanalization of the sinus (*arrow*).

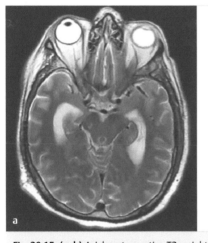
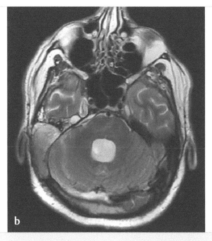
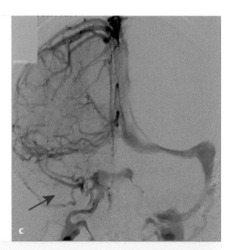

Fig. 20.15 (a, b) Axial postoperative T2-weighted magnetic resonance imaging (MRI) of a patient who underwent surgical resection of a large, right-sided posterior fossa epidermoid via a combined supra- and infratentorial presigmoid retrolabyrinthine approach highlighting the ventriculomegaly that he developed postoperatively (likely secondary to sinus thrombosis) requiring cerebrospinal fluid (CSF) diversion. (c) Postoperative angiogram from this patient showing occlusion of the transverse and sigmoid sinuses on the side of the surgery (right side). Note the venous collaterals which were not adequate (*arrow*).

cortical veins into the sphenoparietal sinuses (▶ Fig. 20.16f). She required no permanent interventions for the sinus occlusion.

20.5 Injury to Venous Sinuses

The venous sinuses are thin-walled structures without any valves. Their walls are kept open by either their attachment to the calvarium, the tentorium, or the falx. They can be lacerated during the drilling and elevation of bone that can be adherent to the sinus wall, especially in older patients.

Therefore, it is important to study the venous anatomy carefully when it is anticipated that there is possibility of injury to the sinus during the surgery. The surgeon can plan for an alternate approach or even prepare to repair the sinus in case of laceration.

Example 1: A 53-year-old man had surgery for a large petroclival meningioma through a right presigmoid retrolabyrinthine approach. Preoperative angiogram showed a dominant transverse and sigmoid sinus preferentially draining the superior sagittal sinus. During drilling of the mastoid bone, there was a laceration of the transverse-sigmoid sinus junction due to

adherence of the bone. The area of the laceration was gently compressed with a cottonoid but no gelfoam was used since it was a large hole and would have got dislodged. Although small tears can be covered with thrombin-soaked gelfoam, large holes necessitate microsurgical repair. After all the edges were adequately defined and prepared, the laceration was repaired directly with 7–0 Prolene sutures (▶ Fig. 20.17a, b). The tumor was then removed in the usual manner. Postoperative MRI venogram showed patency of the sinus although there was a focal stenosis (▶ Fig. 20.17c).

Example 2: A 68-year-old woman underwent a suboccipital craniotomy for decompression of the posterior fossa for an ischemic cerebellar infarct. During the craniotomy, the inferior surface of the torcula was lacerated with the craniotome. There was profuse bleeding that was controlled with elevation of the head and tamponade with cottonoids. Vital signs and end tidal CO_2 were closely monitored for early detection in case of air embolism. Since a portion of the wall was missing, direct repair could not be performed. A patch graft was sewn using a thin piece of acellular dermal graft using 7–0 Prolene sutures (▶ Fig. 20.18a, b). Other autologous graft materials that can be

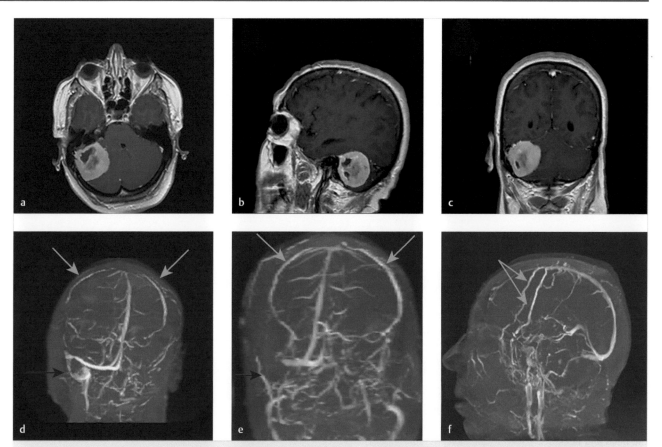

Fig. 20.16 (a) Axial, (b) sagittal, and (c) coronal T1 postcontrast magnetic resonance imaging (MRI) showing the posterior fossa meningioma that was compressing and partially occluding the transverse-sigmoid sinus junction. (d) Coronal three-dimensional reconstruction of the preoperative magnetic resonance venogram (MRV) revealing that the right-sided transverse-sigmoid sinus junction was compressed and partially occluded by the tumor (*blue arrow*) and that the left-sided transverse and sigmoid sinuses were absent. This image also highlights bilateral cortical veins (*green arrows*) that are present preoperatively and assisting with venous drainage. (e) Coronal three-dimensional reconstruction of the postoperative MRV revealing a complete occlusion of the right sigmoid sinus (*blue arrow*), which was her only source of drainage given the absent sinus on the contralateral side. Note, however, that the drainage now is picked up by bilateral cortical veins (*green arrows* which are more robust now in comparison to the preoperative scan when the sigmoid sinus was open). (f) Sagittal three-dimensional reconstruction of the postoperative MRV revealing the bilateral cortical veins (*green arrows*) which now drain the superior sagittal sinus anteriorly through the sphenoparietal sinuses and into the cavernous sinus in order to circumvent the thrombosed sigmoid sinus on the right and the absent transverse sigmoid sinus on the left.

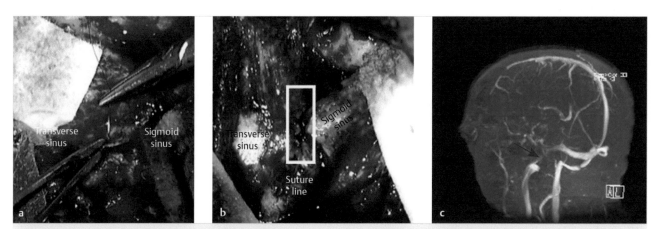

Fig. 20.17 Intraoperative images of a patient who suffered laceration to the dominant transverse sigmoid junction during a presigmoid retrolabyrinthine approach for resection of a large petroclival meningioma. (a) Intraoperative image showing the direct repair of the lacerated edges using 7–0 Prolene sutures. (b) Intraoperative image after repair of the laceration. (c) Three-dimensional reconstruction of postoperative MRV revealing that the transverse sigmoid junction was patent although there was a focal stenosis (*arrow*).

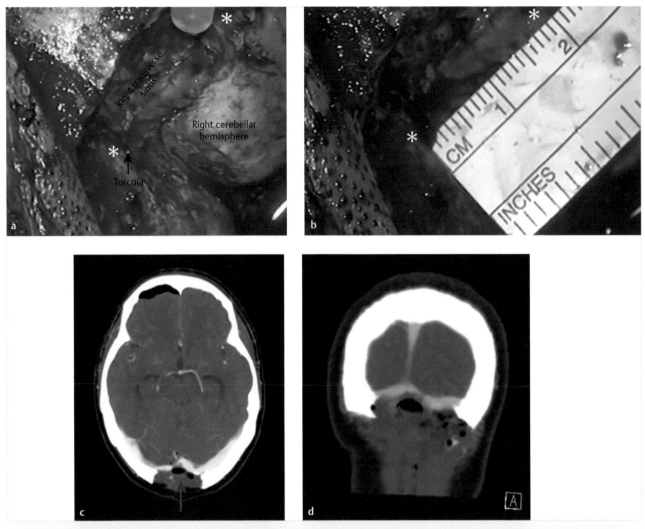

Fig. 20.18 Images of a case where there was a laceration of the inferior portion of the right transverse sinus and torcula during a suboccipital decompression for ischemic cerebellar infarct. **(a)** Intraoperative image of the acellular dermal patch graft (*asterisk to asterisk*) that was sewn in using 7–0 Prolene sutures. **(b)** Intraoperative image showing size (2 cm) of the acellular dermal patch graft. **(c)** Axial and **(d)** coronal postoperative computed tomography venogram (CTV) confirming patency of the torcular and bilateral transverse sinuses (*arrows*).

used for this include pericranium or fascia lata. No systemic anticoagulation was used but the patient was placed on Aspirin after surgery. The postoperative CTV confirmed patency of the torcula and adequate drainage of the superior sagittal sinus into both transverse sinuses (▶ Fig. 20.18c, d).

Example 3: A 34-year-old female had a large, right-sided vestibular schwannoma that was being removed by a translabyrinthine approach. During the temporal bone drilling, the sigmoid sinus was badly lacerated and was sacrificed via suture ligation. While the tumor was being removed, the cerebellum became very swollen and mannitol and hyperventilation were instituted. The surgery was aborted and the patient was taken back to the ICU. No hemorrhage was seen on the CT scan immediately after surgery. The day after surgery she was noted to have severe papilledema. CT showed the ventricles were small. A cerebral angiogram showed that the sigmoid sinus on the right side which was

occluded was the dominant sinus. The left side was small (▶ Fig. 20.19a). She was taken back to the operating room and a saphenous vein was harvested from the lower leg. This was then anastomosed to the side of the transverse sinus while the lower end was anastomosed to the side of the internal jugular vein in the upper cervical area (▶ Fig. 20.19b). The vein was oriented such that the valves were in the direction of the expected flow in an orthograde manner. Postoperative angiogram showed occlusion at the lower end of the vein graft (▶ Fig. 20.19c). This was cannulated retrograde from the internal jugular vein and thrombolysis with urokinase was successfully performed (▶ Fig. 20.19d). However, 2 days later the vein graft occluded again. It was felt that the external soft tissue compression in the neck was the cause of the occlusion. Flow could not be re-established. The patient had a complicated hospital course but ultimately recovered with some neurologic compromise.

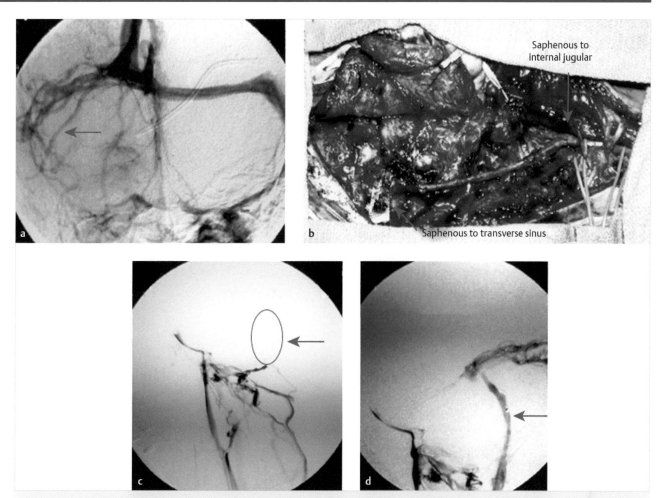

Fig. 20.19 This patient suffered inadvertent laceration and sacrifice of the sigmoid sinus during drilling of the temporal bone in a translabyrinthine approach for a right-sided vestibular schwannoma. The surgery was aborted. **(a)** Postoperative angiogram revealing the right sigmoid sinus occlusion (*arrow*) and a small left sigmoid sinus indicating the right side was dominant. Given these findings, she was taken back to the operating room to place a saphenous vein graft to bridge across the sigmoid occlusion. **(b)** Intraoperative image of the saphenous vein graft that was harvested and anastomosed to the side of the transverse sinus distally and then to the side of the internal jugular vein in the neck proximally. **(c)** Postoperative angiogram showing absence of filling of the saphenous vein graft (*circle and arrow* pointing to the area where the saphenous graft should be filling but is absent) indicating a thrombosis. **(d)** Higher magnification of postoperative angiogram after thrombolysis with urokinase showing filling of the saphenous vein graft (*arrow*).

20.6 Conclusion

Compromise of the normal venous drainage system or alternate drainage pathways that develop secondary to obstructive pathology can have significant consequences. Preoperative imaging, often including formal cerebral DSA, is necessary for a full understanding of the subtleties of the venous drainage in normal and pathologic conditions. The information obtained should be used to plan the appropriate surgery, employ alternate strategies when necessary, and prepare oneself to deal with the complications of iatrogenic direct intraoperative injury or postoperative thrombosis of venous structures.

References

[1] Adachi K, Hasegawa M, Hirose Y. Evaluation of venous drainage patterns for skull base meningioma surgery. Neurol Med Chir (Tokyo). 2017; 57 (10):505–512

[2] Elhammady MS, Heros RC. Cerebral veins: to sacrifice or not to sacrifice, that is the question. World Neurosurg. 2015; 83(3):320–324

[3] Rhoton AL, Jr. The cerebral veins. Neurosurgery. 2002; 51(4) Suppl:S159–S205

[4] Kaku S, Miyahara K, Fujitsu K, et al. Drainage pathway of the superior petrosal vein evaluated by CT venography in petroclival meningioma surgery. J Neurol Surg B Skull Base. 2012; 73(5):316–320

[5] Matsushima K, Matsushima T, Kuga Y, et al. Classification of the superior petrosal veins and sinus based on drainage pattern. Neurosurgery. 2014; 10 Suppl 2:357–367, discussion 367

[6] Matsushima T, Rhoton AL, Jr, de Oliveira E, Peace D. Microsurgical anatomy of the veins of the posterior fossa. J Neurosurg. 1983; 59(1):63–105

[7] Sakata K, Al-Mefty O, Yamamoto I. Venous consideration in petrosal approach: microsurgical anatomy of the temporal bridging vein. Neurosurgery. 2000; 47 (1):153–160, discussion 160–161

[8] Cheng L. Complications after obliteration of the superior petrosal vein: are they rare or just underreported? J Clin Neurosci. 2016; 31:1–3

[9] Koerbel A, Wolf SA, Kiss A. Peduncular hallucinosis after sacrifice of veins of the petrosal venous complex for trigeminal neuralgia. Acta Neurochir (Wien). 2007; 149(8):831–832, discussion 832–833

[10] Liebelt BD, Barber SM, Desai VR, et al. Superior petrosal vein sacrifice during microvascular decompression: perioperative complication rates and comparison with venous preservation. World Neurosurg. 2017; 104:788–794

[11] Masuoka J, Matsushima T, Hikita T, Inoue E. Cerebellar swelling after sacrifice of the superior petrosal vein during microvascular decompression for trigeminal neuralgia. J Clin Neurosci. 2009; 16(10):1342–1344

[12] Narayan V, Savardekar AR, Patra DP, et al. Safety profile of superior petrosal vein (the vein of Dandy) sacrifice in neurosurgical procedures: a systematic review. Neurosurg Focus. 2018; 45(1):E3

[13] Pathmanaban ON, O'Brien F, Al-Tamimi YZ, Hammerbeck-Ward CL, Rutherford SA, King AT. Safety of superior petrosal vein sacrifice during microvascular decompression of the trigeminal nerve. World Neurosurg. 2017; 103:84–87

[14] Perrini P, Di Russo P, Benedetto N. Fatal cerebellar infarction after sacrifice of the superior petrosal vein during surgery for petrosal apex meningioma. J Clin Neurosci. 2017; 35:144–145

[15] Haq IB, Susilo RI, Goto T, Ohata K. Dural incision in the petrosal approach with preservation of the superior petrosal vein. J Neurosurg. 2016; 124(4): 1074–1078

[16] Bayaroğulları H, Burakgazi G, Duman T. Evaluation of dural venous sinuses and confluence of sinuses via MRI venography: anatomy, anatomic variations, and the classification of variations. Childs Nerv Syst. 2018; 34 (6):1183–1188

[17] Bisaria KK. Anatomic variations of venous sinuses in the region of the torcular Herophili. J Neurosurg. 1985; 62(1):90–95

[18] Fukusumi A, Okudera T, Takahashi S, et al. Anatomical evaluation of the dural sinuses in the region of the torcular herophili using three dimensional CT venography. Acad Radiol. 2010; 17(9):1103–1111

[19] Gökçe E, Pınarbaşılı T, Acu B, Fırat MM, Erkorkmaz Ü. Torcular Herophili classification and evaluation of dural venous sinus variations using digital subtraction angiography and magnetic resonance venographies. Surg Radiol Anat. 2014; 36(6):527–536

[20] Benjamin CG, Sen RD, Golfinos JG, et al. Postoperative cerebral venous sinus thrombosis in the setting of surgery adjacent to the major dural venous sinuses. J Neurosurg. 2018:1–7. Online ahead of print

21 Neurophysiologic Monitoring and Its Role During Cerebrovascular Injury

Carla J.A. Ferreira, Katherine Anetakis, Donald J. Crammond, Jeffrey R. Balzer, and Parthasarathy D. Thirumala

Summary

Vascular injury is one of the most feared complications in skull base surgery due to its potential to result in significant morbidity. Immediate feedback concerning cerebral perfusion is crucial for optimized management. This real-time feedback can be provided using multimodality intraoperative neurophysiologic monitoring (IONM). In this chapter, we will review the principles, technical aspects, interpretation, and limitations of each of the different IONM electrophysiological modalities that might be helpful in this context.

Keywords: Neurophysiology, intraoperative neuromonitoring, skull base surgery, vascular injury, cerebral blood flow, ischemia

21.1 Key Learning Points

- Somatosensory evoked potentials (SSEPs) and electroencephalography (EEG) recordings can be obtained continuously in real time during surgery.
- SSEP and EEG are sensitive to changes in cerebral perfusion during surgery.
- Significant changes in SSEPs, an increase in the latency and decrease in amplitude of the cortical responses, can be utilized as a criterion to warn the surgical team of impending neurological injury.
- Significant decrease in the amplitude of the background EEG can serve as an indicator for cerebral perfusion and warn the surgical team.
- SSEP and EEG can serve as a neurophysiological biomarker of cerebral perfusion and postoperative neurological deficits.
- Motor evoked potential (MEP) and brainstem auditory evoked potential (BAEP) are especially useful in subcortical hypoperfusion related to perforator injury.

21.2 Introduction

Skull base surgery faces unique challenges including intimate relationships between tumors and cerebrovascular structures. Resection of tumors located along the path of the internal carotid artery (ICA) carries the risk of injuring the vessel and will be a significant concern. Another example of major arterial risk during skull base tumor resection is the basilar artery. Lesions involving the clivus and foramen magnum may also place the basilar artery, its tributaries, or its branches, at risk. In a similar way, lesions involving the anterior skull base can be intimately related to the anterior communicating artery complex vessels, including the anterior cerebral arteries, and frontopolar and fronto-orbital arteries.[1]

Vascular injury is one of the most feared complications due to its potential for significant morbidity.[2,3,4] Intraoperative neurophysiologic monitoring (IONM) with somatosensory evoked potentials (SSEPs), electroencephalography (EEG), and motor evoked potentials (MEPs) can detect significant cortical and subcortical cerebral hypoperfusion leading to potential corrective action. Real-time information about the functional status of the integrity of the nervous systems secondary to perfusion plays an essential role in the management of vascular complications guiding immediate corrective action before the onset of permanent neurological deficit.[2,5,6,7,8,9]

In addition to direct vascular injury, which can usually be visually identified by the surgical team, other mechanisms can contribute to vascular complications such as cerebral hypoperfusion related to hypotension or hemodilution, and embolic phenomenon associated with vessel manipulation.[7,10] In these cases, an ongoing injury can be overlooked unless continuous functional assessment is in progress.

21.3 Cerebral Perfusion Principles and Neurophysiologic Tools for Measurement

Normal cerebral blood flow (CBF) in awake adults is approximately 50 mL/100 g/minute, with cortical regions requiring higher levels compared with subcortical regions. Animal studies indicate that a decrease in CBF to 16 to 20 mL/100 g/minute results in reversible cellular dysfunction (ischemia) and a significant decrease in neurophysiological response amplitude. CBF below this level risks "electric failure" (functional threshold) and a loss of neurophysiological responses is an immediate precursor of "ion pump failure" and cellular death. The flow threshold for ion pump failure or infarction occurs at 10 to 12 mL/100 g/minute (lesion threshold). This means that there is a time window, as CBF decreases, wherein restoration of flow will avoid permanent injury.[6,7,8]

There is wide variability in the individual susceptibility to hemodynamic changes related to drop in systemic blood pressure, embolic events, direct vascular injury, or arterial cross-clamping. This susceptibility depends on self-regulatory mechanisms, including, but not limited to, the status of the circle of Willis, other collateral circulation, the presence of atherosclerosis, and autoregulation. Thus, during a vascular complication it is often necessary to determine intraoperatively if the hemodynamic situation during the complication is compatible with sufficient cerebral perfusion in each individual.[2,11]

Numerous tools have been proposed that allow for intraoperative assessment of CBF such as Doppler, flow probes, which use ultrasonic measurements, stump pressure, EEG, and SSEPs, among others.[8,11,12] The distinct advantage of neurophysiological methods is the ability to evaluate the consequence of hemodynamic changes while Doppler, flow, and pressure provide local data without information on how it impacts the individual patient.[8,11] Moreover, EEG and SSEP are noninvasive and technically easy to implement and record in the operating room (OR).

The SSEP evaluates the entire somatosensory neural axis which includes the peripheral nerve, spinal cord dorsal columns, the brainstem medial lemniscus pathways to the contralateral thalamus, and connections to the primary somatosensory cortex. These structures are represented by a sequence of scalp recorded SSEP components named according to the polarity (positive [P] or negative [N]) and peak latency. Thus, for the upper limb SSEPs, the N9, N13, and N20/P22 components of the SSEP are generated at the brachial plexus, cervicomedullary junction, and anterior parietal somatosensory cortex, respectively, while for lower limb SSEPs, the equivalent SSEP components are the N20, N30, and N37/P45 components, respectively.[7,13]

Adequate CBF is necessary for the generation of SSEP responses by viable neurons. As stated earlier, decreases in CBF below 16 to 20 mL/100 g/minute causes a reversible decrease in the amplitude of cortical SSEP responses due to desynchronization of cortical neurons and a reduction in the number of functional neurons.[8] Cortical SSEP responses disappear with corresponding CBF values between 12 and 15 mL/100 g/minute as a result of the "electrical failure." Considering that the flow threshold for ion pump failure or infarction occurs at 10 to 12 mL/100 g/minute, these changes in SSEPs can be a precursor of ion pump failure.[6,7,8,14,15,16]

The EEG is a graphical representation of global neuronal electrical activity within the entire cerebral cortex. Physiologically reversible EEG changes such as a decrease in amplitude and frequency alterations also occur with decrease in CBF. For example, decrease in α (8–13 Hz)/β ($\geq$14 Hz) frequencies and increase in θ (5–7 Hz)/δ (0.5–4 Hz) frequencies occur when CBF decreases to $\leq$22 mL/100 g/minute, while isoelectric (i.e., flat) EEG (absence of cerebral activity of over 2 microvolts [μV]) can be observed following more significant reductions in CBF (7–15 mL/100 mg/minute).[8,11,17] To facilitate interpretation and comparison of EEG activity across different time-points during surgery, processed spectral EEG activity can also be used, which use fast Fourier transformation of the raw EEG data.[12]

Other neurophysiologic modalities that may be useful during vascular procedures that pose a risk for vessel injury include brainstem auditory evoked potential (BAEP) and transcranial motor evoked potentials (TcMEPs). BAEPs are generated in response to independent auditory stimulation delivered to the ear and consist of a sequence of deflections called Jewitt Waves I, II, III, IV, and V which originate from the distal cochlear nerve, cochlear nucleus, superior olivary complex, lateral lemniscus (LL), and inferior colliculus (IC), respectively. Thus, the BAEP can assess the integrity of the cochlear nerve and the auditory structures of the brainstem from the pontomedullary junction to the lower midbrain.[6,13,18] Primate studies on the effect of focal brainstem ischemia on BAEPs demonstrate that ischemia increases the latency and reduces the amplitude of BAEP waveforms. The gradient of sensitivity to ischemia where the latency of BAEP responses from the LL was increased at CBF was 12 to 15 mL/100 g/minute, and the CBF was above 20 mL/100 g/minute for inferior colliculus.[6]

TcMEPs assess the integrity of the descending corticospinal tract (CST) from the primary cortex of the frontal, precentral cortex to the skeletal muscles, traversing through the corona radiata, the posterior limb of the internal capsule, the medullary pyramid, the anterior and lateral tracts of the spinal cord, the alpha motor neuron, and the neuromuscular junction. The subcortical CST pathway can be selectively affected by perforating artery injuries which may be undetected as they can occur while other neurophysiologic modalities such as SSEPs and the EEG remain unchanged.[2,22] For example, during clipping of a cerebral aneurysm in the anterior and middle cerebral arteries, inadvertent occlusion of the perforating arteries (e.g., anterior choroidal artery) can lead to change in TcMEPs without significant change in SSEPs and EMPs.

Electromyography (EMG) is another neurophysiological modality which is often used during skull base surgeries for monitoring the motor branches of certain cranial nerves. However, EMG monitoring has no direct role in the management of vascular injury during skull base procedures. For this reason, cranial nerve EMG monitoring is not discussed in this chapter.

Each IONM modality has its strengths and limitations; thus, multimodality monitoring is essential in identifying ischemia during skull base procedures. The selection of IONM modalities should be guided considering the risks of the surgical procedure for each patient and the location of the pathology (▶ Table 21.1).

21.4 IONM Modalities: Technical Considerations

21.4.1 SSEP

SSEPs are recorded in response to stimulation of the median or ulnar nerves at the wrist and the tibial or peroneal nerves at the ankle or fibular head, respectively, using surface or needle electrode pairs placed bilaterally. Subdermal recording electrodes are placed on the scalp at multiple locations, including P3 or CP3, P4 or CP4, Pz, and Fz, according to the international 10–20 system.[20] Cortical SSEP waveforms are recoded using P3–CP3/Fz and P4–CP4/Fz montages for upper extremity stimulation and at Pz/Fz or P4–CP4/P3–CP3 montages for lower extremity stimulation. Subcortical responses are recorded from electrodes placed on the skin surface over C2–C7 spinous process and referenced to scalp electrode Fz. In addition, brachial plexus generated potentials are recorded from electrodes placed over the Erb's point bilaterally and referenced to one another. Interleaved upper and lower extremity stimulation is performed at a rate of 2 to 4 Hz with a pulse duration of 0.2 to 0.3 milliseconds. Typical stimulation intensity ranges from 20 to 40 mA for the upper limbs and from 30 to 60 mA for the lower limbs.[6,7,13,15]

The sensitivity range to display the waveform varies according to the amplitude of the obtained waveforms, which is usually 0.3 to 1 μV. The time base is set at 10 msec/div for upper and lower limbs. Band-pass filters are set from 10 to 300 Hz for cortical recordings and from 30 to 1000 Hz for subcortical and Erb's point recordings. Technical difficulties can be encountered in the collection, display, and analysis of the SSEP waveforms. One problem in stimulation and collection of data is to make sure the electrodes necessary for the process are plugged in appropriate slots in the IONM equipment. Labeling the electrodes can help identify them during the procedure when there is reduced access. Significant noise can be encountered during the collection of the data and averaging SSEPs at either 128 or 256 stimulated trials, depending on the signal quality,[6,7] can alleviate the issue.

Table 21.1 An overview of various modalities utilized during skull base surgery, neurovascular structure evaluation, and advantages and disadvantages of them

Modality	Neurovascular structures evaluation	Advantages	Disadvantages
Somatosensory evoked potential (SSEP)	• Peripheral nerve, dorsal column pathways, ventral thalamus, contralateral somatosensory cortex • Anterior circulation vessels	• Continuous data collection, provides a broad and a specific measure of integrity of various neurovascular structures	• Due to the necessity of averaging, it could take nearly a minute to provide a feedback
Transcranial motor evoked potentials (TcMEPs)	• Corticospinal track • Perforating vessels in the anterior circulation	• Sensitive to changes in perfusion to corticospinal tract	• Cannot be performed continuously during the procedure owing to the movement produced • Risk of seizure, bite injury and arrhythmia • Very susceptible to anesthesia, it demands total intravenous anesthesia
Brainstem auditory evoked potentials (BAEPs)	• Auditory nerve, brainstem auditory pathway • Posterior circulation vessels	• Good resolution about changes in auditory nerve and brainstem perfusion	• Cannot be obtained in patients with hearing loss • Fluid drainage from the surgical site during surgery can reduce the auditory stimulation • Due to the necessity of promediation, it takes several seconds, or even minutes, to provide a feedback
Electroencephalography (EEG)	• Cortical structures	• Easy to set up, real-time information about the changes in cerebral perfusion • Widespread and comprehensive assessment of global cortical function	• Affected by anesthesia, mean arterial pressure, and temperature • Not able to provide information about subcortical structures

21.4.2 EEG

According to the 10–20 international system, 8 to 16 subdermal electrodes are placed on the scalp, and a longitudinal bipolar montage can be assembled to cover the anterior and posterior aspects of each hemisphere adequately. The sensitivity of EEG is partly related to the number of EEG channels and the inter-electrode distances for each channel. Electrode impedance should be below 5 kΩ. The bandpass filter is from 1 Hz to at least 30 Hz, but preferably 70 Hz. A 60 Hz notch filter is generally necessary. Time base is set at 30 mm/second or slower, 15- to 10 mm/second and the sensitivity at 2 to 3 µV/div to better appreciate asymmetries.[5,12,13] Common technical challenges in the collection of the EEG is the placement of electrodes in the head. Due to the intrusion of the surgical field, the placement location can be compromised resulting in two electrodes being too close to each other. Since most of the EEG collection is based on a potential difference between two electrodes, identifying a reference electrode significantly far from the primary electrode will help address the concern.

21.4.3 BAEP

Auditory stimulation is delivered using a click in an alternating fashion using expanding foam earbuds placed in the external auditory canal at 80 to 100 dBpeSPL, at a rate between 10 and 40 Hz, while white noise is applied to the contralateral ear at about 65 dBpeSPL. About 512 to 1,024 responses are averaged for each BAEP epoch depending on the signal quality and signal-to-noise ratio. Recording channels on the scalp include Cz-A1, Cz-A2, A1-A2, and Cz- Cv2, placed as per the international 10–20 system. Amplifier bandpass is 100 to 1000 Hz for all channels.[6,13] Technical concerns secondary to fluid drainage

from the surgical site during surgery can reduce the auditory stimulation. Placing a soft insert in the ear and sealing it will be helpful during the procedure to reduce these conduction problems.

21.4.4 TcMEP

TcMEPs are elicited in response to transcranial electric stimulation using a high-frequency train technique: multipulse stimulation (three to nine stimuli) delivered with a short interstimulus interval (ISI) (2–4 msec), duration of 0.05 to 0.5 msec and an inter-train frequency of 1 to 2 Hz. Subdermal stimulating electrodes are placed at C3, C4, C1, C2, Cz, and 6 cm anterior to Cz allowing multiple montages: C1/C4, C2/C3, C3/C4, C3–C4/Cz and Cz, Cz/Cz+6 cm. The intensity of stimulus usually ranges from 40 to 200 mA. Responses are recorded from muscles in the form of a compound muscle action potential from all four limbs. Muscle recordings are typically from abductor pollicis brevis and abductor hallucis which have optimal cortical representation. Additional muscle groups can be utilized depending on the procedure. Recording parameters include sweep length of 100 msec, bandpass filter from 100 to 2,000 Hz, and a sensitivity of 15 to 500 µV/div according to the amplitude of the obtained responses.[13,21,22,23] In comparison to SSEPs, BAEP, and EEG, which are usually continually monitored throughout the procedure, TcMEPs are usually acquired at certain periodic intervals due to patient movement induced by excessive muscle contraction, and thus they are monitored intermittently. Tongue laceration and seizures have noted to be risks of TcMEPs during a surgical procedure. Placing a soft bite block in between teeth after intubation, and screening patients for preoperative seizures can reduce the risk. Care should be taken to communicate to the anesthesia team about the need for total intravenous anesthesia and use of neuromuscular blocking agents for intubation. This will help the neurophysiology team obtain baseline data before major surgical manipulation and use it as a reference to compare with data collected during surgery.

21.5 Anesthetic Considerations

Effects of anesthesia on IONM modalities are well documented in the literature.[13,16,24,25,26] Theoretically, any drug has some potential to compromise IONM while IONM may be realized under any anesthetic regimen. It depends on the dose used, the stability of the infusion, and the neurophysiologic modalities being used. Therefore, proper interaction between the anesthesiology and neurophysiology teams is crucial.

In general, cortical, polysynaptically generated responses are more affected than subcortical or peripheral responses. Anesthetic changes typically result in a symmetric decrease in the amplitude as well as a prolongation of latency of responses. It is possible, however, for previously damaged pathways to display more pronounced paradoxical, unilateral changes which can be misleading during interpretation of systemic effects of various anesthetic agents.

MEPs are particularly adversely affected by volatile anesthetic agents, while BAEP are least susceptible and SSEPs have intermediate vulnerability. TcMEPs are readily abolished with the use of pharmacological paralytic agents, inhalational agents, barbiturates, and benzodiazepines. Thus, *total intravenous anesthesia* (TIVA) with steady infusion rates of opioid and propofol are recommended when multimodality monitoring will be used as the TIVA technique has the least deleterious effect on MEP and SSEP recordings. Conversely, some drugs can actually enhance the evoked potential responses. These include ketamine, etomidate, or even neuromuscular blocking agents which can improve EEG, SSEP, and BAEP responses by optimizing the signal-to-noise rate due to the reduction of muscle activity.[26,27]

Regarding EEG, at lower anesthetic levels, fast frequencies are common with induction agents, followed by a dose-dependent reduction in frequency and amplitude. The anesthetic-induced fast frequencies are the first to be eliminated during ischemia, which may aid in identification of perfusion asymmetries. Further increase in anesthetic concentrations results in a burst suppressed pattern of EEG and even complete cessation of all EEG activities which precludes accurate analysis of cerebral perfusion.

Of course, not all anesthetic agents follow these general principles. However, details about the effect of specific agents are beyond the scope of this chapter. For further information, targeted literature is recommended.[12,24,25,26,27]

21.6 Interpretation

SSEP recordings are useful to assay both cortical and subcortical cerebral perfusion of structures involved in the generation of the responses. The most accepted alarm criterion for significant SSEP change is a persistent 50% reduction in primary somatosensory cortical amplitude or a latency delay >10% from baseline. This change should persist in more than two

average trials to rule out technical issues like noise as the reason for the change, thus avoiding unnecessary alarm.[7,11,13]

In a study performed by our group involving 976 patients during endoscopic endonasal skull base surgery (ESBS), the positive and negative predictive values of SSEPs to predict neurovascular deficits were 80.00 and 99.79%, respectively.[7] These changes improved or did not worsen with increases in blood pressure and no patient had postoperative neurological deficit.

Another interesting finding in this study was related to the false-positive group. The mean time for recognition of a significant change from the beginning of the procedure was 95 minutes in this group compared to 196 minutes in the true-positive group ($p < 0.05$). Thus, it is prudent to exercise additional caution when recognizing and informing the surgical team of SSEP changes in the early part of the procedure particularly when no clinical correlation can be identified. Anesthesia and position effects should always be considered before alarming the surgical team. Another reason described for false positive is the intraoperative formation of pneumocephalus which was identified on the postoperative CT in one of the cases of false positive reporting in this study.

BAEP recording is particularly useful in detecting brainstem ischemia during manipulation around the vertebrobasilar circulation as is the case for surgery involving petrous or clival tumors. In these cases, significant BAEP changes are best reflected by measuring the amplitude and latency of wave V, considering that vascular complications in skull base procedures typically affect the brainstem at or proximal to the level of superior olivary complex.[5,6] Warning criteria include prolongation of 0.5 to 1 ms of wave V or, more importantly, reduction of its amplitude by >50% in more than two consecutive averaged trials.[5,6,18,28] However, it is recommended that the neurophysiologist dynamically report wave V changes to keep the surgical team aware of progressive changes. Thus, once the change reaches the alarm criteria (or before), immediate corrective action can be taken.

Regarding EEG, a decrease of amplitude or fast activities by >50%, or an increase of slow activities by >50% is indicative of hypoperfusion. Loss of all frequency bands indicates severe hypoperfusion. Regarding quantitative EEG, a 95% spectral edge frequencies (SEF) decrease of more than 50% or a 40 to 50% decrease of total power are considered warning criteria;[11] an example of the change in EEG is discussed in Case 2. These changes are more often ipsilateral to a damaged ICA or middle cerebral artery (MCA), but also can be bilateral or even contralateral owing to suppression of collateral compensation.

EEG is particularly helpful should injury to the internal carotid or its cortical branches occur. These are rare but potentially devastating complications. Should an injury occur, real-time information about distal perfusion provided by EEG combined with cortical SSEP activity will be crucial as a guide for immediate management. Often, bleeding is stopped using pressure applied by packing which can compromise cerebral perfusion. Should the injured vessel need to be sacrificed, a lack of significant EEG and SSEP changes under temporary occlusion can be used as an index of sufficient collateral perfusion. Should significant changes occur, primary repair of the vessel is indicated and measures to provide brain protection, such as burst suppression, can be employed during the repair. It should also be recognized that if changes do not occur it is advisable, prior to permanent vessel sacrifice, that provocative testing be performed with SSEP and EEG guidance. This can be done by decreasing the patient's blood pressure to determine if the IONM tolerates a decrease in cerebral perfusion. This is important as general anesthesia provides a level of brain protection such that cerebral metabolism and consequent CBF is already decreased in this patient population. Only if the patient's IONM data remains completely unchanged during the provocative testing should vessel sacrifice be considered potentially safe.

EEG has some advantages over SSEP-only recording. EEG offers faster feedback since SSEP recording requires averaging which takes nearly a minute to complete and hence is not an instantaneous measure. EEG also provides a more widespread and comprehensive assessment of global cortical function as compared to SSEPs which may inform primarily only about anterior parietal (somatosensory) cortical function. On the other hand, EEG cannot provide information about subcortical structures while SSEP can. No specific studies have compared the diagnostic accuracy of these modalities to detect cerebral hypoperfusion in carotid injury. Based on carotid endarterectomy data, SSEP has a higher mean sensitivity while mean EEG and SSEP specificities are similar.[8,14,17] In the same context, we have demonstrated a higher accuracy for predicting perioperative stroke with the combined use of EEG and SSEP than monitoring with either of these modalities alone.[15]

The lack of consensus about alarm criteria for TcMEPs is a significant limiting factor in its utility. Although some groups only notify the surgeon when the TcMEP is absent, others prefer to report an alert when there is a consistent decrease in amplitude greater than 50 or 80%.[19,22,23,29] However, this last criterion has been associated with a significant number of false-positive alerts. An increase in the threshold stimulus intensity required to elicit the TcMEP or a decrease of its complexity has also been used as alarm criteria, though to be clear, no prospective studies have been done to compare and evaluate any TcMEP alarm criteria. Alarms based on latency changes are generally not useful for TcMEP.

The benefit of using TcMEP in IONM has been demonstrated in a wide range of intracranial procedures, particularly aneurysm clipping,[19,29] but scarce data can be found concerning its value in skull base surgeries. Considering the proportion of only 0.2% of false negative using SSEP during endoscopic endonasal approach (EEA) procedure in our study mentioned above,[7] it is not clear whether the addition of TcMEP would provide additional benefits in all cases. However, one potential benefit of TcMEPs would be to detect internal capsular ischemia secondary to perforating artery vasospasm or occlusion, which cannot be detected by SSEP, EEG, or BAEP monitoring. Another study which evaluated significant changes of multimodality IONM during resection of infratentorial lesions in 305 patients found a sensitivity and a specificity of SSEP and MEP for long tract deficit of 95 and 85%, respectively, with 48% of positive predictive value and 99% of negative predictive value.[10] In this study, the accuracy of SSEP and MEP were combined without an analysis of each one separately.

Considering the different possible mechanisms that can contribute to vascular complications, the monitoring regimen should encompass a strategy that assesses the entire neural axis from the peripheral nerve to the cortex and focuses on the region potentially affected. Once the strengths and limitations of each modality are well understood, the team will be able to interpret the findings adequately. Henceforth, changes in IONM during skull base surgery can provide real-time information about cerebral perfusion and impending but often reversible perioperative neurological deficits. Similarly, the negative predictive values provide us with confidence and reassurance that tumor resection can continue when no IONM changes are observed, increasing the probability of a total resection without new neurological deficits.

21.7 Case Examples

21.7.1 Case 1: IONM as an Indicator of Adequate Brain Perfusion

A 7-year-old boy presented with headache and diplopia related to left CN VI palsy. MRI of brain revealed a large clival lesion, consistent with chordoma, with extension to the petrous bone and parapharyngeal space and adjacent to the petrous and parapharyngeal segments of the ICA (▶ Fig. 21.1a). The patient had endoscopic endonasal transclival, transsellar, and infrapetrous approaches assisted by a transcervical incision for proximal ICA control. Four limb baseline SSEPs were present and symmetric at baseline. During the tumor exposure, the left lacerum segment of the ICA was inadvertently injured with a cutting rongeur. The site of bleeding was packed, and the cervical ICA was clipped without changes in SSEPs (▶ Fig. 21.1b). After removal of the packing, there was brisk back-bleeding from the distal stump of the injured ICA but still no change in the baseline SSEPs, even with induced hypotension. The ICA was sacrificed using bipolar coagulation considering the neurophysiological indicator of adequate cerebral perfusion.

The patient remained hemodynamically and electrophysiologically stable, and it was decided to proceed with the remaining resection. After the surgery, under continued SSEP monitoring, the patient was taken for endovascular evaluation which demonstrated complete occlusion of the left intracranial ICA (▶ Fig. 21.1c). Fortunately, good cross filling of left anterior chamber area (ACA) and MCA was detected via widely patent anterior communicating artery in addition to anomalous connections between external carotid and internal carotid also providing some filling of the ICA branches especially left MCA (▶ Fig. 21.1d). Further protection of the sacrificed ICA was made with proximal coil embolization. Postoperative MRI had no ischemic changes and confirmed complete tumor resection which was allowed by the real-time, intraoperative information about the functional, neurological status provided via IONM.

21.7.2 Case 2: IONM as an Indicator of Insufficient Brain Perfusion

A 39-year-old female presented with clinical and hormonal features consistent with acromegaly. Her MRI with contrast showed a macroadenoma with extension into the right cavernous sinus encasing the ICA and suprasellar extension abutting the optic chiasm. She underwent a transsellar and transcavernous EEA resection. Four limbs baseline SSEPs were present and symmetric. The procedure was complicated by a laceration of the distal cavernous segment of the right ICA. There were sig-

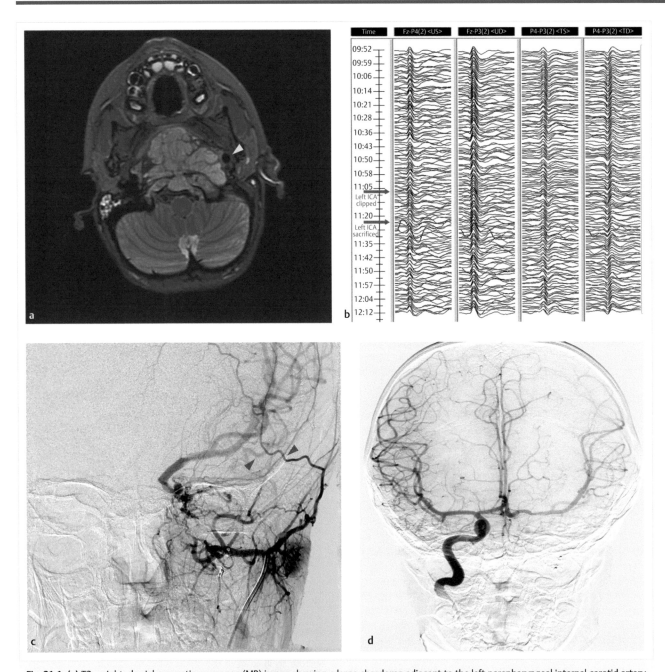

Fig. 21.1 **(a)** T2-weighted axial magnetic resonance (MR) image showing a large chordoma adjacent to the left parapharyngeal internal carotid artery (ICA) (*arrowhead*). **(b)** Waterfall plot showing stable somatosensory evoked potential (SSEP) in the four limbs despite injury and sacrifice of the left ICA. **(c)** Postoperative angiogram showing a left common carotid artery injection demonstrating complete occlusion of the left ICA with anomalous external carotid to internal carotid connections (*arrowheads*) providing some filling of left-sided branches, especially the left middle cerebral artery (MCA). **(d)** Postoperative angiogram showing good cross-filling of left anterior chamber area (ACA) and MCA via a widely patent anterior communicating artery.

nificant difficulties packing the site of bleeding and following attempted aneurysm clip placement and finally packing, a significant reduction of 60 to 70% in the amplitude of right cortical/left limbs SSEPs were noted (▶ Fig. 21.2). These SSEP changes were blood pressure dependent suggesting that an occlusive lesion in the cavernous segment of the ICA could not be tolerated. A Foley balloon was placed, and then the patient was taken urgently to neurointerventional radiology (NIR). Angiography showed near-complete occlusion of the injured

ICA with no cross fill. During the endovascular procedure, there was a fluctuation in the amplitude on the right cortical SSEP worse in the lower limb where the potential was lost at two time points of the early manipulation. EEG was in anesthetic-induced burst suppression and showed only a mild asymmetry with lower amplitudes in the right hemisphere (▶ Fig. 21.3). TcMEPs were not recorded in the OR or in NIR. Three overlapping stents were placed, and the flow in the right ICA was restored. Cortical SSEP responses improved entirely in upper limb

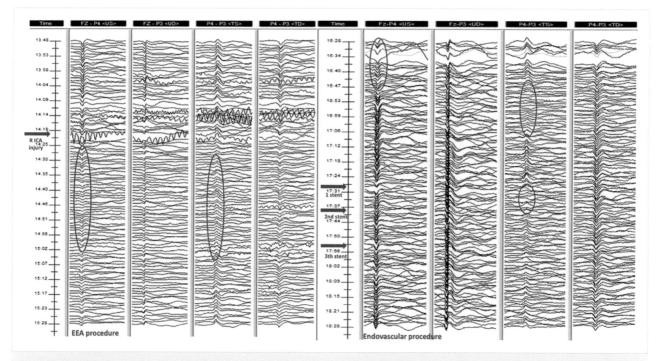

Fig. 21.2 Waterfall plot showing unstable left limbs somatosensory evoked potentials (SSEPs) during endoscopic endonasal surgery (left) and endovascular procedure (right). Critical reduction points in SSEP were encircled. By the end of the endovascular procedure, US SSEP has improved entirely, and TS was in progressive recovery.

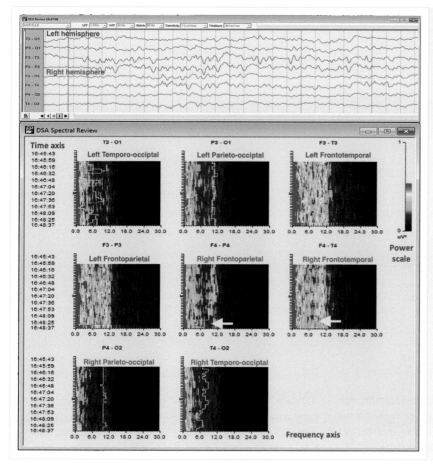

Fig. 21.3 Raw (upper panel) and digital spectral electroencephalography (EEG) (lower panel) exhibiting only slight asymmetry with lower amplitudes in the right hemisphere indicating critical brain hypoperfusion. Warm colors reflect more prominent frequencies while cold colors represent frequencies that are less prominent.

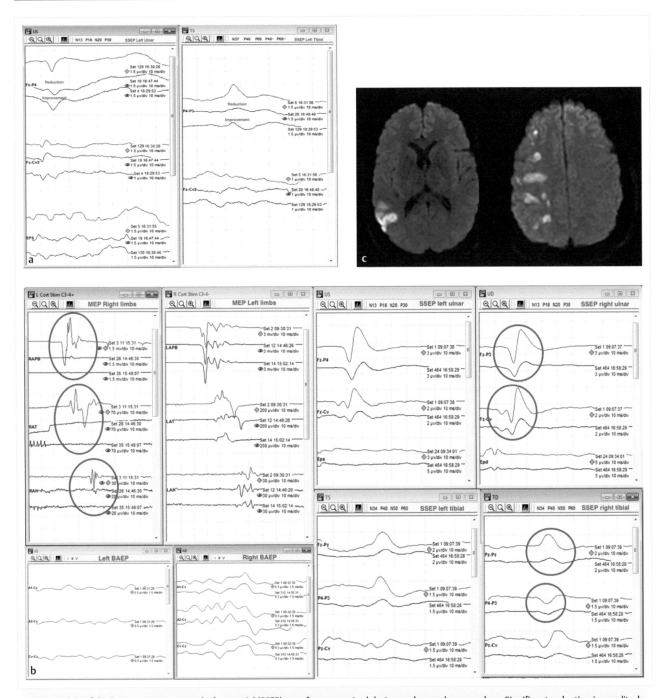

Fig. 21.4 (a) Left limbs somatosensory evoked potential (SSEP) waveforms acquired during endovascular procedure. Significant reduction in amplitude of cortical response followed by improvement after stent placement. **(b)** Angiogram showing right internal carotid artery (ICA) nearly occluded with sluggish filling in the cervical, petrous, and cavernous segments. In the cavernous segment, an area of critical stenosis is seen at the site of the vessel defect. Post cavernous carotid artery segment stenting: the right ICA demonstrates significantly improved flow without any distal filling defects noted. **(c)** Postoperative diffusion-weighted imaging (DWI) magnetic resonance (MR) showing multiple areas of infarction in the anterior and posterior watershed distributions.

and was recovering in the lower limb at the end of the endovascular procedure (▶ Fig. 21.4a, b).

The patient woke up without neurological deficits although postoperative MRI demonstrated small areas of restricted diffusion in the right anterior and posterior watershed distribution (▶ Fig. 21.4c). Residual tumor around the right ICA was treated with gamma knife radiosurgery.

21.7.3 Case 3: IONM as a Predictor of a Large Postoperative Stroke

A 78-year-old woman with recent breast cancer history presented with diplopia and facial numbness. She was found to have a left cavernous sinus mass which was encasing and constricting the left carotid artery. She underwent a transsellar

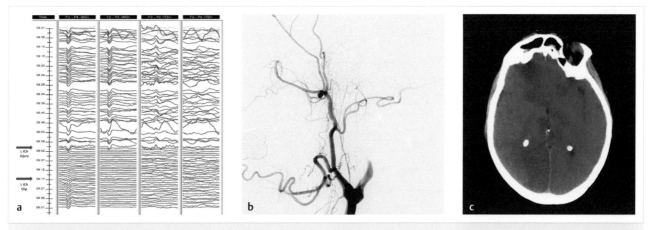

Fig. 21.5 **(a)** A waterfall plot of somatosensory evoked potential (SSEP) responses shows loss of cortical responses of bilateral lower limbs and right upper limb as well as significant but transient reduction of the amplitude of left upper limb. **(b)** Cerebral angiogram of common carotid artery injection showing complete occlusion of the left internal carotid artery (ICA). **(c)** Postoperative computed tomography (CT) confirmed wide infarction involving the entire left cerebral hemisphere as well as the right anterior chamber area (ACA) and posterior cerebral artery (PCA) matching with the intraoperative neurophysiologic findings.

transcavernous endoscopic endonasal biopsy. Four limbs baseline SSEPs were present and symmetric. Following biopsy of the portion of the tumor medial to the left carotid artery, a minimal amount of bleeding was noticed from this area and then packed off. When the surgeon was starting to harvest fat graft for closure, the cortical SSEP responses were lost from the right upper limb, and both the lower limbs besides an 80% reduction of amplitude from the left upper limb (▶ Fig. 21.5a). The left carotid artery began to bleed profusely when packing was removed. New attempts to stop the bleeding were made with cottonoid and a Fogarty balloon without success. The surgeons were forced to sacrifice the artery with two clips despite the neurophysiologic changes. By the end of the surgery, the left upper SSEP had recovered to 60% of the baseline but the SSEP of the other three limbs remained absent.

The patient was rushed to angiogram where she was found to have complete occlusion of the left ICA which supplied the majority of the intracranial vasculature (▶ Fig. 21.5b). Postoperative CT showed catastrophic infarction involving the entire left cerebral hemisphere as well as right ACA and PCA territories matching the neurophysiological findings (▶ Fig. 21.5c). The patient died on the third postoperative day.

21.7.4 Case 4: IONM as a Predictor of a Subcortical Stroke

A 74-year-old woman presented with a history of petroclival meningioma which had a previous retromastoid resection with good debulking but complicated by left hearing loss and left CN VI palsy. The tumor proved to be a WHO grade 2 with high Ki-67 and within few months had rapid growth of the clival

residual portion with significant brainstem compression associated with dysphagia and severe ataxia.

The patient underwent a transclival endoscopic endonasal surgery under multimodality IONM with SSEP, MEP, BAEP, and EMG. Baselines were present and symmetric except for the absent left BAEP. During the resection, while the surgeon was resecting tumor from the left side of the brainstem, the left cortical MEP was lost. Additionally, there was a 60% reduction in the amplitude of the left cortical SSEPs. The right BAEP stayed stable (▶ Fig. 21.6). No bleeding or any other indication of vascular injury was visualized by the surgeon and he decided to complete the tumor debulking without any further extracapsular dissection. There was no improvement at the IONM responses through the end of the procedure. The patient woke up with dense right hemiparesis and a partial right CN VI palsy. Postoperative MRI showed early infarction involving the pons, right occipital pole, and hippocampus compatible with an occlusive event in the posterior circulation (▶ Fig. 21.7).

21.8 Conclusion

Although rare, vascular complications have the potential to have catastrophic clinical consequences. As such, real-time information concerning adequate cerebral perfusion in the form of IONM can optimize its management. IONM can identify impending injury, serve as a guide to interventions, and evaluate their efficacy. For its optimum use, multimodality IONM should be tailored to each case considering the risks related to the lesion topography and the surgical approach as well as having a fundamental understanding of the strengths and limitations of specific IONM modalities.

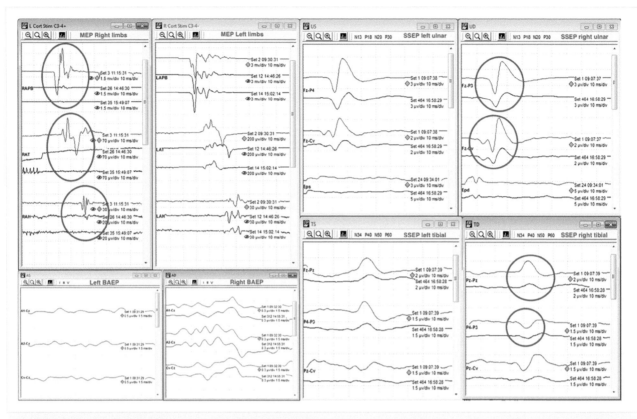

Fig. 21.6 The graphics show loss of left cortical motor evoked potential (MEP) in addition to significant reduction of amplitude in the left cortical somatosensory evoked potential (SSEP) (baselines are in red and the last potentials in black); the changed potentials are circled. **MEP**: L cort Stim C3–4 + : right hemibody and R cort Stim C3–4 + : left hemibody; **BAEP**: AS: left and AD: right; **SSEP**: TD, right tibial; TS, left tibial; UD, right ulnar; US, left ulnar.

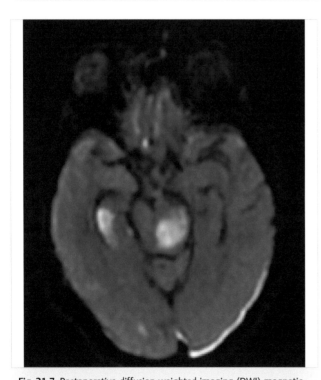

Fig. 21.7 Postoperative diffusion-weighted imaging (DWI) magnetic resonance imaging (MRI) showing areas of interval early infarction involving the left pons, right occipital pole, and right hippocampus compatible with an embolic mechanism or vasospasm.

References

[1] Rhoton AL, Jr. The supratentorial arteries. Neurosurgery. 2002; 51(4) Suppl: S53–S120

[2] Gardner PA, Tormenti MJ, Pant H, Fernandez-Miranda JC, Snyderman CH, Horowitz MB. Carotid artery injury during endoscopic endonasal skull base surgery: incidence and outcomes. Neurosurgery. 2013; 73(2) Suppl Operative:ons261–ons269, discussion ons269–ons270

[3] Kassam AB, Prevedello DM, Carrau RL, et al. Endoscopic endonasal skull base surgery: analysis of complications in the authors' initial 800 patients. J Neurosurg. 2011; 114(6):1544–1568

[4] Inamasu J, Guiot BH. Iatrogenic carotid artery injury in neurosurgery. Neurosurg Rev. 2005; 28(4):239–247, discussion 248

[5] Singh H, Vogel RW, Lober RM, et al. Intraoperative neurophysiological monitoring for endoscopic endonasal approaches to the skull base: a technical guide. Scientifica (Cairo). 2016; 2016:1751245

[6] Thirumala PD, Kodavatiganti HS, Habeych M, et al. Value of multimodality monitoring using brainstem auditory evoked potentials and somatosensory evoked potentials in endoscopic endonasal surgery. Neurol Res. 2013; 35(6): 622–630

[7] Thirumala PD, Kassasm AB, Habeych M, et al. Somatosensory evoked potential monitoring during endoscopic endonasal approach to skull base surgery: analysis of observed changes. Neurosurgery. 2011; 69(1) Suppl Operative:ons64–ons76, discussion ons76

[8] Florence G, Guerit J-M, Gueguen B. Electroencephalography (EEG) and somatosensory evoked potentials (SEP) to prevent cerebral ischaemia in the operating room. Neurophysiol Clin. 2004; 34(1):17–32

[9] Elangovan C, Singh SP, Gardner P, et al. Intraoperative neurophysiological monitoring during endoscopic endonasal surgery for pediatric skull base tumors. J Neurosurg Pediatr. 2016; 17(2):147–155

[10] Slotty PJ, Abdulazim A, Kodama K, et al. Intraoperative neurophysiological monitoring during resection of infratentorial lesions: the surgeon's view. J Neurosurg. 2017; 126(1):281–288

[11] Guérit J-M. Intraoperative monitoring during carotid endarterectomy. In: Nuwer MR, ed. Intraoperative Monitoring of Neural Function. Vol. 8. Elsevier; 2008:776–790

[12] Griessenauer CJ, Fisher WS III. Techniques of regional cerebral blood flow measurement and relationship of rCBF to other monitoring methods. In: Loftus CM, Biller J, Baron EM, eds. Intraoperative Neuromonitoring. McGraw-Hill Education; 2014

[13] Simon MV. Neurophysiologic test used in the operating room. In: Intraoperative Neurophysiology. New York: Demos Medical; 2010:1–46

[14] Nwachuku EL, Balzer JR, Yabes JG, Habeych ME, Crammond DJ, Thirumala PD. Diagnostic value of somatosensory evoked potential changes during carotid endarterectomy: a systematic review and meta-analysis. JAMA Neurol. 2015; 72(1):73–80

[15] Thirumala PD, Natarajan P, Thiagarajan K, et al. Diagnostic accuracy of somatosensory evoked potential and electroencephalography during carotid endarterectomy. Neurol Res. 2016; 38(8):698–705

[16] Markand ON. Continuous assessment of cerebral function with EEG and somatosensory evoked potential techniques during extracranial vascular reconstruction. In: Loftus CL, Biller J, Barron EM, eds. Intraoperative Neuromonitoring. McGraw-Hill Education; 2014:23–45

[17] Thirumala PD, Thiagarajan K, Gedela S, Crammond DJ, Balzer JR. Diagnostic accuracy of EEG changes during carotid endarterectomy in predicting perioperative strokes. J Clin Neurosci. 2016; 25:1–9

[18] American Clinical Neurophysiology Society. Guideline 9C: guidelines on short-latency auditory evoked potentials. J Clin Neurophysiol. 2006; 23(2): 157–167

[19] Szelényi A, Kothbauer K, de Camargo AB, Langer D, Flamm ES, Deletis V. Motor evoked potential monitoring during cerebral aneurysm surgery: technical aspects and comparison of transcranial and direct cortical stimulation. Neurosurgery. 2005; 57(4) Suppl:331–338, discussion 331–338

[20] Klem GH, Lüèders HO, Jasper HH, Elger C. The ten±twenty electrode system of the International Federation. In: Recommendations for the Practice of Clinical Neurophysiology: Guidelines of the International Federation of Clinical Physiology (EEG Suppl. 52). Elsevier Science B.V.; 1999:3–6

[21] Szelényi A, Kothbauer KF, Deletis V. Transcranial electric stimulation for intraoperative motor evoked potential monitoring: stimulation parameters and electrode montages. Clin Neurophysiol. 2007; 118(7):1586–1595

[22] Macdonald DB, Skinner S, Shils J, Yingling C, American Society of Neurophysiological Monitoring. Intraoperative motor evoked potential monitoring—a position statement by the American Society of Neurophysiological Monitoring. Clin Neurophysiol. 2013; 124(12):2291–2316

[23] Legatt AD, Emerson RG, Epstein CM, et al. ACNS guideline: transcranial electrical stimulation motor evoked potential monitoring. J Clin Neurophysiol. 2016; 33 (1):42–50

[24] Jäntii V, Sloan TB. EEG and anesthetic effects. In: Nuwer MR, ed. Intraoperative Monitoring of Neural Function. Vol. 8. Elsevier B. V.; 2008:77–93

[25] Sloan TB, Jäntii V. Anesthesic effects on evoked potentials. In: Nuwer MR, ed. Intraoperative Monitoring of Neural Function. Vol. 8. Elsevier B. V.; 2008:94–126

[26] James ML. Anesthetic considerations. In: Hussain A, ed. A Practical Approach to Neurophysiologic Intraoperative Monitoring. Demos; 2008:55–66

[27] Simon MV. The effects of anesthetics on intraoperative neurophysiology studies. In: Simon MV, ed. Intraoperative Clinical Neurophysiology. New York: Demos Medical; 2010:325–334

[28] Thirumala PD, Carnovale G, Habeych ME, Crammond DJ, Balzer JR. Diagnostic accuracy of brainstem auditory evoked potentials during microvascular decompression. Neurology. 2014; 83(19):1747–1752

[29] Szelényi A, Langer D, Beck J, et al. Transcranial and direct cortical stimulation for motor evoked potential monitoring in intracerebral aneurysm surgery. Neurophysiol Clin. 2007; 37(6):391–398

22 Simulation and Training—Preparing for Vascular Injury

Rowan Valentine and Peter-John Wormald

Summary

Vascular injury is perhaps the most challenging complication of skull base surgery to manage. Given that most skull base pathologies are centered around major vascular structures, surgical training on their management is critical. Surgical simulators create a vehicle for the development and teaching of surgical skill acquisition and excellence. Recently there has been a range of vascular injury simulators developed, predominantly synthetic, cadaveric, or live animal simulators. Each model has its own advantages such as portability, anatomical accuracy, or hemostatic physiology. Most importantly, simulated training of endoscopic skull base surgeons has allowed the development of the surgical techniques required to control the surgical field and identify methods and technologies that reliably achieve rapid hemostasis in this setting. Simulated training improves surgeon's confidence and skill during vascular events, resulting in superior outcomes for patients.

Keywords: Vascular injury, carotid artery, endoscopic, skull base surgery, simulation, surgical training

22.1 Key Learning Points

- Preparing and training for a major vascular event through simulation is imperative.
- Controlling the surgical field is the first vital step; "if you can't see then you can't do."
- Animal simulation models provide surgical confidence in hemostatic techniques with physiological accuracy.
- Simulation and training for vascular injury improves patient outcomes.

22.2 Introduction

Over the last few decades there has been a universally accepted paradigm shift from traditional external approaches to endoscopic endonasal approaches (EEAs) for many areas of the skull base. The benefits of the endonasal corridor over traditional approaches include reduced hospital admission times, improved visualization, minimized surgical morbidity by avoiding sacrifice of intervening structures, and avoidance of external skin incisions and brain retraction.[1] This change in direction has been driven by technological innovations and the development of new and improved surgical instrumentation. Vitally important (as with all new surgical corridors) is improved understanding of endoscopic endonasal anatomy, especially the course of the internal carotid artery (ICA). However, surgical technique advances rely not only on improved surgical instrumentation and anatomic understanding but also on surgeon's training and experience.

Endonasal transphenoidal pituitary surgery has become universally accepted and is commonplace, with a low estimated ICA injury rate of 0.3%.[2] Ciric et al performed an interesting postal questionnaire survey involving over 900 microscopic transsphenoidal neurosurgeons, enquiring about their complication profile. Surgeons with an experience of over 500 transsphenoidal pituitary approaches had a 50% chance of intraoperative ICA injury.[3] This highlights that increasing subspecialization of endoscopic pituitary surgery will increase the chance that the team will need to know how to manage a carotid artery catastrophe.[4] Additionally, endoscopic management of advanced skull base pathologies centering on the ICA come with a greater risk of ICA rupture. Endoscopic resections of craniopharyngiomas, clival chordomas, and chondrosarcomas have a vascular injury rate of up to 2 to 9%.[5,6,7]

Vascular injury, during either endoscopic endonasal or open surgery, is perhaps the most challenging complication of skull base surgery to manage. It creates immediate confusion and panic among the skull base team and is incredibly anxiety provoking. Ordered systematic thought during the chaos of a vascular injury is virtually impossible, leading to a need for prospective training of skull base teams in its management. Training of specialist skull base surgical teams on how to manage this challenging event will help to improve patient outcomes.

It is not surprising to see that there is a lack of high-quality research in the field of appropriate techniques and protocols for the management of major vascular injuries. Surgeons are reluctant to publish their experience with vascular injuries and articles that are published are typically case reports only without scientific prospective research into the best surgical techniques required.

22.3 Simulation Training

Simulation of a real-world scenario allows the users to gain experience and to observe and interact with the simulation via realistic visual, auditory, or tactile cues.[8] This is usually done in the form of a device or model. Experience with simulators began with flight simulation, used for improving aviation safety and pilot training. Both aviation disasters and major vascular injuries during surgery are unpredictable and uncommon. This makes traditional skill acquisition via the apprentice model of teaching not possible. Surgical simulation creates a vehicle for research and development, to develop and teach surgical skill acquisition and excellence and to transfer these learned techniques to the operating room.[9]

Surgical simulators each have their own advantages and disadvantages, with a range of different types existing. Bench top-based models are easily portable and cheap, and require no specific supervision but are the least realistic and inanimate. Cadavers have the advantages of anatomical accuracy and high fidelity; however, they can be expensive with limited availability of material. Cadaver models are excellent for surgical field training but are limited for hemostatic evaluation, requiring pump perfusion for a realistic simulation.[10] Virtual reality provides the opportunity for reusable simulation with anatomical accuracy, with immediate objective feedback but sense of realism varies greatly and it may also appear inanimate.

Animal models have been used for many years, with experience as far back as 600 bc.[11] They play an important role in surgical education and training in the medical field. Live animals have a high level of fidelity, and offer the most realistic experience with regard to major vascular injuries and tissue hemostasis due to the similarities in tissue construct and blood constituents. Major disadvantages, however, are ethical issues, animal welfare laws, anatomical differences, high costs, and requirement of special facilities.

22.4 Vascular Injury Simulation

Surgical skill simulation improves operating room skill, proficiency, and surgical confidence. The development of the ideal intraoperative vascular injury simulator is challenging. It needs to be able to show attributes such as standardization, validation, and reproduction, allowing its use in research and training. Research and development rely on accurate reproducibility of the vascular injury simulator every time it is used.

Creating familiarity is perhaps the most important attribute of a surgical simulator if training in vascular injuries is to be effective. Surgeons need to be immediately familiar with the surgical environment and instrumentation that they will be using to manage the vascular event. This eliminates one major hurdle in skill acquisition. If special instrumentation or materials are required, simulation exercises provide the opportunity for the surgeon to develop familiarity for those rare events when they are employed.

Each scenario of a vascular injury has a unique set of challenging circumstances or constraints. The ideal surgical simulator should be able to recreate these challenges and circumstances. For example, surgical exposure at the site of injury may range from limited such as during a sphenoidotomy during endoscopic sinus surgery to wide surgical exposure during an expanded skull base resection. An endonasal vascular injury also occurs down a narrow nasal corridor where even a small amount of blood may immediately disorientate the surgeon and obscure the surgical field.

Not all vascular injury configurations are the same and will depend on the surgical instrument that caused the injury. Padhye et al[12] investigated various hemostatic techniques in a range of injury configurations. Injury types investigated included a 3 mm punch injury, a 4 mm linear injury, and a 4-mm stellate injury. This study identified that the linear injury type was associated with the greatest volume of blood loss and the longest time to achieving hemostasis, hence the most challenging to manage. Clearly the size of the injury also has major impact on the ability to and options for control.

Challenging vascular injury scenarios may have different pressure and volume characteristics. High-flow/low-pressure scenarios such as cavernous sinus bleeding are considered easier to control during endoscopic approaches as the surgical field is less threatened. Visualization of the defect site is easier in low pressure scenarios and easier for the surgical team to act accordingly. In contrast, high-flow/high-pressure injuries such as the ICA create a pulsatile blood stream that rapidly fills the surgical field, making visualization of the injury site much more difficult. In an animal model, rapid exsanguination from an ICA rupture may occur, which will change the vascular

event rapidly from a high-flow/high-pressure scenario to the high-flow/low-pressure scenario. Thus, rapid active resuscitation is important during ICA vascular injury simulation to maintain the more challenging high-flow/high-pressure vessel injury characteristics.

Vascular injuries can also have short-term and long-term vessel complications such as secondary bleed, pseudoaneurysm formation, and vascular occlusion. Minimizing morbidity following a carotid artery injury relies primarily on achieving hemostasis, but secondarily on maintaining vascular patency. The ongoing assessment of the injury site over time is important but often overlooked in simulating vascular injuries to allow analysis of the incidence of these complications and determine the best management algorithm.

The working environment should also closely simulate the clinical scenario as much as possible, which has been shown to improve skill acquisition.[13] The use of anesthetic machines, monitoring equipment, pressure bag resuscitation, and the ability to monitor blood pressure and pulse parameters immediately recreates the familiarity of a working operating room. Perhaps most important is the recreation of the "life or death" pressure scenario, placing the trainee in immediate and obvious surgical stress. As such, large animals are ideal in vascular catastrophe simulation as they have a similar blood volume to humans, have similar blood pressure, and pulse characteristics and are robust.

22.5 Cadaver Models of Endoscopic Vascular Injury

Recently there have been a number of endoscopic vascular injury cadaver models that offer a range of advantages and disadvantages. These models have the advantage of anatomical accuracy for endonasal surgery[12,13] and Pacca et al even used an aortic balloon pump to recreate the pulsatile nature of blood flow.[10] These models are very useful for training surgeons in surgical field control techniques and improving surgeon's confidence. The less significant operational cost of these models improves accessibility. The main downsides to these models, however, are the lack of physiological hemostatic accuracy and absence of feedback to the surgeon regarding delayed outcomes of successful hemostatic technique.

22.6 The Sheep Model of Vascular Injury

Animal models of vascular injury provide accurate feedback and confidence to surgeons regarding the use of different hemostatic techniques. Sheep have the advantage of being a robust animal with a similar blood volume to humans and similar-sized carotid artery to the human ICA at the skull base. All sheep are weighed to ensure a weight greater than 20 kg. This minimum size ensures an accurate comparison to the caliber of the intracavernous ICA in humans. Coagulation profiling and full blood count is performed preoperatively. All sheep are fasted 12 to 18 hours before surgery. General anesthesia is induced and performed via injection with sodium thiopentone (19 mg/kg body weight) into the left jugular vein. Endotracheal

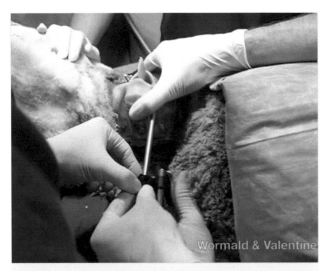

Fig. 22.1 The model is fixed to the operating table with vessel sited within the model.

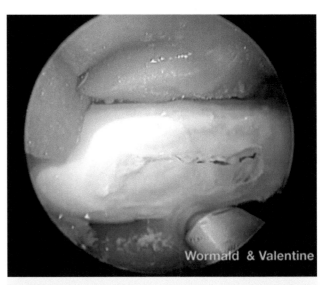

Fig. 22.2 A drill is used to thin the plastic cover over the carotid artery.

intubation then follows with maintenance anesthesia maintained by inhalation of 1.5 to 2.0% isoflurane, to a depth that allows spontaneous ventilation and minimizes hypotension.

The sheep are positioned on their backs and a midline neck incision is performed from the thyroid cartilage to the base of the neck, through the superficial layer of the deep cervical fascia to the anterior tracheal wall. The visceral fascia is then dissected from the lateral tracheal wall to reveal the right carotid sheath. The right common carotid artery is then dissected free for a length of 15 cm from the angle of the mandible to the base of the neck. The left carotid artery is also dissected and identified as described above. The left carotid artery is then cannulated to allow for continuous invasive arterial pressure monitoring and the left internal jugular vein is cannulated with a rapid infusion catheter exchange set (Arrow International Inc., Reading, Pennsylvania) to allow for rapid fluid resuscitation.

The Sinus Model Otorhino Neuro Trainer (SIMONT, Prodelphus, Brazil) is added onto the sheep model and simulates the endoscopic environment so that carotid injuries can be managed with the anatomical accuracy of the limitations and confines seen in the human nasal vestibule, nasal cavity, and sphenoid sinus. This model is an accurate reconstruction of the anatomical features of the human nasal cavity and paranasal sinuses. Surgical neoderma is a specifically patented material that recreates the colors, consistency, and elasticity of the nasal mucosa and paranasal sinus bony architecture. This model allows the use of routine sinus and skull base surgical instrumentation and provides the realistic tissue resistances encountered during endonasal surgery. Bilateral large sphenoidotomies and partial middle turbinectomies are performed. A detachable posterior sphenoid sinus wall has been designed to allow the placement of the freely dissected carotid artery into the sphenoid sinus. A plastic cover is placed over the vessel that mimics the thin bony covering over the carotid artery. A specific fastener system has been developed that allows this vessel to be held within the model and prevents blood leaking around the back of the model, allowing blood to run out through the nares of the model. Absence of carotid compression on entry and exit

of the carotid artery into and out of the model is confirmed visually and by observing no change in the mean arterial pressure between the left and right carotid arteries. The model construction is then fixed to the operating table and onto the neck of the sheep to prevent displacement during surgical intervention (▶ Fig. 22.1). Importantly, this model has also been modified to allow the use of the internal jugular vein of the sheep, creating a less challenging low-pressure/high-flow vascular injury scenario. This provides stepwise skill acquisition from a less challenging situation to the carotid blowout scenario.

A standard skull base burr and 0-degree endoscope are used to drill away the plastic plate which simulates the thin bony covering of the carotid siphon within the sphenoid sinus (▶ Fig. 22.2). As is standard for some surgeons when exposing the carotid artery, a Hajek punch can then be utilized to expose the carotid artery creating a bony window, revealing the underlying vessel (▶ Fig. 22.3). This allows for the variable bony exposure that may be experienced during an unanticipated vascular event. An 11-blade scalpel can be used to create an approximately 4 mm longitudinal incision through the anterior wall of the carotid artery (▶ Fig. 22.4). Rapid bleeding occurs immediately, obstructing the surgical view (▶ Fig. 22.5).

Simultaneous fluid resuscitation with warmed normal saline is commenced at approximately 200 mL/minute. Rapid resuscitation with a pressure bag continues in order to maintain a mean arterial pressure at the preinjury level. Aggressive simultaneous fluid resuscitation ensures the maintenance of a high-flow, high-pressure vascular injury model. The adverse effects of hypothermia on the coagulation cascade are prevented by ensuring constant temperature control with the use of a thermal blanket (**Video 22.1**).[14]

22.7 Surgical Field Visualization and Control

Central to bleeding control is visualization. "If you can't see, then you can't do." Endoscopic endonasal control of a bleeding

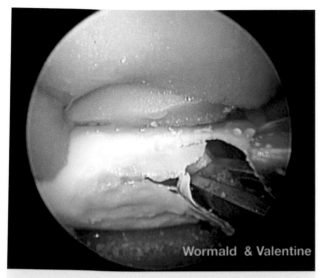

Fig. 22.3 A Hajek punch is used to expose the vessel within the sphenoid sinus.

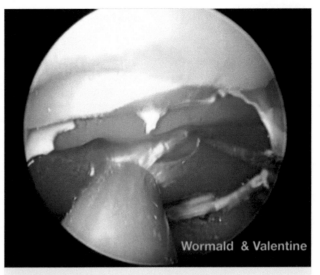

Fig. 22.4 A controlled 4 mm linear injury is created.

surgical field is more challenging due to the narrow confines of the nasal cavity. With a major arterial bleeding scenario in endoscopic surgery there is regular loss of vision and soiling of the endoscope, the so-called "red out." Visualization of the injury site is necessary to make decisions in regard to appropriate hemostatic techniques. Using the sheep model, Valentine and Wormald were able to simulate a total of 42 carotid and 25 venous injuries in the endoscopic environment and describe critical steps for control.[15,16]

A team-based approach to the management of vascular injury is critical. The two-surgeon technique permits one surgeon to navigate and clear the endoscope while the other has two hands free to manage bleeding. Multiple surgical instruments and suctions can be employed in the nasal cavity at the same time. The pulsatile jet of blood tends to favor one side of the nasal cavity over the other. As a result, vision is best gained by placing the endoscope on the side of the nasal cavity that is more protected, and using the posterior edge of the nasal septum as a shield to prevent constant soiling of the endoscope tip.

An endoscopic lens cleaning system is also a valuable asset as it prevents the constant need for removing the endoscope from the nasal cavity in order clean it, and allows the team to maintain their anatomical bearings and positioning of surgical instruments within the surgical field.

The larger the suction size, the greater the volume of blood that can be evacuated at any one time. A size of 12 French suction or larger is recommended. Sometimes a second suction is required due to the volume of blood, or to manipulate a nasoseptal flap or other tissue that may have "floated" into the surgical field. The suction tip can also be used to manipulate the stream of blood away from the endoscope. It is for this reason that suction placement down the nostril contralateral to the endoscope is important. The suction should hover directly above the site of injury to maintain visualization. These recommendations give the surgical team the best chance of maintaining visualization.

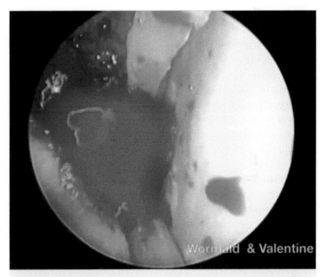

Fig. 22.5 A high-flow/high-pressure vascular injury is created.

22.8 Hemostatic Techniques in Simulated Vascular Injury

Although visualization is imperative, it is only one component of management. Definitive control and success are largely dependent on the hemostatic technique employed. A literature review reveals a range of hemostatic agents that have been used. Valentine et al performed the first scientific trial of different hemostatic agents in the setting of carotid bleeding.[17] The use of a flowable hemostatic matrix or oxidized regenerated cellulose resulted in a failure of primary hemostasis. Chitosan gel was effective in 50% of cases initially but failed to maintain hemostasis for the entire duration of the procedure. In contrast, a crushed muscle patch and U-clip anastomotic device (Medtronic, Jacksonville, FL) were both able to gain and maintain hemostasis in 100% of cases.

A follow-up study looked at different hemostatic agents and techniques and their effectiveness for different injury subtypes. Both short-term and long-term vessel complications were evaluated. Bipolar electrocautery has been described in the literature in case reports but had mixed results in gaining hemostasis. By contrast, the crushed muscle patch and aneurysm clip were able to gain primary hemostasis reliably in 100% of cases regardless of injury type. Crushed muscle had a low risk of destabilization and pseudoaneurysm formation and was the only hemostatic material associated with a 100% rate of long-term carotid patency. The aneurysm clip had no incidence of pseudoaneurysm and long-term preservation of blood flow depended on its placement. In addition to the U-clip and aneurysm clip, Padhye et al have investigated the Anastoclip (LeMaitre, Burlington, MA).[18] This device was able to gain primary hemostasis in 100% of cases and had a very low risk of pseudoaneurysm when compared to other techniques.

22.9 Outcomes of Vascular Simulation Training

A patient is at high risk of morbidity or mortality during an inadvertent ICA injury despite intraoperative management; complications such as stroke, pseudoaneurysm formation, and carotico-cavernous fistula may still occur. Pseudoaneurysms may have fatal consequences if these rupture, with a reported incidence of up to 60% after ICA injury.[15] Review of the current literature discovered 89 cases of published ICA injury, with a reported mortality rate of 15% and a permanent morbidity rate of 26%.[15]

An endoscopic ICA injury simulator has allowed for the trial of management techniques, but perhaps most importantly been employed in workshops to help train surgeons worldwide. Skull base teams are now able to practice the communication, teamwork, and hemostatic techniques required to confidently manage a carotid injury during endoscopic endonasal surgery.

Padhye et al recently reviewed the value of vascular injury training[16] in a retrospective case series study of endoscopic vascular trained surgeons and their cases of major endoscopic arterial hemorrhage. A total of nine cases were reported; eight were ICA injuries and one was a basilar artery injury. Free crushed muscle graft was used in each case at the injury site to successfully gain primary hemostasis. After initial intervention, there were two cases of carotid stenosis or occlusion and one pseudoaneurysm. In each instance, the patient underwent successful endovascular intervention and made otherwise unremarkable recoveries. In this series of endoscopic vascular trained surgeons, there was no mortality and no major morbidity, providing the evidence for the value of vascular training in this potentially devastating situation.

22.10 Conclusion

Vascular injury during skull base surgery can have disastrous complications. Increasing experience with endonasal and open skull base approaches and the development of specialist skull base teams mean that these teams need to be familiar with the techniques required to manage a major vascular injury. Perfused cadaver models can replicate the anatomic challenges with simulated bleeding, and live large animal surgical simulation accurately replicates the challenging physiological scenario of endoscopic surgical management of a high-flow/high-pressure vascular injury. Simulated training of endoscopic and open skull base surgeons has allowed the development of the surgical techniques required to control the surgical field and identify methods and technologies that reliably achieve rapid hemostasis. Simulated training improves surgeon's confidence and skill during vascular events, resulting in superior outcomes for patients.

References

[1] Kassam AB, Snyderman C, Gardner P, Carrau R, Spiro R. The expanded endonasal approach: a fully endoscopic transnasal approach and resection of the odontoid process: technical case report. Neurosurgery. 2005; 57(1) Suppl:E213–, discussion E213

[2] Gardner PA, Tormenti MJ, Pant H, Fernandez-Miranda JC, Snyderman CH, Horowitz MB. Carotid artery injury during endoscopic endonasal skull base surgery: incidence and outcomes. Neurosurgery. 2013; 73(2) Suppl Operative:ons261–ons269, discussion ons269–ons270

[3] Ciric I, Ragin A, Baumgartner C, Pierce D. Complications of transsphenoidal surgery: results of a national survey, review of the literature, and personal experience. Neurosurgery. 1997; 40(2):225–236, discussion 236–237

[4] Rowan NR, Turner MT, Valappil B, et al. Injury of the carotid artery during endoscopic endonasal surgery: surveys of skull base surgeons. J Neurol Surg B Skull Base. 2018; 79(3):302–308

[5] Couldwell WT, Weiss MH, Rabb C, Liu JK, Apfelbaum RI, Fukushima T. Variations on the standard transsphenoidal approach to the sellar region, with emphasis on the extended approaches and parasellar approaches: surgical experience in 105 cases. Neurosurgery. 2004; 55(3):539–547, discussion 547–550

[6] Frank G, Sciarretta V, Calbucci F, Farneti G, Mazzatenta D, Pasquini E. The endoscopic transnasal transsphenoidal approach for the treatment of cranial base chordomas and chondrosarcomas. Neurosurgery. 2006; 59(1) Suppl 1: ONS50–ONS57, discussion ONS50–ONS57

[7] Gardner PA, Kassam AB, Snyderman CH, et al. Outcomes following endoscopic, expanded endonasal resection of suprasellar craniopharyngiomas: a case series. J Neurosurg. 2008; 109(1):6–16

[8] Rosen JM, Long SA, McGrath DM, Greer SE. Simulation in plastic surgery training and education: the path forward. Plast Reconstr Surg. 2009; 123(2): 729–738, discussion 739–740

[9] Davies J, Khatib M, Bello F. Open surgical simulation—a review. J Surg Educ. 2013; 70(5):618–627

[10] Pacca P, Jhawar SS, Seclen DV, et al. "Live cadaver" model for internal carotid artery injury simulation in endoscopic endonasal skull base surgery. Oper Neurosurg (Hagerstown). 2017; 13(6):732–738

[11] Limberg AA. The planning of local plastic operations on the body surface: theory and practice. Lexington, MA: DC Heath and Company; 1984

[12] Padhye V, Valentine R, Paramasivan S, et al. Early and late complications of endoscopic hemostatic techniques following different carotid artery injury characteristics. Int Forum Allergy Rhinol. 2014; 4(8):651–657

[13] Stefanidis D, Sevdalis N, Paige J, et al. Association for Surgical Education Simulation Committee. Simulation in surgery: what's needed next? Ann Surg. 2015; 261(5):846–853

[14] Valentine R, Wormald PJ. A vascular catastrophe during endonasal surgery: an endoscopic sheep model. Skull Base. 2011; 21(2):109–114

[15] Valentine R, Wormald PJ. Carotid artery injury after endonasal surgery. Otolaryngol Clin North Am. 2011; 44(5):1059–1079

[16] Padhye V, Valentine R, Sacks R, et al. Coping with catastrophe: the value of endoscopic vascular injury training. Int Forum Allergy Rhinol. 2015; 5(3): 247–252

[17] Valentine R, Boase S, Jervis-Bardy J, Dones Cabral JD, Robinson S, Wormald PJ. The efficacy of hemostatic techniques in the sheep model of carotid artery injury. Int Forum Allergy Rhinol. 2011; 1(2):118–122

[18] Padhye V, Murphy J, Bassiouni A, Valentine R, Wormald PJ. Endoscopic direct vessel closure in carotid artery injury. Int Forum Allergy Rhinol. 2015; 5(3): 253–257

Index

Note: Page numbers set **bold** or *italic* indicate headings or figures, respectively.